Atlas of Signs in Radiology

J. B. Lippincott Company

Philadelphia

London   Mexico City   New York
St. Louis   São Paulo   Sydney

Atlas

of Signs

WITHDRAWN

in

Radiology

Ronald L. Eisenberg, M.D.

Professor and Chairman, Department of Radiology
Louisiana State University School of Medicine
Shreveport, Louisiana

Acquisitions Editor: William Burgower
Sponsoring Editor: Darlene D. Pedersen
Manuscript Editor: Martha Hicks-Courant
Indexer: Pamela W. Fried
Art Director: Maria S. Karkucinski
Designer: Arlene Putterman
Production Supervisor: N. Carol Kerr
Production Assistant: George V. Gordon
Compositor: Ruttle, Shaw and Wetherill, Inc.
Printer/Binder: Halliday Lithograph

3   5   6   4   2

Eisenberg, Ronald Lee.
    Atlas of signs in radiology.

    Bibliography: p.
    Includes index.
    1. Diagnosis, Radioscopic.   I. Title.   [DNLM:
1. Radiology—Atlases.   2. Technology, Radiologic—Atlases.
WN 17 E36a]
RC78.E53   1983   616.07′572   83-16255
ISBN 0-397-50592-2

To Zina, Avlana, and Cherina

Preface

Signs are the spices of medicine. Some are basic and used by the novice and expert alike, whereas others are so subtle and rare that they can be savored only by the diagnostic gourmet. Signs serve as shorthand phrases, a few words that convey a complete picture and often a specific or limited differential diagnosis. They are almost a secret language, identifying the user as a knowledgeable member of a medical specialty.

In this single volume, I have attempted to bring together a large number of radiologic signs that have been scattered throughout the medical literature. The first four chapters are arranged according to organ system, the last three by imaging modality. The signs are listed in alphabetical order for easy accessibility, and each is followed by a short bibliography and one or more illustrations.

At last count, there were 455 signs spanning the entire spectrum of radiology. Nevertheless, some special signs dear to readers of this book may have been overlooked. Therefore, I extend an open invitation to all readers to send illustrations and references for their favorite signs. These additional signs will be included in any subsequent editions and their contributors appropriately acknowledged.

Ronald L. Eisenberg, M.D.

Acknowledgments

I want to express my thanks to Betty DiGrazia for the many hours she spent in the arduous task of typing and retyping the manuscript. I greatly appreciate the efforts of James Kendrick of George Washington University and the Medical Communications Department at Louisiana State University School of Medicine in Shreveport for skillfully photographing the many illustrations. Thanks should also go to the residents and staff of the Radiology Department at LSU, who were continually on the lookout for new and exotic signs. And, of course, I am grateful to the many physicians who have kindly allowed me to use their published material as illustrations in this book. Finally, I acknowledge the unceasing support and encouragement of William Burgower, Senior Editor, and the entire staff at J.B. Lippincott Company, who always make the immense technical problems of preparing a book as painless as possible.

Contents

1. Gastrointestinal   1

2. Genitourinary

3. Chest

4. Bone

5. Angiography and Myelography — 407

6. Ultrasound — 433

7. Computed Tomography 465

Index 487

1

Gastrointestinal

Abdominal Fat Necrosis Sign

A mottled pattern of speckled radiolucencies, representing normal fat interspersed with the water density of hydrolyzed or saponified fat, has been reported to be pathognomonic of acute pancreatitis (Fig. 1-1). The mottled density almost always includes the pancreatic area but may extend some distance from it. Clinically, the radiographic pattern of fat necrosis is often concurrent with a precipitous fall in serum calcium level, probably as a result of mobilization of calcium into the necrotic areas in the form of calcium soaps. Although the pattern may superficially resemble a collection of fecal material, peritoneal fat necrosis does not follow the distribution of the colon, nor does the pattern change from day to day as it does with stool (Fig. 1-2). In addition, the radiolucent component is significantly blacker in the case of stool or gas in an abdominal abscess (Fig. 1-3). Although infrequently seen, the abdominal fat necrosis sign is diagnostic of acute pancreatitis and is associated with a high mortality rate.

BIBLIOGRAPHY
Berenson JE, Spitz HB, Felson B: The abdominal fat necrosis sign. Radiology 100:567–571, 1971

FIG. 1-1. (*Left*) Excretory urogram shows mottled lucencies in the left midabdomen in a patient with pancreatitis and fat necrosis. Residue in the colon is from a previous barium enema examination. (*Right*) Upper gastrointestinal series shows a large mass displacing the stomach and occluding the duodenum. The mottled lucencies in the left midabdomen are again visible. (Berenson JE, Spitz HB, Felson B: The abdominal fat necrosis sign. Radiology 100:567–571, 1971)

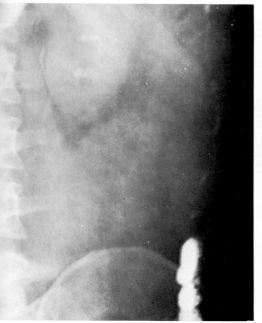
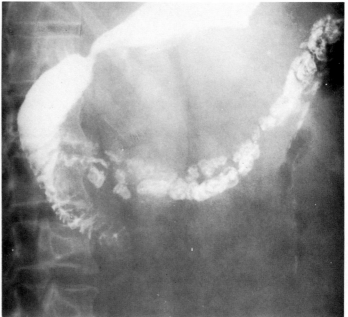

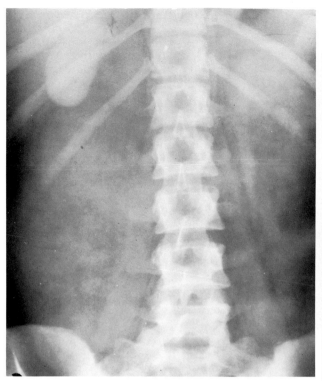

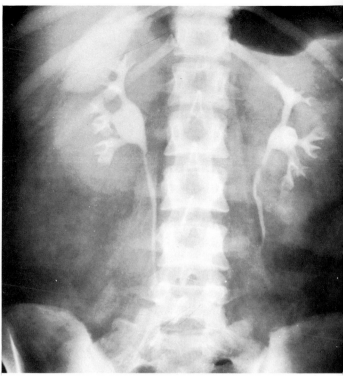

FIG. 1-2. (*Left*) A questionable mass is present in the right midabdomen with faint mottled lucencies within it. The gallbladder is opacified 24 hr after an intravenous cholangiogram, and the upper right psoas shadow appears blurred. (*Right*) The mass and mottling are now more definite in this patient, whose pancreatitis resolved after supportive therapy. The excretory urogram is normal. The gallbladder remained opacified for 16 days. (Berenson JE, Spitz HB, Felson B: The abdominal fat necrosis sign. Radiology 100:567–571, 1971

FIG. 1-3. Gas abscess of the pancreas. The bubbles here are much blacker than those in Figures 1-1 and 1-2. (Berenson JE, Spitz HB, Felson B: The abdominal fat necrosis sign. Radiology 100:567–571, 1971)

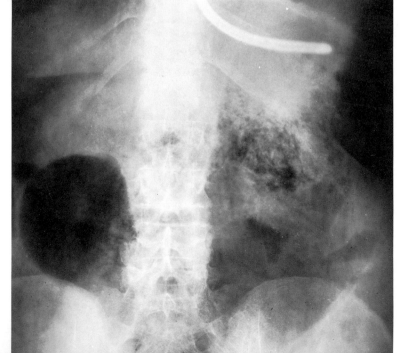

Absent Gastric Air Bubble Sign

On upright films of patients with achalasia, the air bubble of the gastric fundus is usually small or totally absent (Fig. 1-4). Therefore, absence of the gastric air bubble has been reported to be strongly suggestive of achalasia, especially if there is concomitant widening of the mediastinum, often with an air–fluid level, due to dilatation and tortuosity of the esophagus.

FIG. 1-4. (*Top*) Frontal and (*bottom, left*) lateral chest radiographs demonstrate absence of the gastric air bubble. (*Bottom, right*) Contrast study demonstrates narrowing of the distal esophagus with proximal dilatation which is characteristic of achalasia.

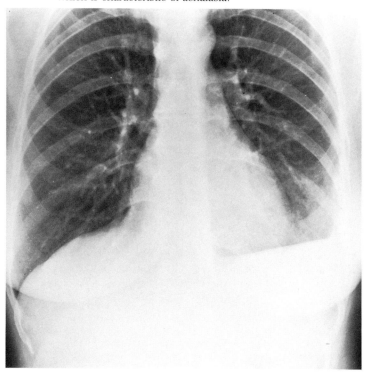

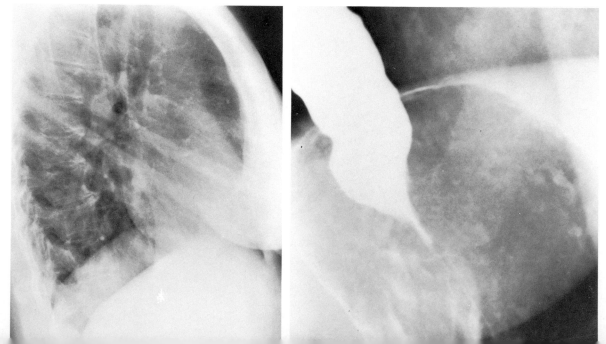

Absent Liver Sign

Identification of bowel gas within the right hemithorax permits the diagnosis of a congenital diaphragmatic hernia. However, in cases with herniation of the liver only, the diagnosis is often missed. On chest radiographs of the neonate, the combination of opacification in the right hemithorax and the presence of intestinal gas in the right upper abdominal quadrant (absent liver sign) should suggest the possibility of intrathoracic hepatic herniation (Fig. 1-5).

BIBLIOGRAPHY
Riggs W, Herschman A: Absent liver sign in congenital diaphragmatic hernia. South Med J 63:265–267, 1979

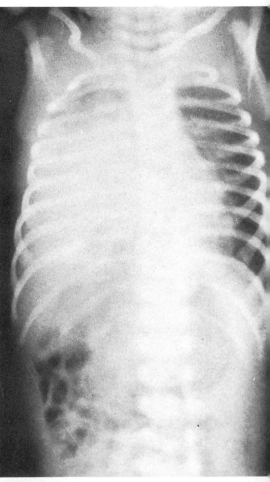

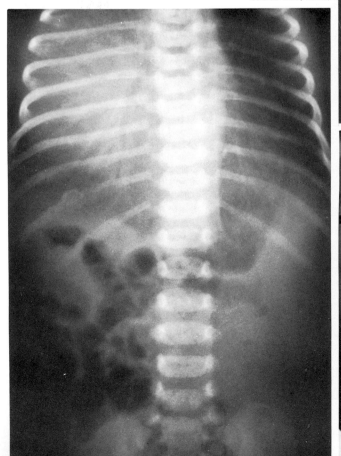

FIG. 1-5 Three different patients with congenital diaphragmatic hernia. Note the thoracic opacification and intestinal gas in the right upper abdomen. The normal soft-tissue density of the liver is missing in the upper abdomen. (Riggs W, Herschman A: Absent liver sign in congenital diaphragmatic hernia. South Med J 63:265–267, 1979)

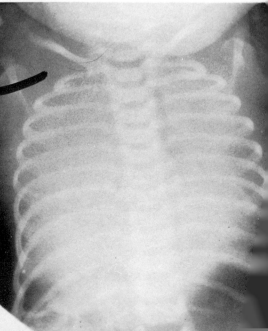

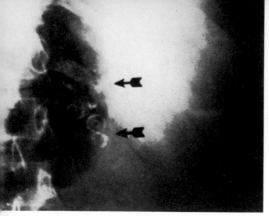

FIG. 1-6 Accordion sign (**arrows**) in a patient with a left upper quadrant mass. (Shuster D, Palayew MJ: Accordion-like compression of a clacified splenic artery: A plain film roentgenographic sign of splenic enlargement. AJR 116:423–425, 1972. Copyright 1972. Reproduced by permission)

FIG. 1-7. Abdominal radiograph obtained 8 months before Figure 1-6 demonstrates that the course and position of the markedly calcified splenic artery (**arrows**) are normal. (Shuster D, Palayew MJ: Accordion-like compression of a calcified splenic artery: A plain film roentgenographic sign of splenic enlargement. AJR 116:423–425, 1972. Copyright 1972. Reproduced by permission)

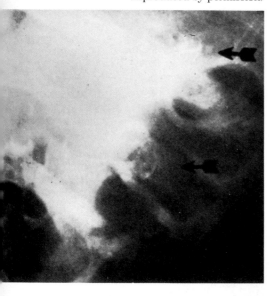

Accordion Sign

Accordion-like compression and medial displacement of a calcified splenic artery seen on plain abdominal radiographs are a sign of splenic enlargement (Fig. 1-6). The accordion sign is of special value if previous radiographs are available for comparison (Fig. 1-7). Development of the accordion sign following trauma suggests the diagnosis of subcapsular splenic hemorrhage or rupture.

BIBLIOGRAPHY
Shuster D, Palayew MJ: Accordion-like compression of a calcified splenic artery: A plain film roentgenographic sign of splenic enlargement. AJR 116:423–425, 1972

Signs of Adenomyomatosis

Adenomyomatosis is a proliferation of surface epithelium with gland-like formations and outpouchings of the mucosa into or through the thickened muscular layer. An adenomyoma is a single filling defect in the gallbladder that reflects a localized form of adenomyomatosis rather than a true neoplasm. This intramural mass projects into the gallbladder and often contains an opaque central speck of contrast medium representing umbilication of the mound. Opaque dots representing intramural diverticula can often be seen at the periphery of the nodule.

The various radiographic appearances of adenomyomas have given rise to several colorful signs. The *omega sign* is a crescent-shaped defect with a central crater (Fig. 1-8). The *life buoy sign* is a totally circumscribed intraluminal adenomyoma that appears as a rounded filling defect containing a relatively dense dot in its center (Fig. 1-9). Filling of multiple intramural diverticula around the periphery of an adenomyoma produces multiple specks of contrast within the lucent mass, giving an appearance of bullet marks around the eye of a target (*target practice sign*) (Fig. 1-10). An adenomyoma of semilunar shape at the tip of the gallbladder may contain a funnel-shaped spot of contrast within a diverticulum or umbilication, producing a design similar to an organ point in musical notation (*organ point sign*) (Fig. 1-11). An adenomyoma may be extraluminal and separated from the body of the opacified gallbladder by a congenital fold or localized thickening of the gallbladder wall. The central crater in such a lesion is filled with opaque material and surrounded by a circular series of little dots corresponding to the communicating diverticula. This characteristic rosette appearance is termed the *Cromlech sign* because of its resemblance to the ancient monument of that name in Brittany (Fig. 1-12).

BIBLIOGRAPHY
Jutras JA: Hyperplastic cholecystoses. AJR 83:795–827, 1960

FIG. 1-8. Series of diagrammatic illustrations demonstrates the development of a gradually enlarging central crater in the fundus of the gallbladder culminating in the omega sign of adenomyomatosis. (Jutras JA: Hyperplastic cholecystoses. AJR 83:795–827, 1960. Copyright 1960. Reproduced by permission)

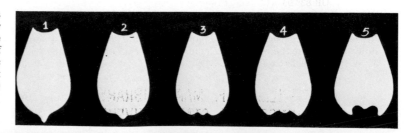

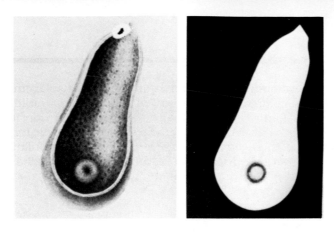

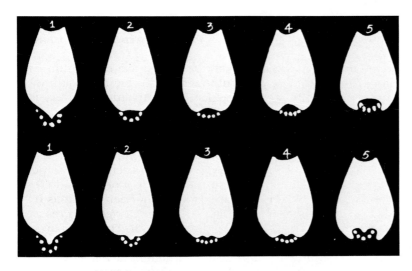

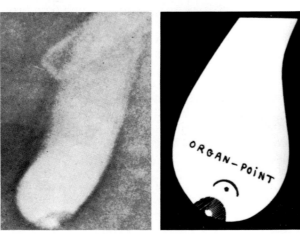

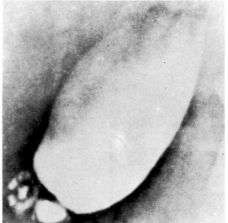

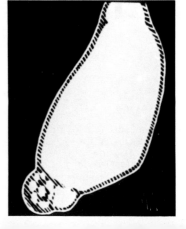

FIG. 1-9. Life buoy sign. (Jutras JA: Hyperplastic cholecystoses. AJR 83:795–827, 1960. Copyright 1960. Reproduced by permission)

FIG. 1-10. Target practice sign. (Jutras JA: Hyperplastic cholecystoses. AJR 83:795–827, 1960. Copyright 1960. Reproduced by permission)

FIG. 1-11. (*Left*) Radiograph and (*right*) diagram demonstrate contrast within a diverticulum associated with a semilunar adenomyoma at the tip of the gallbladder, producing the organ point sign. (Jutras JA: Hyperplastic cholecystoses. AJR 83:795–827, 1960. Copyright 1960. Reproduced by permission)

FIG. 1-12. Cromlech sign. (*Top*) Cholangiogram and (*bottom*) corresponding line drawing illustrate the rosette appearance of an extraluminal adenomyoma. (Jutras JA: Hyperplastic cholecystoses. AJR 83:795–827, 1960. Copyright 1960. Reproduced by permission) ▶

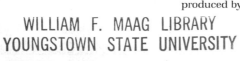
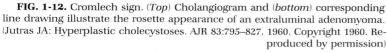

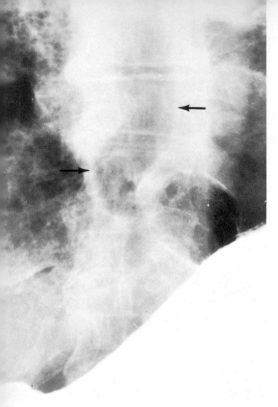

Air Esophagram Sign

The presence on an erect lateral chest film of an air-filled esophagus, without distention and without an air–fluid level, has been described as suggestive, if not typical, of scleroderma (Fig. 1-13). This phenomenon is attributed to smooth muscle dysfunction, which is reflected in diminished peristalsis and limited collapsibility of the esophageal walls. Air in a dilated esophagus associated with a prominent air–fluid level suggests distal obstruction, such as a tumor, stricture, or achalasia (Fig. 1-14), and is frequently associated with no air in the gastric fundus. Infrequently reported causes of the air esophagram sign include thoracic surgery, mediastinal inflammatory disease, total laryngectomy in persons who practice esophageal speech, and endotracheal intubation and positive-pressure ventilation in infants with an H type of tracheoesophageal fistula. Several authors have reported that air in the esophagus is a frequent radiographic finding on routine chest films in normal patients (Fig. 1-15). Although this usually appears as transitory segmental collections of air, air occupying almost the entire length of the esophagus has also been reported in normal patients (Fig. 1-16). Therefore, although the air esophagram sign is suggestive of scleroderma, achalasia, or other esophageal abnormality, it may be seen in normal persons as well.

BIBLIOGRAPHY

Cimmino CV: A roentgenologic study in mediastinal anatomy afforded by air in the mid-esophagus. AJR 94:333–336, 1965

Dinsmore RE, Goodman D, Dreyfuss JR: The air esophagram: A sign of scleroderma involving the esophagus. Radiology 87:348–349, 1966

House AJS, Griffiths GJ: The significance of an air oesophagogram visualized on conventional chest radiographs. Clin Radiol 28:301–305, 1977

Martinez LO: Air in the esophagus as a sign of scleroderma (differential diagnosis with some other entities). J Can Assoc Radiol 25:234–237, 1974

Proto AV, Lane EJ: Air in the esophagus: A frequent radiographic finding. AJR 129:433–440, 1977

Smith WL, Franken EA, Smith JA: Pneumoesophagus as a sign of H type tracheoesophageal fistula. Pediatrics 58:907–909, 1976

FIG. 1-15.

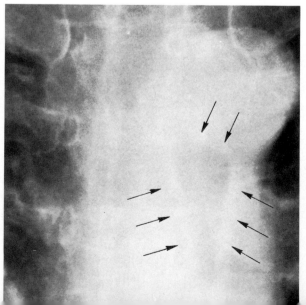

FIG. 1-13. (*Top*) Frontal and (*bottom*) lateral views of the chest demonstrate an air-filled nondistended esophagus (**arrows**) in two patients with scleroderma. (Martinez LO: Air in the esophagus as a sign of scleroderma [differential diagnosis with some other entities]. J Can Assoc Radiol 25:234–237, 1974)

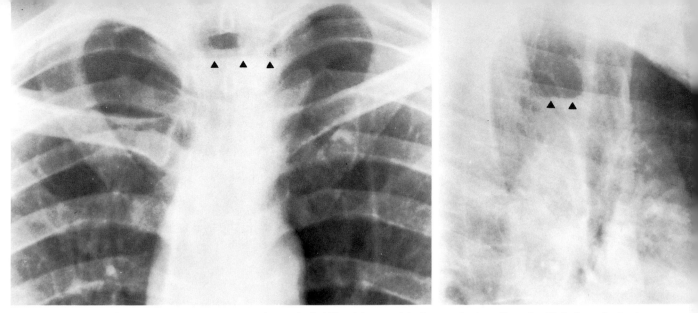

FIG. 1-14. Prominent air–fluid level (**arrows**) in the proximal portion of a dilated esophagus in a patient with achalasia. (*Left*) Frontal view. (*Right*) Lateral view.

FIG. 1-15. (*Opposite page*) Radiograph of a normal patient without esophageal disease demonstrates a typical triangular appearance (**arrows**) of esophageal air below the aortic knob. (Proto AV, Lane EJ: Air in the esophagus: A frequent radiographic finding. AJR 129:433–440, 1977. Copyright 1977. Reproduced by permission)

FIG. 1-16. (*Left*) Chest radiograph demonstrates esophageal air (**arrows**) occupying a long length of esophagus below the level of the aortic knob. (*Right*) Chest radiograph demonstrates esophageal air (**arrows**) occupying almost the entire length of the esophagus above and below the aortic knob. (Proto AV, Lane EJ: Air in the esophagus: A frequent radiographic finding. AJR 129:433–440, 1977. Copyright 1977. Reproduced by permission)

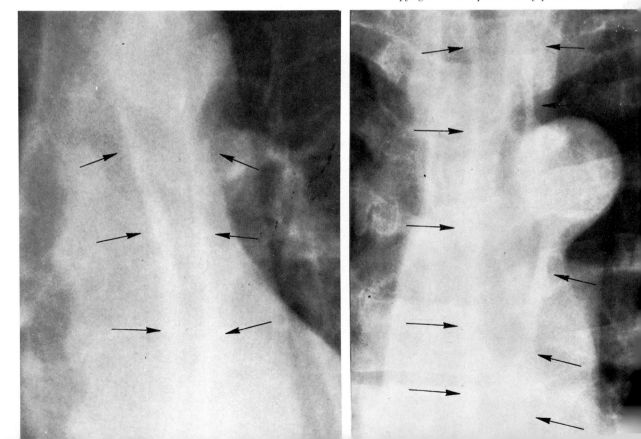

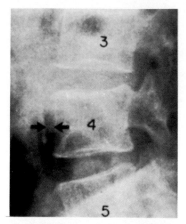

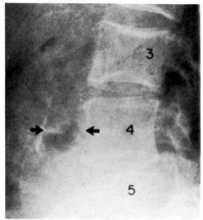

Anteriorly Migrating Abdominal Aorta Sign ▬▬▬▬

Demonstration on lateral radiographs of interval anterior migration of the calcified abdominal aorta from the lumbar spine is an indication of a mass in the retroperitoneal space (Fig. 1-17). Because the abdominal aorta is a central structure, the serial views need not be strictly lateral to form a valid comparison. The change in position between two examinations is much more important than the absolute distance between the calcified abdominal aorta and the lumbar spine.

BIBLIOGRAPHY

Cimmino CV: The anteriorly migrating abdominal aorta: A sign of retroperitoneal tumor. Radiology 94:149–150, 1970

FIG. 1-17. There is a substantial difference in the distance between aorta and spine on lateral abdominal radiographs performed (*top*) in 1958 and in 1962 (*bottom*) in this patient with widespread metastases from bronchogenic carcinoma. (Cimmino CV: The anteriorly migrating abdominal aorta: A sign of retroperitoneal tumor. Radiology 94:149–150, 1970)

Antral Pad Sign

The antral pad sign originally referred to splaying of rugal folds in the antrum due to a mass directly posterior to this portion of the stomach. In recent years, the term has been applied to an extrinsic indentation on the posteroinferior aspect of the antrum with associated draping of rugae over the mass. The sign is usually due to lesions arising from the head or body of the pancreas (Fig. 1-18). A similar pattern may be produced by normal structures, such as the gallbladder (Fig. 1-19) or colon, which indent the gastric antrum.

BIBLIOGRAPHY

Case JP: Roentgenology of pancreatic disease. AJR 44:485–518, 1940
Smeets R, Op den Orth JO: Gallbladder: Common cause of antral pad sign. AJR 132:571–573, 1979

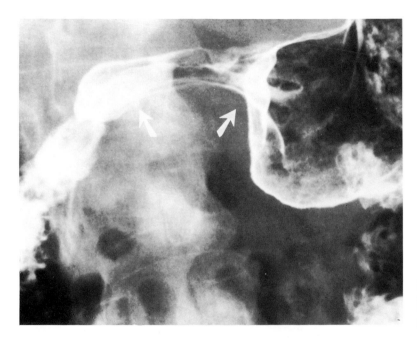

FIG. 1-18. Antral pad sign (**arrow**) caused by adenocarcinoma of the pancreas. (Eisenberg RL: Gastrointestinal Radiology: A Pattern Approach. Philadelphia, JB Lippincott, 1983)

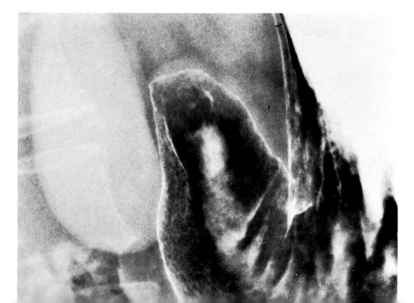

FIG. 1-19. Antral pad sign produced by indentation of a normal gallbladder on the greater curvature side of the antrum. (Smeets R, Op den Orth JO: Gallbladder: Common cause of antral pad sign. AJR 132:571–573, 1979. Copyright 1979. Reproduced by permission)

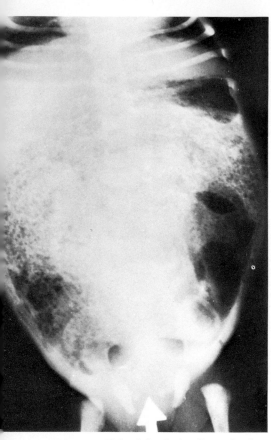

Applesauce Sign

Meconium ileus is a cause of distal small bowel obstruction in infants, in whom the thick and sticky meconium cannot be readily propelled through the bowel. The excessive viscosity of meconium, which is frequently associated with mucoviscidosis, results from the lack of normal pancreatic and intestinal gland secretions during fetal life. The abnormal obstructing meconium, mixed with gas, produces a characteristic "applesauce," or "soap bubble," radiographic pattern (Fig. 1-20).

BIBLIOGRAPHY
Tucker AS, Izant RJ: Problems with meconium. AJR 112:135–142, 1971

FIG. 1-20. Plain abdominal radiograph of an infant with meconium ileus demonstrates massive distention of the small bowel and a profound soap bubble effect of air mixed with meconium (**arrow**). (Swischuk LE: Radiology of the Newborn and Young Infant. Baltimore, Williams & Wilkins, 1980)

Arrowhead Sign

The arrowhead sign is a manifestation of segmental dilatation of bile ducts with areas of rapid peripheral tapering (Fig. 1-21). The sign is a cholangiographic finding in patients with cholangiohepatitis (recurrent pyogenic hepatitis), a major cause of acute abdomen in the Far East.

BIBLIOGRAPHY

Ho CS, Wesson DE: Recurrent pyogenic cholangitis in Chinese immigrants. AJR 122:368–384, 1974

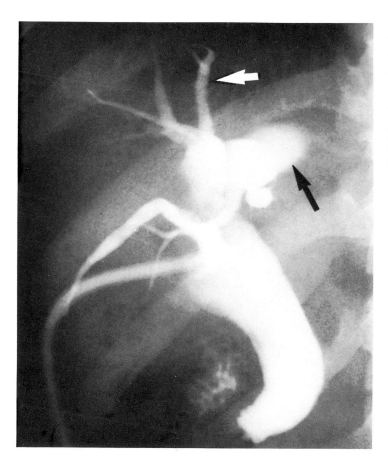

FIG. 1-21. Segmental dilatation of bile ducts with areas of rapid peripheral tapering in a patient with cholangiohepatitis (recurrent pyogenic cholangitis). There is a dilatation of the common bile duct and interhepatic ducts (**lower arrow**). The **upper arrow** shows a moderately dilated bile duct with short branches arising at right angles to the duct. (Ho CS, Wesson DE: Recurrent pyogenic cholangitis in Chinese immigrants. AJR 122:368–374, 1974. Copyright 1974. Reproduced by permission)

Bird's Beak Sign

When a barium enema is performed in a patient with sigmoid volvulus, the flow of contrast ceases at the level of the obstruction, and the rectum becomes distended. The lumen tapers toward the site of stenosis, producing a pathognomonic bird's beak sign (Fig. 1-22). If barium passes the stenosis and the proximal part of the torsion is also tapered, the appearance resembles that of two birds with their beaks together.

BIBLIOGRAPHY

Frimann-Dahl J: Roentgen Examinations in Acute Abdominal Diseases. Springfield, IL, Charles C Thomas, 1974

FIG. 1-22. "Bird's beak" configuration (**arrow**). (Eisenberg RL: Gastrointestinal Radiology: A Pattern Approach. Philadelphia, JB Lippincott, 1983)

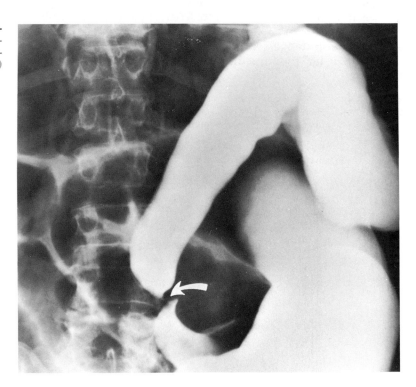

Border Sign

Diverticula seen *en face* rather than in profile can appear to lie within the lumen, rather than projecting beyond it, and can be difficult to distinguish from polyps. Although rotation of the patient usually demonstrates that the diverticulum truly extends beyond the colonic lumen, a barium-coated, gas-filled diverticulum sometimes remains superimposed on the lumen of the bowel on multiple projections. Polyps and diverticula can sometimes be differentiated by evaluation of the quality of the barium coating their borders. The barium coating a polyp usually has a smooth and well-defined inner border (where it abuts the mucosal surface of the polyp) but a less well defined outer surface (where it is in contact with the fecal stream) (Fig. 1-23*A*). In contrast, the ring of barium coating a diverticulum tends to have a smooth, well-defined outer border (where it is in contact with the diverticular mucosa) but an irregular inner surface (Fig. 1-23*B*).

BIBLIOGRAPHY

Welin S: Über die roentgenologische Untersuchung des Dickdarmes mit der Doppelkontrastmethode: Die Malmomodifikation. Radiologie (Berlin) 2:87–100, 1962

Youker JE, Welin S: Differentiation of true polypoid tumors of the colon from extraneous material: A new roentgen sign. Radiology 84:610–615, 1965

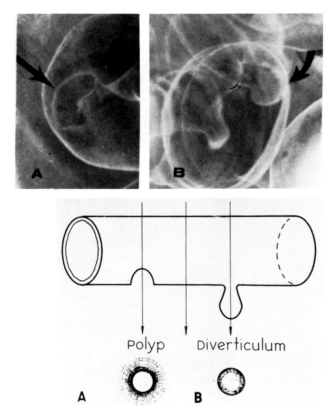

FIG. 1-23. (**A**) The barium encircling this sessile polyp (**arrow**) has a sharp inner border and a less well defined outer border. (**B**) The barium confined within this diverticulum (**arrow**) has a sharp outer border and a poorly defined inner border. A second diverticulum shows a gas–fluid level. (Youker JE, Welin S: Differentiation of true polypoid tumors of the colon from extraneous material: A new roentgen sign. Radiology 84:610–615, 1965)

Carman Meniscus Sign

The Carman meniscus sign is diagnostic of a specific type of ulcerated gastric malignancy. When examined in profile using compression, the ulcer is seen to have a semicircular (meniscoid) configuration (Fig. 1-28). The inner margin of the barium trapped within the ulcer is usually regular. It is always convex toward the lumen, in contrast to the crescent sign of benign gastric ulcers, in which the inner margin is concave toward the lumen (see Fig. 1-37). The base (outer margin) of the barium collection trapped within this malignant neoplasm is almost always located where the gastric wall would normally be. This is the case because the underlying tumor has relatively little intraluminal mass other than the elevated rim of tissue at the periphery of the lesion.

BIBLIOGRAPHY

Carman RD: A new roentgen-ray sign of ulcerating gastric cancer. JAMA 77:990–992, 1921

Kirklin BR: The meniscus complex in the roentgenologic diagnosis of ulcerating carcinoma of the stomach. AJR 47:571–583, 1942

Nelson SW: The discovery of gastric ulcers and the differential diagnosis between benignancy and malignancy. Radiol Clin North Am 5–25, 1969

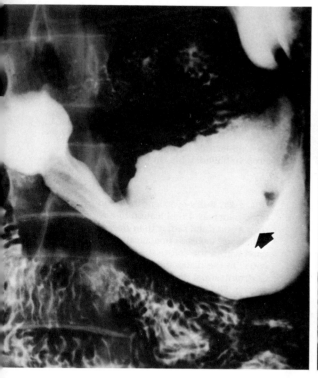
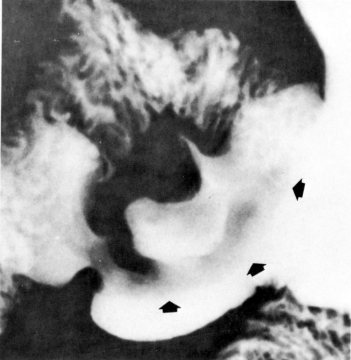

FIG. 1-28. (*Left*) Huge ulcer with a semicircular configuration and an inner margin convex toward the lumen (**arrow**) in a patient with gastric lymphoma. (*Right*) The combination of such a Carman-type ulcer and the radiolucent shadow of the elevated ridge of neoplastic tissue that surrounds it (**arrows**) forms the Kirklin complex in a patient with adenocarcinoma of the stomach. (Eisenberg RL: Gastrointestinal Radiology: A Pattern Approach. Philadelphia, JB Lippincott, 1983)

Coffee Bean (Kidney Bean) Sign ▬▬▬▬

An obstructed closed loop bent on itself may assume the shape of a coffee bean or kidney bean (Figs. 1-29 and 1-30).

BIBLIOGRAPHY

Frimann-Dahl J: Roentgen Examinations in Acute Abdominal Diseases. Springfield, IL, Charles C Thomas, 1974

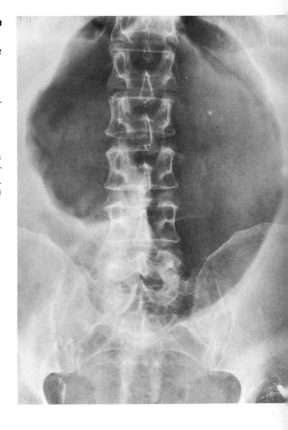

FIG. 1-29. In this patient with cecal volvulus, the distended, gas-filled cecum is displaced upward and to the left, assuming the shape of a coffee bean or kidney bean. (Eisenberg RL: Gastrointestinal Radiology: A Pattern Approach. Philadelphia, JB Lippincott, 1983)

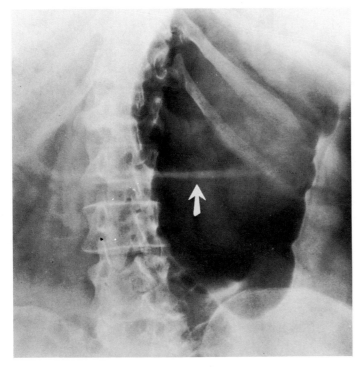

FIG. 1-30. The dilated, gas-filled cecum in this patient with cecal volvulus has a shape suggesting a coffee bean or a kidney bean. The double width of the apposed cecal walls and the torqued and thickened mesentery mimic the cleft of the bean (**arrow**). (Eisenberg RL: Gastrointestinal Radiology: A Pattern Approach. Philadelphia, JB Lippincott, 1983)

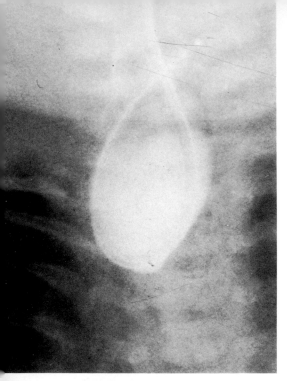

Coiled Tube Sign

Tube coiling has been described as a sign of obstruction in both the esophagus and the small bowel. In the neonate, coiling of a feeding tube in the upper esophagus is diagnostic of esophageal atresia with a blind proximal esophageal pouch (Fig. 1-31). In the small bowel, coiling of a long tube is a sign of obstruction. As the leading end of the long tube reaches the point of obstruction, further progress is prevented. Continued peristaltic activity carries additional tubing into the area of obstruction, thus forcing the leading end of the tube to turn backward upon itself. As more tubing enters the area of obstruction, the tube begins to coil and may continue to do so until it fills the dilated intestinal lumen (Fig. 1-32). This coiled tube sign permits accurate localization of the site of small bowel obstruction; in some instances, the diameter of the dilated small bowel can be inferred from the size or diameter of the bolus of coiled tubing.

BIBLIOGRAPHY

Figiel LS, Figiel SJ: Coiling of the long tube in the small intestine: A sign of intestinal obstruction. AJR 87:721–723, 1962

FIG. 1-31. This neonate has coiling of the esophageal tube, indicative of esophageal atresia. The injection of contrast permits definition of the caudal limit of the blind esophageal pouch.

FIG. 1-32. (*Left*) Abdominal radiograph demonstrates a long tube with the opaque mercury portion in the pelvic cavity. (*Center*) Abdominal radiograph made on the next day demonstrates identical orientation of the coiled tubing. (*Right*) Following the administration of barium through the tube, there is obvious dilatation of the small bowel containing the coiled tubing. (Figiel LS, Figiel SJ: Coiling of the long tube in the small intestine: A sign of intestinal obstruction. AJR 87:721–723, 1962. Copyright 1962. Reproduced by permission)

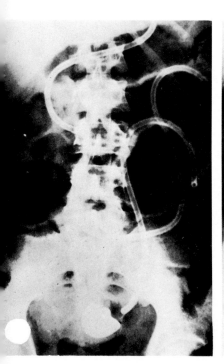
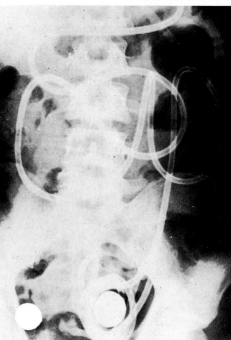
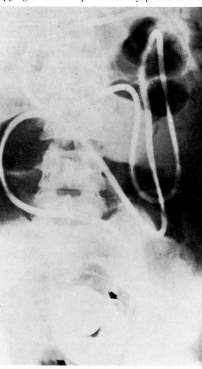

Colon Cut-Off Sign

The colon cut-off sign, though infrequently seen, is often considered highly suggestive of acute pancreatitis. The cut-off is not in the proximal transverse colon, as originally thought; rather, it has become apparent that pancreatitis more commonly causes gaseous distention of the right and entire transverse colon, so that the cut-off of the gas column occurs abruptly at the splenic flexure (Fig. 1-33). The mechanism for this phenomenon probably depends on the anatomic position of the transverse mesocolon, which connects the transverse colon with the anterior surface of the pancreas and permits inflammatory exudate from acute pancreatitis to spread to involve the transverse colon. Although the colon cut-off sign is suggestive of acute pancreatitis, it is nonspecific; a similar appearance may be caused by colonic obstruction at the splenic flexure, mesenteric vascular thrombosis, and ischemic colitis.

BIBLIOGRAPHY
Brascho DJ, Reynolds TN, Zanca P: The radiographic "colon cut-off sign" in acute pancreatitis. Radiology 79:763–768, 1962

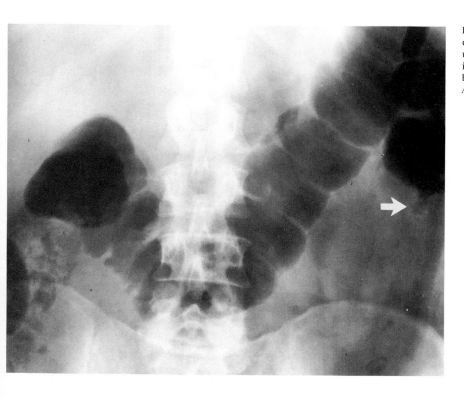

FIG. 1-33. Plain abdominal radiograph demonstrates abrupt cut-off of the colon gas column just distal to the splenic flexure (**arrow**) in a patient with acute pancreatitis. (Eisenberg RL: Gastrointestinal Radiology: A Pattern Approach. Philadelphia, JB Lippincott, 1983)

Contrast Bubble Sign

Extraluminal bubbles formed during studies with water-soluble agents have been reported to represent contrast medium bubbling through a small perforation in the gastrointestinal tract (Fig. 1-34). Although the walls of the bubbles may be radiodense, the presence of contrast material may be impossible to detect if the bubbles are small and dilute contrast material is used. Extraluminal bubble formation by contrast material may identify and localize a small perforation in the gut when other findings are inconclusive (Fig. 1-35).

BIBLIOGRAPHY

Cipel L, Gyepes MT: "Contrast bubble": A sign indicating perforation of the digestive tract. AJR 133:97–101, 1979

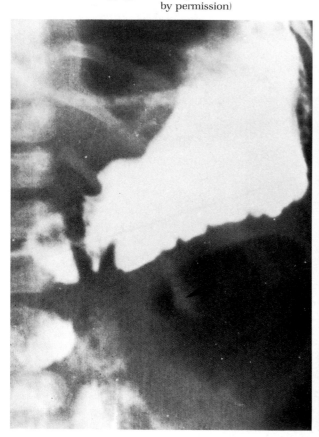 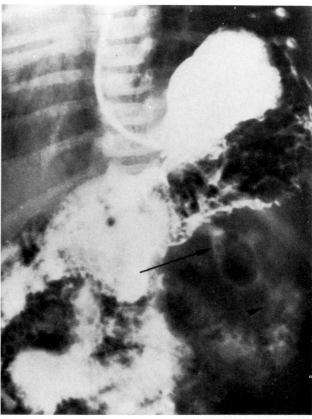

FIG. 1-34. (*Left*) Extravasation of contrast material (**arrow**) on an early film from an upper gastrointestinal series. (*Right*) Small bubbles (**arrow**) close to the stomach and away from small bowel loops (**arrowhead**). (Cipel L, Gyepes MT: "Contrast bubble": A sign indicating perforation of the digestive tract. AJR 133:97–101, 1979. Copyright 1979. Reproduced by permission)

FIG. 1-35. (*Left*) During the first injection of contrast material, small bubbles are seen in the right upper chest (**arrow**). No definite extravasation of contrast seen. (*Right*) A second, more forceful injection clearly demonstrates the perforation. Ideally, the tip of the tube should be higher. (Cipel L, Gyepes MT: "Contrast bubble": A sign indicating perforation of the digestive tract. AJR 133:97–101, 1979. Copyright 1979. Reproduced by permission)

Converging Lines Sign

On supine abdominal radiographs of patients with sigmoid volvulus, there are often three dense, curved lines running downward and converging toward the point of stenosis (Fig. 1-36). These lines appear to end in a small tumor-like density that corresponds to the twisted mesenteric root. The central and most constant line is a dense midline crease produced by the two walls of the torqued loop lying pressed together. The other two lines, less frequently seen, are made up of the outer margins of the closed loop joined with the medial walls of the cecum on the right and the descending colon on the left.

BIBLIOGRAPHY

Frimann-Dahl J: Roentgen Examinations in Acute Abdominal Diseases. Springfield, IL, Charles C Thomas, 1974

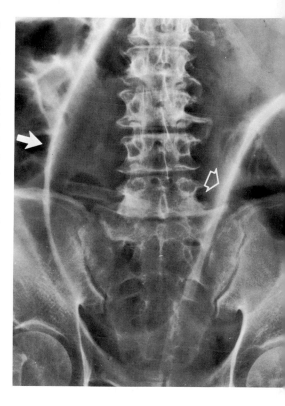

FIG. 1-36. Two of the characteristic three dense lines are seen running downward and converging toward the point of stenosis in this patient with sigmoid volvulus. The central line (**open arrow**) is produced by the two walls of the torqued loop lying pressed together. The right line (**solid arrow**) consists of the outer margin of the closed loop joined with the medial wall of the cecum. The left line is not clearly seen, because there is no gas within the lower descending colon. (Eisenberg RL: Gastrointestinal Radiology: A Pattern Approach. Philadelphia, JB Lippincott, 1983)

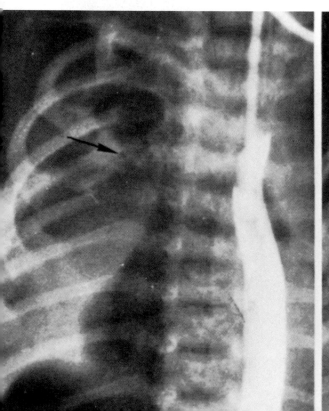
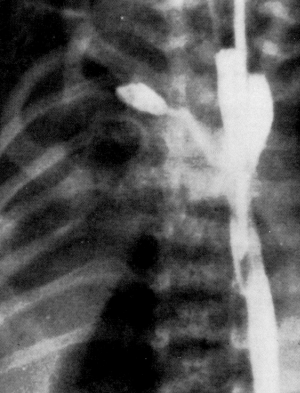

Crescent (Quarter-Moon) Sign

An unusually large, benign ulcer located on the greater curvature of the antrum of the stomach may have a crescent-shaped or quarter-moon appearance with concavity toward and convexity away from the gastric lumen (Fig. 1-37). The collection of barium seen in the crescent sign of a benign gastric ulcer is produced by the mound of overhanging mucosa around the orifice of the ulcer. Unlike Carman's meniscus sign of a malignant ulcer, in which the inner margin of the crater is usually irregular, with its convexity toward the lumen (see Fig. 1-28), the crescent sign of a benign gastric ulcer has a smooth inner margin, with its concavity toward the lumen.

BIBLIOGRAPHY

Han SY, Witten DM: Benign gastric ulcer with "crescent" (quarter moon) sign. Radiology 113:573–575, 1974

Nelson SW: A crescent-shaped collection of residual cholecystographic contrast material: A new sign of benign gastric ulcer? AJR 116:293–303, 1972

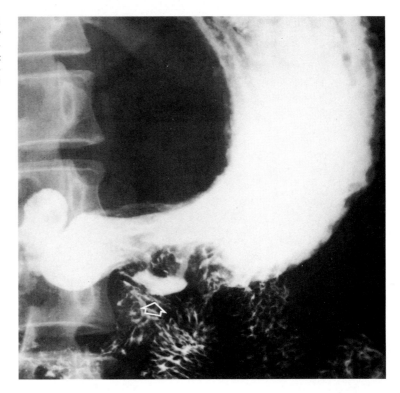

FIG. 1-37. A crescentic collection of barium (**arrow**) with concavity toward and convexity away from the gastric lumen represents a benign greater curvature ulcer. (Eisenberg RL: Gastrointestinal Radiology: A Pattern Approach. Philadelphia, JB Lippincott, 1983)

Dilated Transverse Colon Sign

Dilatation of the transverse colon, an empty cecum and ascending colon, and, often, an abrupt zone of demarcation between the two areas have been described as a sign of acute appendicitis (Fig. 1-38). Because the sign has not been seen in nonperforated appendicitis, it is believed to be one of the earliest, if not the earliest, radiographic sign of perforation. The dilated transverse colon sign apparently results from a combination of paralytic ileus of the transverse colon and spasm of the ascending colon. This appearance must be distinguished from that of normal transverse colon gas accumulations, in which the ascending colon usually contains gas or fecal material (Fig. 1-39), as well as from the dilated transverse colon associated with pancreatitis, in which the clinical findings are usually somewhat different.

BIBLIOGRAPHY
Swischuk LE, Hayden CK: Appendicitis with perforation: The dilated transverse colon sign. AJR 135:687–689, 1980

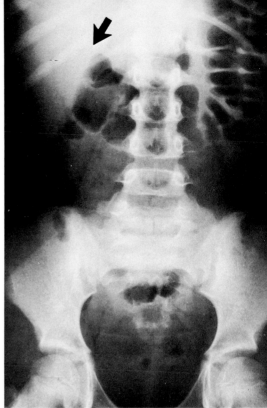

FIG. 1-38. Distended transverse colon and empty ascending colon in a patient with a perforated appendix. Note the sharp demarcation between these two parts of the colon (**arrow**). (Swischuk LE, Hayden CK: Appendicitis with perforation: The dilated transverse colon sign. AJR 135:687–689, 1980. Copyright 1980. Reproduced by permission)

FIG. 1-39. Although the demarcation between the transverse and ascending colon is relatively sharp (**arrow**), fecal material is present in the hepatic flexure in this normal child with chronic constipation. Residual barium is seen in the rectum. (Swischuk LE, Hayden CK: Appendicitis with perforation: The dilated transverse colon sign. AJR 135:687–689, 1980. Copyright 1980. Reproduced by permission)

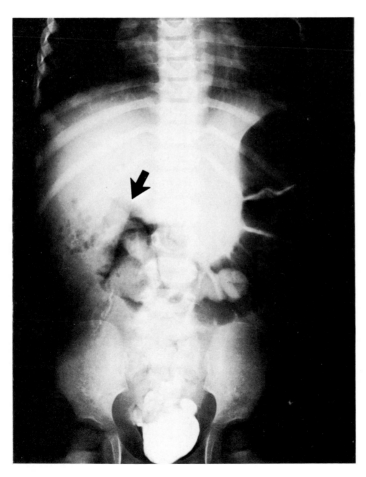

Distended Common Bile Duct Sign

A distended common bile duct may produce a tubular impression on the immediate postbulbar portion of the duodenum (Fig. 1-40). This sign is not specific for a distended bile duct, however; enlarged lymph nodes or other masses in the immediate vicinity of the duodenohepatic ligaments can produce an identical appearance.

BIBLIOGRAPHY

Hodes PJ, Pendergrass EP, Winston NJ: Pancreatic, ductal and Vaterian neoplasms: Their roentgen manifestations. Radiology 62:1–15, 1954

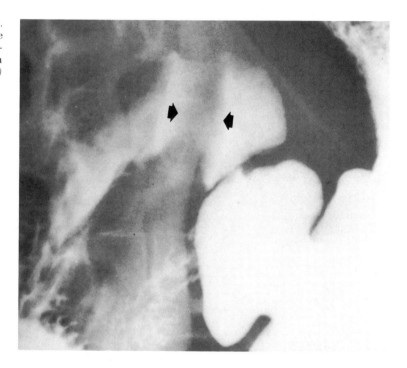

FIG. 1-40. Distended common bile duct sign. The **arrows** show a tubular impression on the duodenum near the apex of the bulb. (Eisenberg RL: Gastrointestinal Radiology: A Pattern Approach. Philadelphia, JB Lippincott, 1983)

Dog's Ears Sign

When the patient is in the supine position, free blood in the peritoneal cavity gravitates to the dependent portions of the pelvis and accumulates within the pelvic peritoneal reflections (Fig. 1-41). Filling of the recesses on both sides of the bladder produces a symmetric density resembling dog's ears (Fig. 1-42).

BIBLIOGRAPHY
McCort JJ: Radiological examination in blunt abdominal trauma. Radiol Clin North Am 2:121–143, 1964

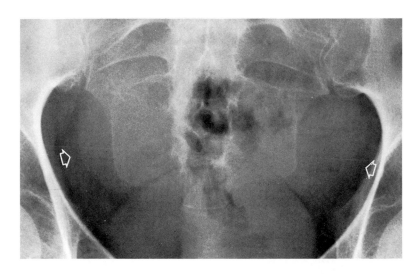

FIG. 1-41. Supine abdominal radiograph demonstrates accumulation of a large amount of ascitic fluid within the pelvic peritoneal reflections (**arrows**).

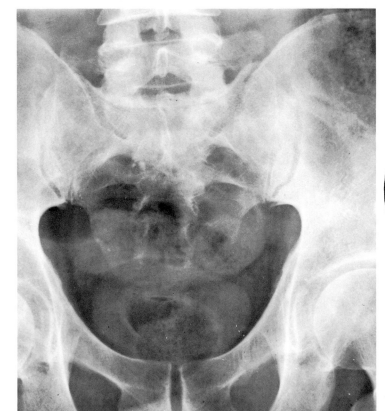

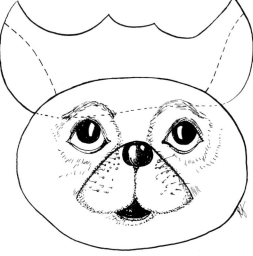

FIG. 1-42. (*Left*) Following traumatic fracture of the spleen, a supine lower abdominal radiograph demonstrates free blood in the peritoneum gravitating to the dependent pelvic portions and filling the recesses on both sides of the rectum and bladder, producing the "dog's ears" sign graphically depicted in the figure (*right*). (McCort JJ: Radiological examination in blunt abdominal trauma. Radiol Clin North Am 2:121–143, 1964)

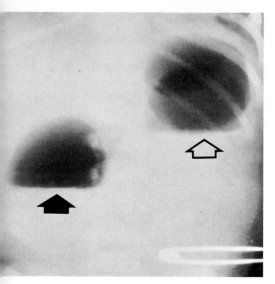

Double Bubble Sign

The classic radiographic finding of duodenal obstruction in newborn infants is the double bubble sign (Fig. 1-43). This appearance reflects large amounts of gas both in a markedly dilated stomach (left bubble) and in that portion of the duodenum that is proximal to the obstruction (right bubble). In duodenal atresia, there is complete obstruction of the duodenum and therefore a total lack of gas within the small and large bowel distal to the level of the lesion. Demonstration of even small amounts of gas distal to a duodenal obstruction rules out the possibility of duodenal atresia and suggests a high-grade, but incomplete, congenital stenosis such as annular pancreas or midgut volvulus (Fig. 1-44).

BIBLIOGRAPHY

Fonkalsrud EW, DeLorimier AA, Hays DM: Congenital atresia and stenosis of the duodenum. A review compiled from the members of the surgical section of the American Academy of Pediatrics. Pediatrics 43:79–83, 1969

FIG. 1-43. Duodenal atresia with the double bubble sign. The left bubble (**open arrow**) represents gas in the stomach; the right bubble (**solid arrow**) reflects duodenal gas. There is no gas in the small or large bowel distal to the level of the complete obstruction. (Eisenberg RL: Gastrointestinal Radiology: A Pattern Approach. Philadelphia, JB Lippincott, 1983)

FIG. 1-44. Congenital duodenal stenosis. The presence of small amounts of gas distal to the obstruction indicates that the stenosis is incomplete. (Eisenberg RL: Gastrointestinal Radiology: A Pattern Approach. Philadelphia, JB Lippincott, 1983)

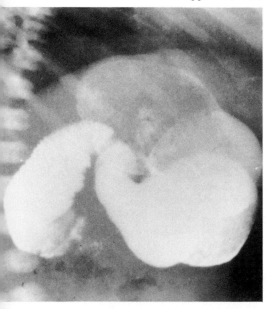

Double Condom Sign

One of the most ingenious schemes for smuggling narcotics is that of placing drugs in condoms, folding the condoms to form 3-cm balls, and then swallowing them before crossing international borders. The contraband is thus safely hidden in the gastrointestinal tract of the smuggler during transport. After arriving at his destination, the smuggler carefully watches his stools until all the narcotic-filled balls are recovered. Although the major narcotics are not radiopaque, they can be detected radiographically in the gastrointestinal tract by virtue of the way in which they are "packaged" in the condoms. To prevent intoxication of the carrier and to protect the valuable contents, each narcotic ball is doubly wrapped in two condoms, each folded on itself three times (Fig. 1-45). The gas trapped between the individual layers of the two condoms produces a pathognomonic lucent ring shadow (double condom sign) on abdominal radiographs (Fig. 1-46).

BIBLIOGRAPHY
Pinsky MF, Ducas J, Ruggere MD: Narcotic smuggling: The double condom sign. J Can Assoc Radiol 29:79–81, 1978

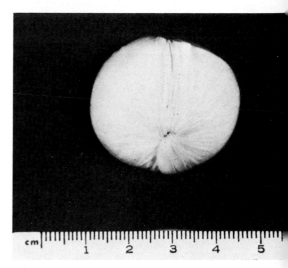

FIG. 1-45. Example of a condom ball containing narcotics. (Pinsky MF, Ducas J, Ruggere MD: Narcotic smuggling: The double condom sign. J Can Assoc Radiol 29:79–81, 1978)

FIG. 1-46. Several lucent ring shadows (**arrows**) can be identified within the transverse and sigmoid colon. Sixteen condom balls containing cocaine were recovered from this patient. (Pinsky MF, Ducas J, Ruggere MD: Narcotic smuggling: The double condom sign. J Can Assoc Radiol 29:79–81, 1978)

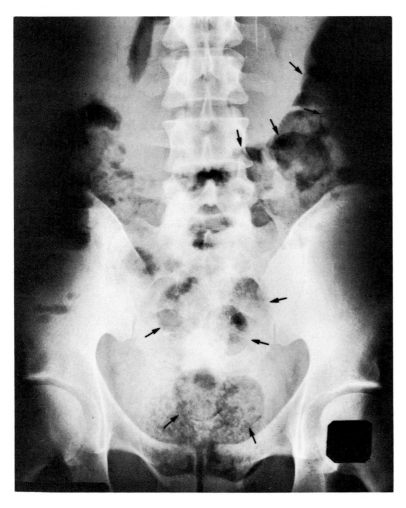

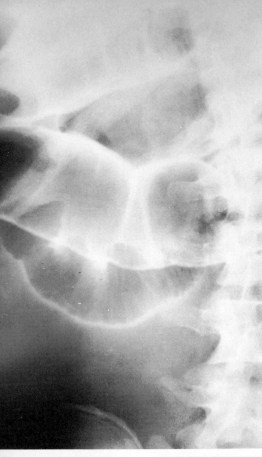

Double Wall Sign

Demonstration of the outer as well as the inner wall of loops of bowel is a virtually pathognomonic sign of pneumoperitoneum (Fig. 1-47). The double wall sign is seen on supine abdominal radiographs and is of special value in very ill patients who cannot assume an upright or decubitus position. An appearance similar to the double wall sign has been reported to result from two loops of distended intestine lying in contact with each other in patients without pneumoperitoneum (Fig. 1-48).

BIBLIOGRAPHY

de Lacey G, Bloomberg T, Wignall BK: Pneumoperitoneum: The misleading double wall sign. Clin Radiol 28:445–448, 1977

Rigler LG: Spontaneous pneumoperitoneum: A roentgenologic sign found in the supine position. Radiology 37:604–607, 1941

FIG. 1-47. Pneumoperitoneum demonstrated on supine abdominal radiographs. Large quantities of free intraperitoneal gas may be diagnosed indirectly in these two patients because the gas permits visualization of the outer margins of the intestinal wall. (Eisenberg RL: Gastrointestinal Radiology: A Pattern Approach. Philadelphia, JB Lippincott, 1983)

FIG. 1-48. Loops of distended bowel lying in contact with each other simulate the double wall sign in this patient with small bowel obstruction and no free intraperitoneal gas. (Eisenberg RL: Gastrointestinal Radiology: A Pattern Approach. Philadelphia, JB Lippincott, 1983)

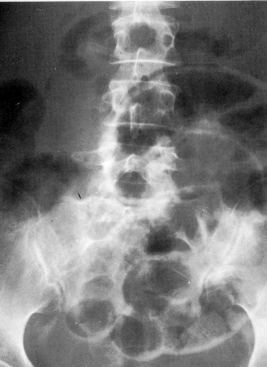

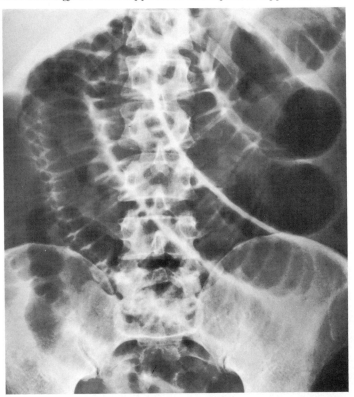

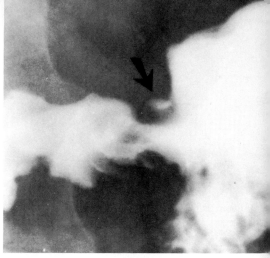

Ellipse Sign

When a persistent collection of barium is seen during radiographic examination of the upper gastrointestinal tract, differentiation of acute ulceration from nonulcerating entities (diverticulum, pseudodiverticulum, postoperative deformity) is sometimes difficult. However, when the persistent collection of barium has an elliptical configuration, the orientation of the long axis of the ellipse can be an indicator of the nature of the pathologic process. If the long axis is parallel to the lumen, the collection represents an acute ulceration (Fig. 1-49). Conversely, if the long axis is perpendicular to the lumen, the collection represents a deformity without acute ulceration (Fig. 1-50).

BIBLIOGRAPHY
Eisenberg RL, Hedgcock MW: The ellipse sign: An aid in the diagnosis of acute ulcers. J Can Assoc Radiol 30:26–29, 1979

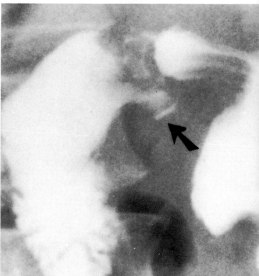

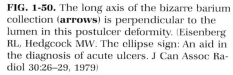

FIG. 1-49. Two benign gastric ulcers are seen as persistent barium collections (**arrows**) running parallel to the lumen. (Eisenberg RL, Hedgcock MW: The ellipse sign: An aid in the diagnosis of acute ulcers. J Can Assoc Radiol 30:26–29, 1979)

FIG. 1-50. The long axis of the bizarre barium collection (**arrows**) is perpendicular to the lumen in this postulcer deformity. (Eisenberg RL, Hedgcock MW: The ellipse sign: An aid in the diagnosis of acute ulcers. J Can Assoc Radiol 30:26–29, 1979)

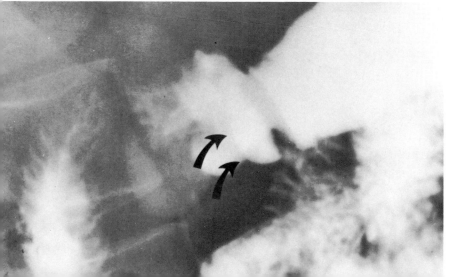

Falciform Ligament Sign

Presence of the outline of the falciform ligament on a supine abdominal radiograph is a sign of pneumoperitoneum (Fig. 1-51). The falciform ligament is a sickle-shaped sagittal fold of peritoneum that helps attach the liver to the diaphragm, separates the right and left lobes of the liver, and extends from the coronary ligament of the liver behind to the umbilicus in front. Because the falciform ligament is outlined radiographically only when there is gas on both sides of it, demonstration of a characteristic curvilinear water density shadow in the upper abdomen to the right of the spine is an important sign of free intraperitoneal gas.

BIBLIOGRAPHY

Schultz EH: An aid to the diagnosis of pneumoperitoneum from supine abdominal films. Radiology 70:728–731, 1958

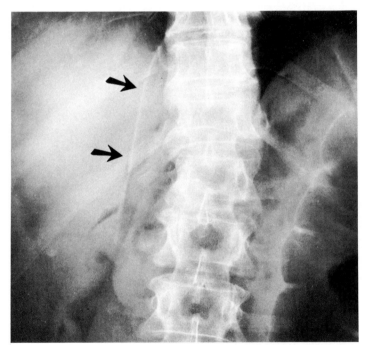

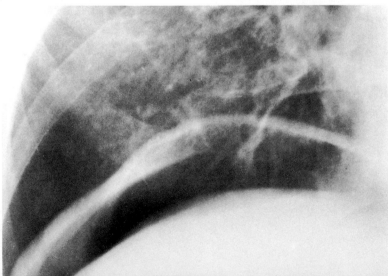

FIG. 1-51. (*Top*) On the supine view, the falciform ligament appears as a curvilinear water density shadow (**arrows**) in the upper abdomen to the right of the spine. This implies that there is a pneumoperitoneum with gas on both sides of the ligament. (*Bottom*) An upright view clearly demonstrates free intraperitoneal gas under the right hemidiaphragm. (Eisenberg RL: Gastrointestinal Radiology: A Pattern Approach. Philadelphia, JB Lippincott, 1983)

Fat Sign

The thickened and inflamed wall of a chronically infected gall-bladder frequently contains abundant deposits of fat. The radiographic demonstration of a crescentic shadow or halo of fat density measuring 4 mm or more in thickness at any point has been reported as a sign of acalculous gallbladder disease (Fig. 1-52). Because of confusing shadows in the gallbladder area, the fat sign may be difficult to appreciate without a cholecystogram (Fig. 1-53) or the presence of gallstones (Fig. 1-54) to localize the gallbladder.

BIBLIOGRAPHY
Russell JGB, Keddie NC, Gough AL et al: Radiology of acalculous gallbladder disease—A new sign. Br J Radiol 49:420–424, 1976

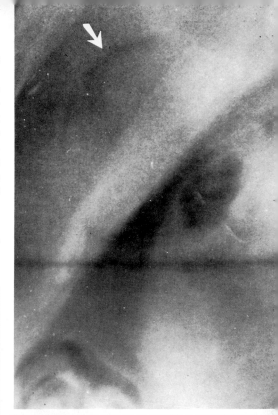

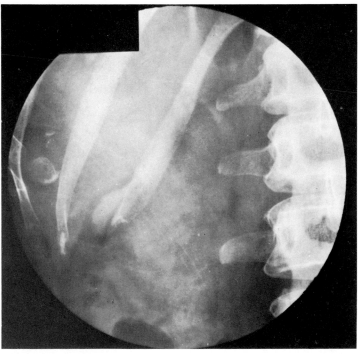

FIG. 1-52. Film from an oral cholecystogram demonstrating a crescentic halo of fat density along the right border of the opacified gallbladder. The diagnosis of acalculous gallbladder disease was confirmed at surgery. (Russell JGB, Keddie NC, Gough AL et al: Radiology of acalculous gallbladder disease—A new sign. Br J Radiol 49:420–424, 1976)

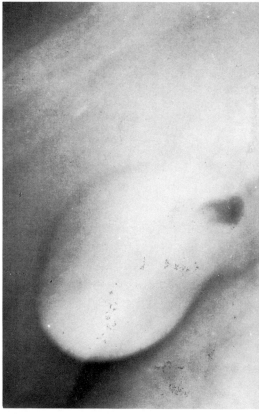

FIG. 1-53. (*Top*) Plain radiograph demonstrates a fine crescentic lucency in the right upper abdomen (**arrow**). (*Bottom*) Cholecystography reveals that the crescent-shaped lucency is the gallbladder wall in this patient with acalculous cholecystitis. (Russell JGB, Keddie NC, Gough AL et al: Radiology of acalculous gallbladder disease—A new sign. Br J Radiol 49:420–424, 1976)

FIG. 1-54. (*continues on overleaf*)

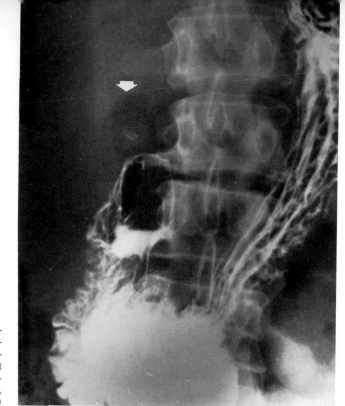

FIG. 1-54. A halo of mural fat (**arrow**) confirms that the calcification above the duodenal bulb represents a gallstone in the gallbladder. (Russell JGB, Keddie NC, Gough AL et al: Radiology of acalculous gallbladder disease—A new sign. Br J Radiol 49:420–424, 1976)

FIG. 1-55. Normal right flank stripe (*). The lateral margin of the lucent flank stripe represents the fascia transversalis and its medial margin, the parietal peritoneum. The mucosal surface of the lateral wall of the colon is identified through the presence of gas and fecal material. The soft-tissue density between the medial margin of the flank stripe and the mucosal surface of the ascending colon (**arrowheads**) is the parietal peritoneum. (Harris JH, Harris WH: The Radiology of Emergency Medicine. Baltimore, Williams & Wilkins, 1981)

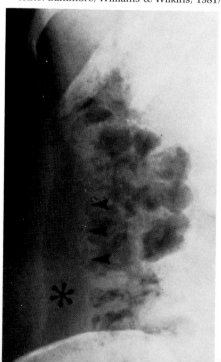

Flank Stripe Sign

The term *flank stripe* refers to the extraperitoneal fat situated between the parietal peritoneum and the inner wall of the abdominal cavity (fascia of the transverse abdominal muscle). In normal patients, there is a 1-mm to 2-mm-wide line of soft-tissue density between the fat density flank stripe and the gas- or feces-filled colon (Fig. 1-55). This soft-tissue density consists of the lateral wall of the colon and the peritoneum. A collection of blood or ascitic fluid in the flank causes medial displacement of the colon and widening of the soft-tissue density (positive flank stripe sign; Fig. 1-56). Because the parietal peritoneum constitutes the medial border of the flank stripe, the presence of peritoneal inflammation and edema may cause the medial margin of the flank stripe to become indistinct (Fig. 1-57).

BIBLIOGRAPHY
Frimann-Dahl J: Roentgen Examinations in Acute Abdominal Diseases. Springfield, IL, Charles C Thomas, 1960

FIG. 1-56. Positive flank stripe sign in a patient with hemoperitoneum following traumatic liver laceration. There is a wide soft-tissue density separating the lateral wall of the gas- and feces-filled ascending colon (**open arrows**) from the extraperitoneal fat (**closed arrows**).

FIG. 1-57. (*Left*) Irregular density of the retroperitoneal flank stripe in a patient with peritonitis. In some portions, the lateral margin of the flank stripe is faintly visible. The medial margin is completely obscured. (*Right*) Radiographic appearance of the same patient's flank stripe (**arrows**) 2 years earlier. (Harris JH, Harris WH: The Radiology of Emergency Medicine. Baltimore, Williams & Wilkins, 1981)

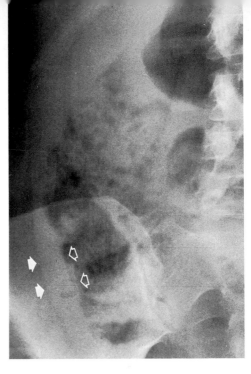

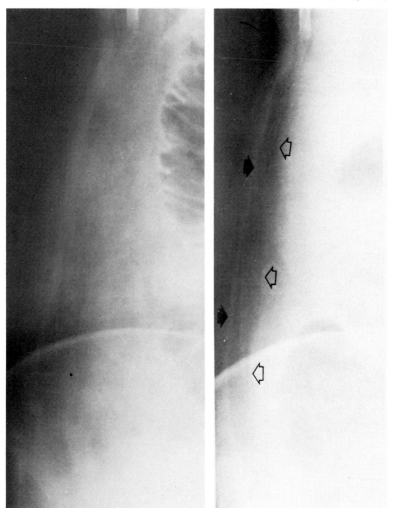

Fleischner Sign ▬▬▬▬▬▬

The term *Fleischner sign* refers to the wide gaping of the ileocecal valve associated with narrowing of the immediately adjacent ileum (Fig. 1-58). Although the resulting umbrella-like deformity has been described as characteristic of tuberculous infection, a similar appearance can be produced in patients with severe Crohn's disease.

BIBLIOGRAPHY

Carrera GF, Young S, Lewicki AM: Intestinal tuberculosis. Gastrointest Radiol 1:147–155, 1976

Fleischner FG: Die Darmtuberculose im Roentgenbild. Ergeb Med Strahlenforsch 3:359–423, 1923

Gershon-Cohen J, Kremens Z: X-ray studies of the ileocecal valve in ileocecal tuberculosis. Radiology 62:251–254, 1954

Short WF, Smith BD, Hoy RJ: Roentgenologic evaluation of the prominent or the unusual ileocecal valve. Med Radiogr Photogr 52:2–26, 1976

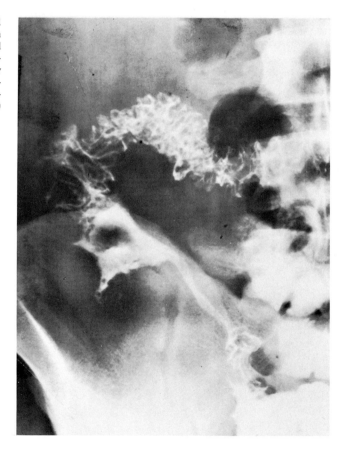

FIG. 1-58. Severe distortion of the ileocecal valve and narrowing of the terminal ileum have caused the valve to have an "inverted umbrella" appearance in this patient with ileocecal tuberculosis. (Short WF, Smith BD, Hoy RJ: Roentgenologic evaluation of the prominent or the unusual ileocecal valve. Med Radiogr Photogr 52:2–26, 1976)

Football Sign

Pneumoperitoneum in children can be manifest as greater than normal radiolucency of the entire abdomen. This radiolucency often assumes an oval configuration similar in appearance to a football as a result of the accumulation of large amounts of free gas in the uppermost (anterior) portion of the peritoneal cavity when the child is supine (Fig. 1-59). Confirmation of the presence of a pneumoperitoneum can be made by demonstration of the soft-tissue shadow of the falciform ligament outlined by gas on both sides of the ligament, or by the demonstration of gas under the hemidiaphragms on an erect view.

BIBLIOGRAPHY
Miller RE: Perforated viscus in infants: A new roentgen sign. Radiology 74:65–67, 1960

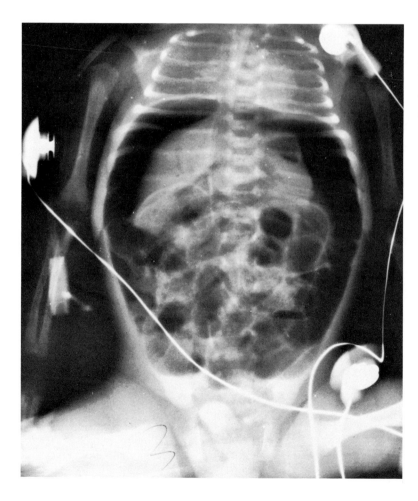

FIG. 1-59. A massive pneumoperitoneum in an infant appears as a large oval lucency on this supine radiograph of the abdomen. The falciform ligament is seen overlying the liver to the right of the spine. Portal venous gas can also be noted. (Wind ES, Pillare GP, Lee WJ: Lucent liver in the newborn: A roentgenographic sign of pneumoperitoneum. JAMA 237:2218–2219, 1977)

Frostberg's Inverted 3 Sign

The inverted 3 sign of Frostberg is an indication of disease involving the region of the medial wall of the descending duodenum and the adjacent head of the pancreas (Fig. 1-60). Although often considered diagnostic of pancreatic carcinoma, the inverted 3 sign of Frostberg is nonspecific. It is seen in fewer than 10% of patients with pancreatic carcinoma (Fig. 1-61) and is actually more common in persons with inflammatory disorders, such as acute pancreatitis (Fig. 1-62) and postbulbar ulcer disease (Fig. 1-63).

The central limb of the "3" represents the point of fixation of the duodenal wall at which the pancreatic and common bile ducts insert into the papilla. The impressions above and below this point reflect either edema of the minor and major papillae or smooth muscle spasm and edema in the duodenal wall.

BIBLIOGRAPHY

Frostberg N: Characteristic duodenal deformity in cases of different kinds of perivaterial enlargement of the pancreas. Acta Radiol 19:164–173, 1938

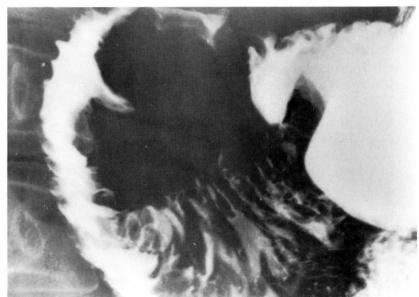

FIG. 1-60. Frostberg's inverted 3 sign in a patient with severe acute pancreatitis. (Eisenberg RL: Gastrointestinal Radiology: A Pattern Approach. Philadelphia, JB Lippincott, 1983)

FIG. 1-61. Frostberg's inverted 3 sign (**arrow**) in a patient with carcinoma of the head of the pancreas. (Eisenberg RL: Gastrointestinal Radiology: A Pattern Approach. Philadelphia, JB Lippincott, 1983)

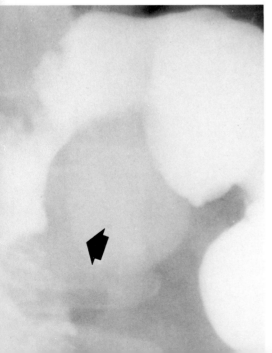

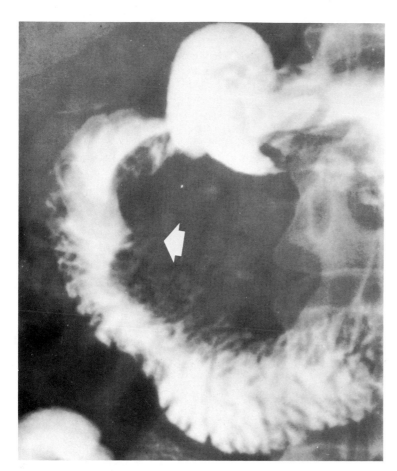

FIG. 1-62. Frostberg's inverted 3 sign (**arrow**) in a patient with acute pancreatitis and no evidence of malignancy. (Eisenberg RL: Gastrointestinal Radiology: A Pattern Approach. Philadelphia, JB Lippincott, 1983)

FIG. 1-63. Frostberg's inverted 3 sign in a patient with a large postbulbar ulcer (**arrow**) and no evidence of malignancy. (Eisenberg RL: Gastrointestinal Radiology: A Pattern Approach. Philadelphia, JB Lippincott, 1983)

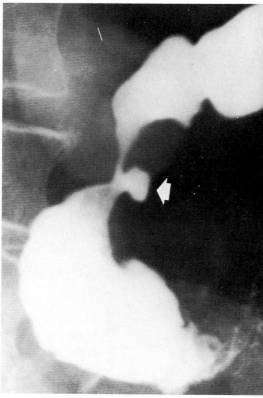

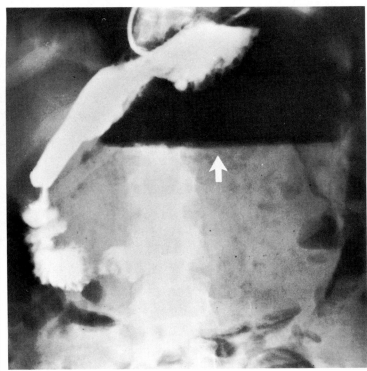

FIG. 1-64. On an upright projection, the gas–fluid interface in the stomach has a fuzzy or blurred appearance.

FIG. 1-65. (*Left*) Plain abdominal radiograph and (*right*) film from a barium study demonstrate a huge lesser sac abscess with a prominent, sharp gas–fluid level (**arrows**). (Eisenberg RL: Gastrointestinal Radiology: A Pattern Approach. Philadelphia, JB Lippincott, 1983)

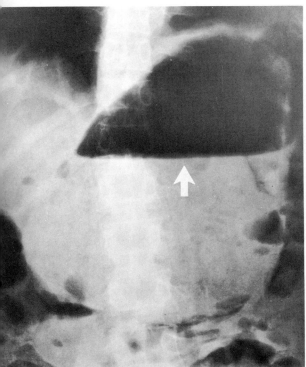

Fuzzy Fluid Level Sign

The radiographic appearance of the gas–fluid interface in an upper abdominal structure has been reported to be of diagnostic value. On upright projections, the gas–fluid interface seen in the stomach has been described as almost always having a fuzzy or blurred appearance with an irregular gradual transition from water density to gas density (Fig. 1-64). This is in contrast to extragastric fluid levels (*e.g.*, fluid levels in other portions of the intestine, abscess cavities, hydropneumoperitoneum), which are sharp and straight, with an abrupt change from fluid to gas density (Fig. 1-65). The presence of a sharp fluid level in the left upper quadrant thus suggests a lesser sac abscess, left subphrenic abscess, or infected pancreatic pseudocyst, rather than a normal stomach. However, both the gastric gas–fluid interface (Fig. 1-66) and the gas–fluid levels within abscesses (Fig. 1-67) may appear fuzzy on one film and sharp on a companion stereoradiograph. Because the appearance depends on the alignment of the x-ray beam with respect to the surface of the fluid rather than on the chemical composition or location of the fluid in the abdomen, the fuzzy fluid level sign does not appear to have diagnostic significance.

BIBLIOGRAPHY
Caruso RD, Berk RN: The fuzzy fluid level sign. Radiology 98:369–372, 1971
Mettler FA, Ghahremani GG: The fuzzy fluid level sign: Reappraisal of its cause and diagnostic value. Radiology 105:509–511, 1972

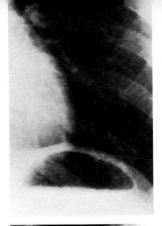

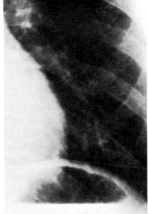

FIG. 1-66. On this pair of chest stereoradiographs of the same patient, the gastric gas–fluid interface appears fuzzy on one film (*top*) and sharp on the other (*bottom*). (Mettler FA, Ghahremani GG: The fuzzy fluid level sign: Reappraisal of its cause and diagnostic value. Radiology 105:509–511, 1972)

FIG. 1-67. Changing appearance of the gas–fluid interface in a subphrenic abscess on posteroanterior (**A,B**) and right lateral (**C,D**) stereoradiographs. (Mettler FA, Ghahremani GG: The fuzzy fluid level sign: Reappraisal of its cause and diagnostic value. Radiology 105:509–511, 1972)

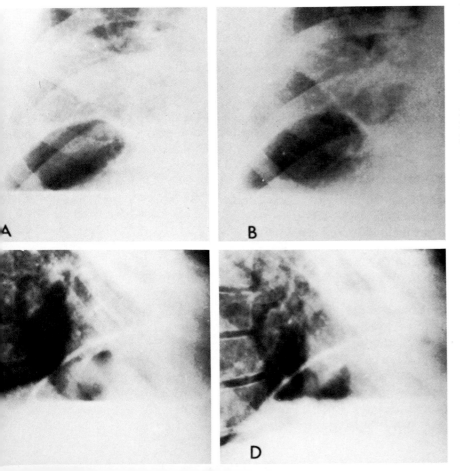

Gallbladder Inertia Sign

Absent or minimal contraction of the gallbladder in response to a fatty meal has been reported as an early sign of celiac sprue. The abnormality is reversible by a gluten-free diet. This phenomenon is most likely due to impaired cholecystokinin release by the damaged small bowel mucosa leading to sequestration of bile in the inert gallbladder. The gallbladder inertia sign may be radiographically evident before clinical features of malabsorption become apparent.

BIBLIOGRAPHY
Delamarre J, Dupas JL, Capron JP et al: Gallbladder inertia: "Early" radiologic sign of celiac disease? AJR 133:563, 1979
Low-Beer TS, Heaton KW, Heaton ST et al: Gallbladder inertia and sluggish enterohepatic circulation of bile-salt in coeliac disease. Lancet 1:991–994, 1971

Gasless Abdomen Sign

A relative lack of gas in the abdominal cavity has been reported to be an indication of several different disease entities (Fig. 1-68). Bowel ischemia, particularly with mesenteric venous occlusion, may produce huge quantities of intraluminal fluid and cause a "gasless abdomen," which suggests strangulation of bowel. A similar appearance has been described in patients with acute pancreatitis and in patients with high intestinal obstruction, as well as in normal persons.

FIG. 1-68. Essentially complete lack of gas in the abdominal cavity in a patient with severe acute pancreatitis.

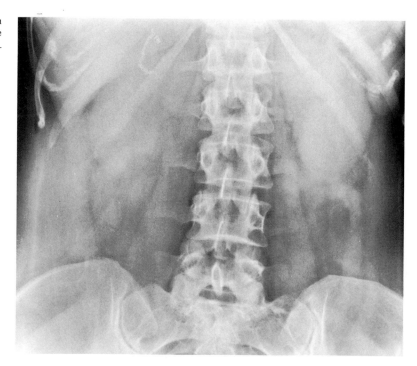

Gastric Cannonball Sign ▬▬▬▬▬▬▬

The term *gastric cannonballs* has been applied to a radiographic appearance of diffuse hepatic metastases in which multiple persistent rounded filling defects are seen within the body of the stomach (Fig. 1-69). The filling defects are fixed in position and are noncompressible, and they demonstrate smooth contours with intact, nonulcerated surface mucosa. The uncommon radiographic appearance of multiple round gastric filling defects may also be seen in such unusual conditions as multiple submucosal leiomyomas or neurofibromas, impressions from multiple hepatic cysts, gastric serosal metastases, intramural varicosities, and hematomas.

BIBLIOGRAPHY
Doss JC, Ferrucci JT: Gastric cannonballs: A roentgen sign of hepatic metastases. Gastroenterology 67:519–520, 1974

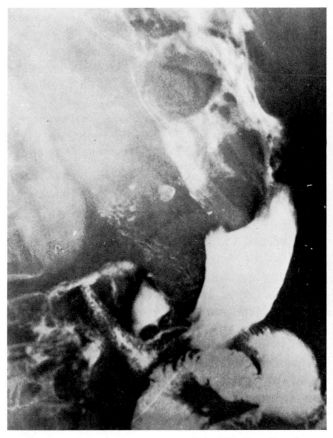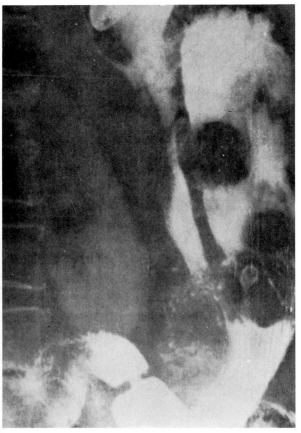

FIG. 1-69. Two films from an upper gastrointestinal series demonstrate multiple smoothly rounded filling defects in the body of the stomach reflecting diffuse hepatic metastases from undifferentiated carcinoma. The intact, nonulcerated surface mucosa and the discrete contours of the masses suggest intramural or adherent serosal masses. Note the displacement of the stomach by the left lobe of the liver. The vertical linear lucency along the lesser curvature was not satisfactorily explained. (Doss JC, Ferrucci JT: Gastric cannonballs: A roentgen sign of hepatic metastases. Gastroenterology 67:519–520, 1974)

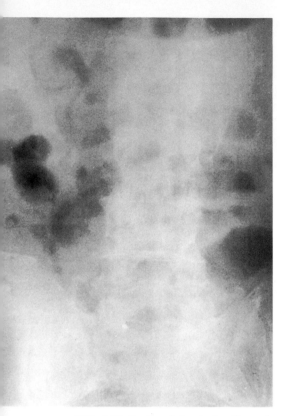

Ground-Glass Sign

Massive ascites produces a "ground-glass" appearance on abdominal radiographs that results from loss of visibility of discrete organ outlines in the abdominal cavity (Fig. 1-70). The degree of radiographic contrast seen is severely decreased as a result of both the increased amount of water density material (ascitic fluid) that must be penetrated by the x-ray beam and the associated invisibility of fat planes infiltrated by water density edema fluid.

BIBLIOGRAPHY
Keeffe EJ, Gagliardi RA, Pfister RC: The roentgenographic evaluation of ascites. AJR 101:388–396, 1967
Nelson SW, Freimanis AK, Wiot J (eds): Gastrointestinal Tract Disease Syllabus, Set 4. Chicago, American College of Radiology, 1973

FIG. 1-70. Supine abdominal radiograph demonstrates general abdominal haziness ("ground-glass" appearance) in this patient with ascites. (Eisenberg RL: Gastrointestinal Radiology: A Pattern Approach. Philadelphia, JB Lippincott, 1983)

FIG. 1-72.

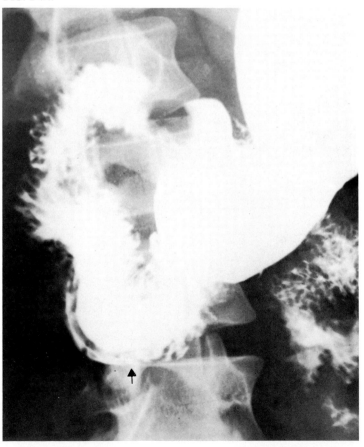

Halo Sign

An intraluminal duodenal diverticulum is a sac of duodenal mucosa originating in the second portion of the duodenum near the papilla of Vater. It is probably due to ballooning of a congenital duodenal web or diaphragm as a result of such mechanical factors as forward pressure by food and strong peristaltic activity (Fig. 1-71). When filled with barium, the intraluminal duodenal diverticulum appears as a finger-like sac separated from contrast within the duodenal lumen by a radiolucent band representing the wall of the diverticulum (Fig. 1-72). Because of its characteristic configuration, the appearance of an intraluminal duodenal diverticulum has also been described as the *comma, teardrop* (Fig. 1-73), and *windsock* signs.

BIBLIOGRAPHY

Heilbrun N, Boyden EA: Intraluminal duodenal diverticula. Radiology 82:887–894, 1964

Laudan JCH, Norton GI: Intraluminal duodenal diverticulum. AJR 90:756–760, 1963

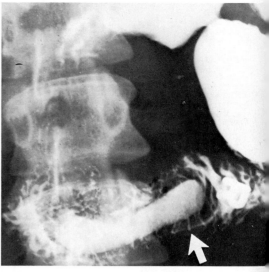

FIG. 1-71. An intraluminal duodenal diverticulum appears as a sac-like collection of contrast surrounded by a lucent halo (**arrow**). (Heilbrun N, Boyden EA: Intraluminal duodenal diverticula. Radiology 82:887–894, 1964)

FIG. 1-72. Characteristic radiographic appearance of intraluminal duodenal diverticula in two patients (**arrows**). Note the radiolucent band representing the wall of the diverticulum separating contrast in the diverticulum from contrast in the duodenal lumen. (Heilbrun N, Boyden EA: Intraluminal duodenal diverticula. Radiology 82:887–894, 1964)

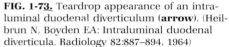

FIG. 1-73. Teardrop appearance of an intraluminal duodenal diverticulum (**arrow**). (Heilbrun N, Boyden EA: Intraluminal duodenal diverticula. Radiology 82:887–894, 1964)

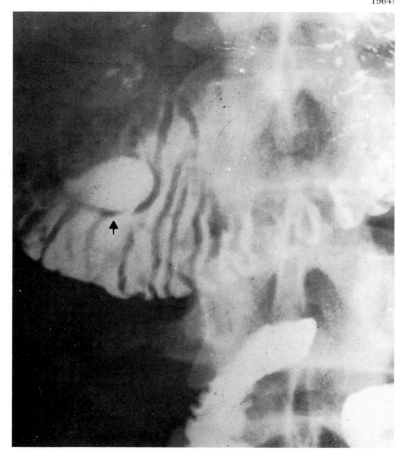

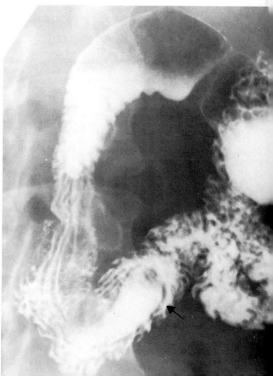

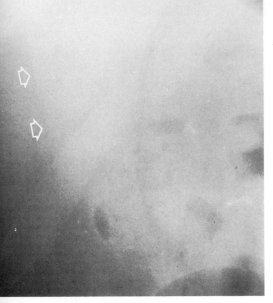

Hellmer's Sign

Medial displacement of the lateral border of the liver on abdominal radiographs is generally considered pathognomonic of ascites. Because of the relative difference in density between the liver and ascitic fluid collected lateral to it, the free intraperitoneal fluid appears as a lucent zone between the liver and the costal margin (Hellmer's sign; Fig. 1-74). A similar pattern of a medially displaced lateral liver edge has also been reported in a patient with a large extraperitoneal fluid collection (Fig. 1-75), indicating that Hellmer's sign may reflect a pathologic process in either the intra- or the extra-peritoneal space.

BIBLIOGRAPHY

Hellmer H: Die Konturen des rechten Leberascites. Acta Radiol 23:533, 1942

Wixson D, Kazam E, Whalen JP: Displaced lateral surface of the liver (Hellmer's sign) secondary to an extraperitoneal fluid collection. AJR 127:679–682, 1976

FIG. 1-74. Abdominal radiograph demonstrates medial displacement of the lateral border of the liver (**arrows**) as a result of ascites. The free intraperitoneal fluid appears as a lucent zone lateral to the liver.

FIG. 1-75. (*Left*) Abdominal radiograph demonstrates medial displacement of the lateral border of the liver (**arrows**), suggesting the presence of ascites. (*Top, right*) Transverse sonogram performed with the patient in the supine position shows a large echo-free collection surrounding the medially located liver (**L**). (*Bottom, right*) Transverse sonogram performed with the patient in the left lateral decubitus position shows no change in the shape or position of the collection, thereby excluding the diagnosis of free intraperitoneal fluid. Surgery revealed an extraperitoneal (posterior pararenal) fluid collection with extension into the right lateral abdominal wall. (Wixson D, Kazan E, Whalen JP: Displaced lateral surface of the liver [Hellmer's sign] secondary to an extraperitoneal fluid collection. AJR 127:679–682, 1976. Copyright 1976. Reproduced by permission)

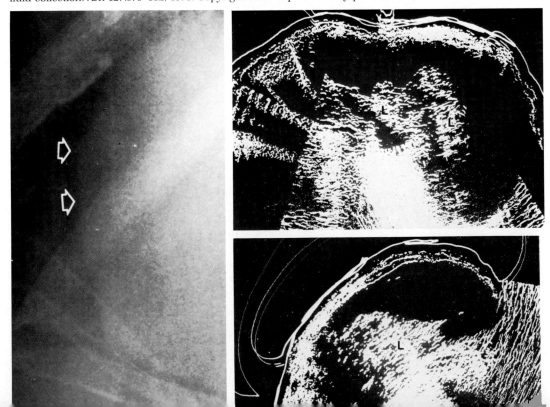

Hepatic Angle Sign

The inferior and right lateral margins of the liver are commonly identified on routine abdominal films (Fig. 1-76, *left*). The radiographic lateral border of the liver actually represents the liver and parietal peritoneum bordered by extraperitoneal fat. The lower edge of the liver may be visualized depending upon its proximity to the greater omentum and pericolic fat and is best appreciated in its most lateral portion (the hepatic angle). An accumulation of sufficient intraperitoneal fluid in this area may insinuate itself between the lower edge of the liver and the omental fat, effectively obscuring the hepatic angle (Fig. 1-76, *right*).

The hepatic angle sign is of limited value as an indication of intraperitoneal fluid; nonvisualization of the hepatic angle has been demonstrated in up to one third of normal healthy adults, especially on radiographs of poor technical quality. However, if the extraperitoneal fat lateral to the liver is clearly seen, the hepatic angle should also be well outlined. If it is not, the presence of intraperitoneal fluid should be suspected.

BIBLIOGRAPHY

Keeffe EJ, Gagliardi RA, Pfister RC: The roentgenographic evaluation of ascites. AJR 101:388–396, 1967

Margulies M, Stoane L: Hepatic angle in roentgen evaluation of peritoneal fluid. Radiology 88:51–56, 1967

Moskowitz M: The psoas sign, hepatic angle, normal patients, and everyday practice. Gut 14:308–310, 1973

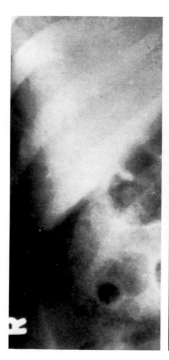
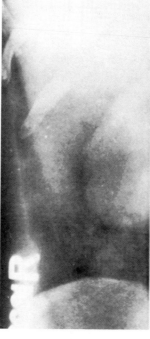

FIG. 1-76. (*Left*) Plain abdominal radiograph of a patient admitted to the hospital following a stab wound to the left flank demonstrates a normal hepatic angle outlined by fat. Abdominal paracentesis at this time was negative. Eighteen hours later, a repeat paracentesis yielded gross blood, and at laparotomy, a lacerated spleen was removed. The pancreas was accidentally incised during the resection. (*Right*) Radiographic examination 4 days later, after signs of peritonitis have developed, demonstrates obliteration of the hepatic angle. Note also the positive flank stripe sign, which is not present in the previous radiograph. (Margulies M, Stoane L: Hepatic angle in roentgen evaluation of peritoneal fluid. Radiology 88:51–56, 1967)

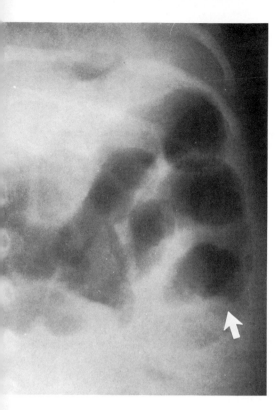

Hump Sign

In *Ascaris* infestation, conglomerate masses of the roundworms may be identified on plain abdominal radiographs. With the patient erect, the worm bolus often demonstrates an irregularity or nodularity that distorts the gas–fluid level, producing a hump (Fig. 1-79). This sign is accentuated when the hump contains irregular gas bubbles or linear radiolucent shadows (Fig. 1-80).

BIBLIOGRAPHY
Ellman BA, Wynne JM, Freeman A: Intestinal ascariasis: New plain film features. AJR 135:37–42, 1980

FIG. 1-79. Distention of loops of small bowel with the hump sign produced by a bolus of worms intruding into the lumen (**arrow**). (Ellman BA, Wynne JM, Freeman A: Intestinal ascariasis: New plain film features. AJR 135:37–42, 1980. Copyright 1980. Reproduced by permission)

FIG. 1-80. Hump sign (**solid arrow**) with a bolus of worms clearly seen below (**open arrow**). (Ellman BA, Wynne JM, Freeman A: Intestinal ascariasis: New plain film features. AJR 135:37–42, 1980. Copyright 1980. Reproduced by permission)

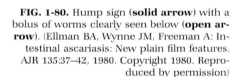
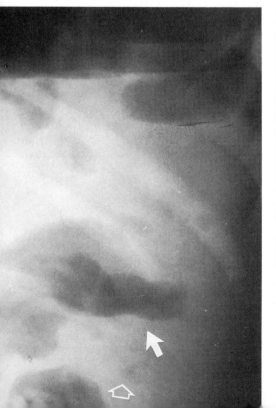

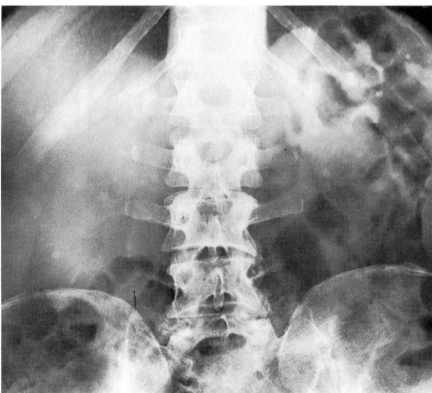

FIG. 1-81. Multiple nodular densities projected over the abdomen are skin lesions on the abdominal wall in a patient with neurofibromatosis. Note that most are well defined with complete borders.

Incomplete Border Sign

The radiographic appearance of the border of an abdominal mass can aid in the determination of whether the lesion lies within the abdominal wall or is situated within the abdomen or on the skin. A mass on the skin (Fig. 1-81) or within the abdomen is well defined with a complete border. In contrast, a mass within the abdominal wall, such as a hernia, is characterized by an incomplete border, because at some point in its contour its boundary merges with the adjacent soft-tissue densities (Fig. 1-82).

BIBLIOGRAPHY
Mendelson E: Abdominal wall masses: The usefulness of the incomplete border sign. Radiol Clin North Am 2:161–166, 1964

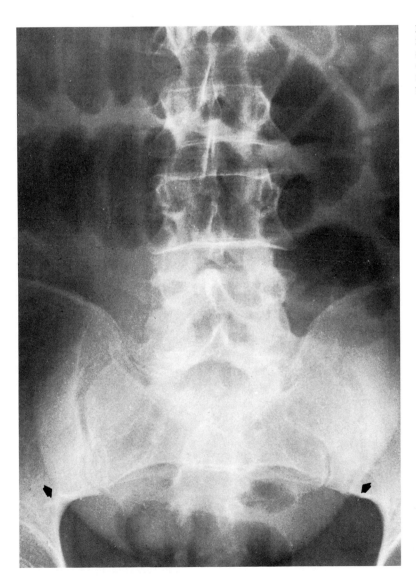

FIG. 1-82. A large soft-tissue mass (**arrows**) in the midabdomen and upper pelvis is characterized by an incomplete border. This indicates that the mass, which represents a large umbilical hernia, lies within the abdominal wall.

Incomplete Ring Sign

A small collection of residual cholecystographic contrast in the configuration of an incomplete ring can occasionally be identified in the right upper abdomen medial and posterior to the gallbladder (Fig. 1-83, *top*). On upper gastrointestinal series, the contrast collection is seen to be located in a peptic ulcer of the duodenal bulb or postbulbar duodenum (Fig. 1-83, *bottom*). The cholecystographic incomplete ring sign, though uncommon, is reported to be fairly specific for duodenal ulcer and suggests the need for an appropriate barium examination.

BIBLIOGRAPHY
Sickles EA: Cholecystographic diagnosis of duodenal ulcer: The incomplete ring sign. Radiology 124:27–30, 1977

FIG. 1-83. (*Top*) Prone film from an oral cholecystogram shows a small, incomplete, ring-shaped collection of retained contrast material medial to the normally opacified gallbladder and superior to the hepatic flexure of the colon (**arrow**). (*Bottom*) Subsequent barium study in the same radiographic projection demonstrates a postbulbar duodenal ulcer crater (**arrow**). Note that this crater is identical in size and location to the collection of retained contrast. (Sickles EA: Cholecystographic diagnosis of duodenal ulcer: The incomplete ring sign. Radiology 124:27–30, 1977)

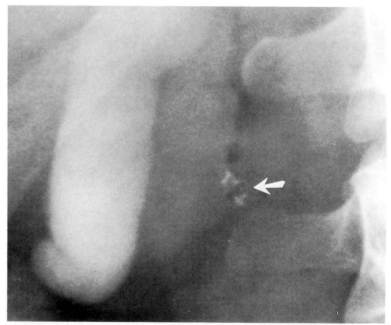

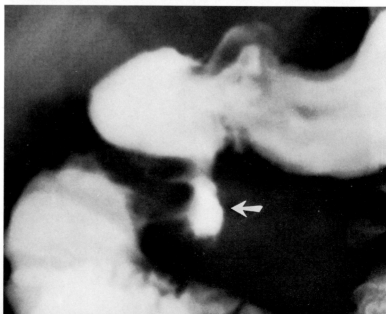

Intrahepatic Gas Sign ▬▬▬▬▬▬

In a patient suffering thoracic or abdominal injury, the demonstration of unexplained gas in the substance of the liver may be of value in calling attention to unsuspected hepatic trauma (Fig. 1-84). The intrahepatic gas is of unexplained origin; it may have been driven into the biliary tree from the upper gastrointestinal tract at the time of injury. Other causes of gas in the region of the liver (abscess, portal vein) can usually be eliminated on the basis of the history and clinical presentation.

BIBLIOGRAPHY
Wolfel DA, Brogdon BG: Intrahepatic air: A sign of trauma. Radiology 91:952–953, 1968

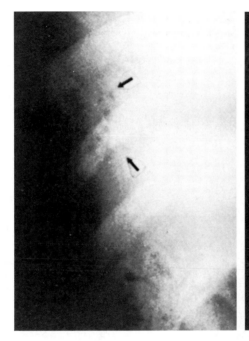 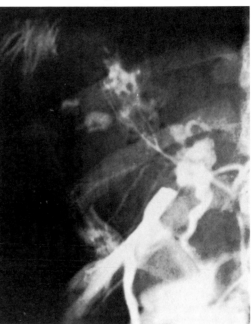

FIG. 1-84. (*Left*) Small collections of gas (**arrows**) are present in the right lobe of the liver. (*Right*) Operative cholangiogram demonstrates rupture of small branches of the right hepatic duct with extravasation of contrast material. (Opaque drains are seen in the subdiaphragmatic and subhepatic spaces.) (Wolfel BA, Brogdon BG: Intrahepatic air: A sign of trauma. Radiology 91:952–953, 1968)

Inverted U Sign

A long, redundant loop of sigmoid colon can undergo a twist on its mesenteric axis and form a closed-loop obstruction. In sigmoid volvulus, the greatly inflated sigmoid loop appears as a characteristic inverted U-shaped shadow that rises out of the pelvis vertically or obliquely and can even reach the level of the diaphragm (Fig. 1-85).

BIBLIOGRAPHY

Love L: Large bowel obstruction. Semin Roentgenol 8:299–322, 1973

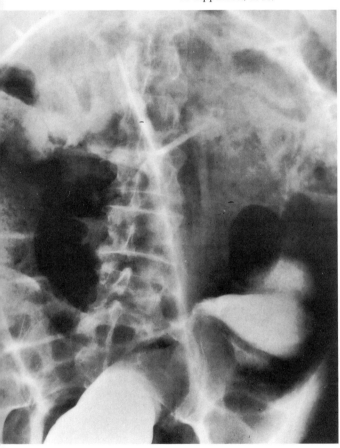
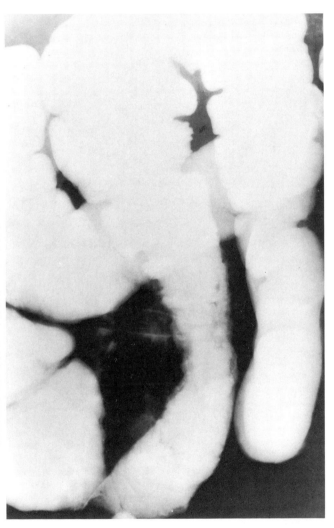

FIG. 1-85. *(Left)* A massively dilated loop of sigmoid appears as an inverted U-shaped shadow rising out of the pelvis in this patient with sigmoid volvulus. *(Right)* A barium enema examination following reduction of the volvulus demonstrates a severely ectatic sigmoid colon. (Eisenberg RL: Gastrointestinal Radiology: A Pattern Approach. Philadelphia, JB Lippincott, 1983)

Inverted V Sign

Free gas outlining the lateral umbilical ligaments makes these structures visible in the lower abdomen, where they form an inverted "V" as they course inferiorly and laterally from the umbilicus (Fig. 1-86). The ligaments, which contain the umbilical arterial remnants, may be unilaterally or fractionally visualized. The inverted V sign, which strongly suggests a pneumoperitoneum, is seen on supine abdominal radiographs performed in patients who are too ill for erect films.

BIBLIOGRAPHY
Weiner CI, Diaconis JN, Dennis JM: The "inverted V": A new sign of pneumoperitoneum. Radiology 107:47–48, 1973

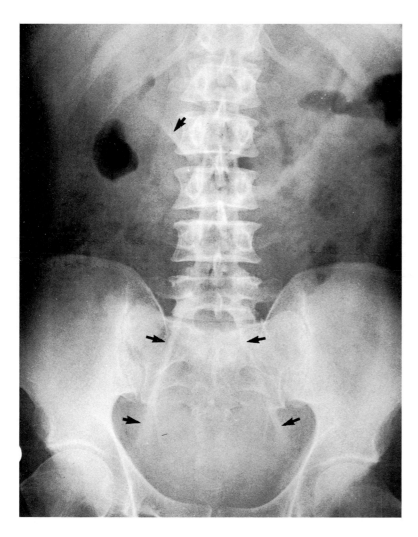

FIG. 1-86. Supine abdominal radiograph shows the lateral umbilical ligaments (**lower arrows**) diverging from the umbilicus, implying the presence of a pneumoperitoneum. Free intraperitoneal gas also makes the falciform ligament visible (**upper arrow**). (Weiner CI, Diaconis JN, Dennis JM: The "inverted V": A new sign of pneumoperitoneum. Radiology 107:47–48, 1973)

Jet Phenomenon

The term *jet phenomenon* refers to the appearance of the barium column as it is vigorously propelled through a relatively narrow opening in an esophageal web (Fig. 1-87). The presence of a jet suggests that the degree of stenosis is more marked than usually encountered with a web; the width of the jet immediately below the level of the web indicates the size of the orifice. At times, the jet phenomenon stimulates a long stenosing lesion in the esophagus.

BIBLIOGRAPHY

Shauffer IA, Phillips HE, Sequeira J: The jet phenomenon: A manifestation of esophageal web. AJR 129:747–748, 1977

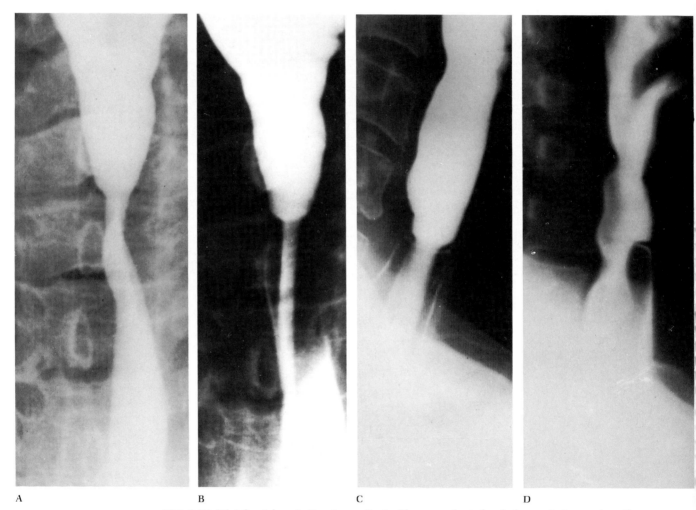

A   B   C   D

FIG. 1-87. **(A)** A frontal projection in a patient with an esophageal web demonstrates an abruptly narrowed barium column simulating a long stenosing lesion in the upper esophagus. **(B)** The double-contrast effect below the web shows the width of the jet and the normal caliber of the esophagus below the web. **(C)** The lateral projection better illustrates the annular constriction of the esophagus produced by the web. **(D)** Further opacification of the esophagus more graphically delineates the web. (Shauffer IA, Phillips HE, Sequeira J: The jet phenomenon: A manifestation of esophageal web. AJR 129:747–748, 1977. Copyright 1977. Reproduced by permission)

Keyhole Sign

Pseudolesions in the duodenal bulb are produced by barium surrounding and entrapped in contiguous parallel duodenal folds (Fig. 1-88, *left*). As peristalsis progresses, a characteristic "keyhole" appearance is produced (Fig. 1-88, *right*). The pseudolesion disappears with peristalsis or with distention of the duodenal bulb with gas.

BIBLIOGRAPHY

Seymour EQ: Duodenal pseudolesions: The key hole sign. Rev Int Radiol 4:189–191, 1979

FIG. 1-88. (*Left*) Concentric rugal folds with entrapped barium (**arrow**) are seen before development of a duodenal pseudolesion. (*Right*) With the duodenal bulb partially emptied by peristalsis, a pseudolesion presenting the characteristic "keyhole" appearance is now evident (**arrow**). (Seymour EQ: Duodenal pseudolesions: The key hole sign. Rev Int Radiol 4:189–191, 1979)

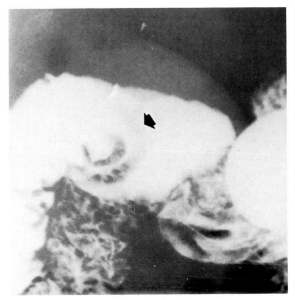

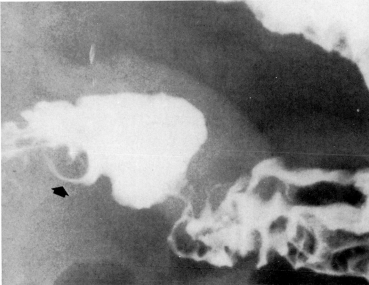

Lollipop-Tree Sign

In both Caroli's disease and congenital hepatic fibrosis, T-tube or operative cholangiography demonstrates large or small cystic spaces communicating with the intrahepatic bile ducts, producing a "lollipop-tree" appearance of the biliary system (Fig. 1-89).

BIBLIOGRAPHY

Unite I, Maitern A, Bagnasco FM et al: Congenital hepatic fibrosis associated with renal tubular ectasis. Radiology 109:565–570, 1973

FIG. 1-89. Operative cholangiogram demonstrates the "lollipop-tree" appearance of the biliary system in a patient with congenital hepatic fibrosis. (Unite I, Maitern A, Bagnasco FM et al: Congenital hepatic fibrosis associated with renal tubular ectasis. Radiology 109:565–570, 1973)

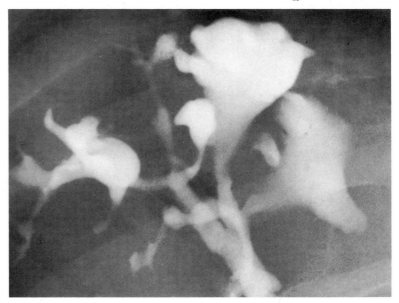

Lucent Liver Sign

On abdominal radiographs in the newborn, the density of the liver should be the same as the density of adjacent deep soft tissues, which in effect act as an internal control. When relatively small amounts of free intraperitoneal gas are trapped between the anterior surface of the liver and the peritoneum, lucencies varying from streaks or bubbles to a homogeneous appearance may be visualized (Fig. 1-90). The contrast between the density of the deep soft tissues of the muscles in the lateral abdominal wall and that of the gas-covered liver provides the lucent liver sign of pneumoperitoneum. Rarely, a similar appearance is due to interposition of gas-containing bowel or a fatty liver; however, demonstration of the lucent liver sign in an appropriate clinical setting should suggest the need for upright or left lateral decubitus views to confirm the presence of free intraperitoneal gas.

BIBLIOGRAPHY

Wind ES, Pillari GP, Lee WJ: Lucent liver in the newborn: A roentgenographic sign of pneumoperitoneum. JAMA 237:2218–2219, 1977

FIG. 1-90. (*Left*) On the frontal view of the abdomen, the lucent liver is the only radiographic manifestation of pneumoperitoneum. The umbilical venous catheter is superficially placed. (*Right*) A lateral view of the abdomen shows free intraperitoneal gas anterior to the liver. (Wind ES, Pillari GP, Lee WJ: Lucent liver in the newborn: A roentgenographic sign of pneumoperitoneum. JAMA 237:2218–2219, 1977. Copyright 1977, American Medical Association)

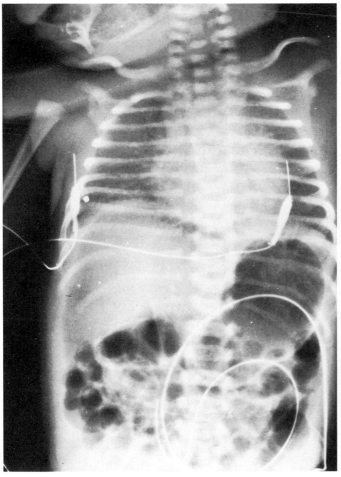
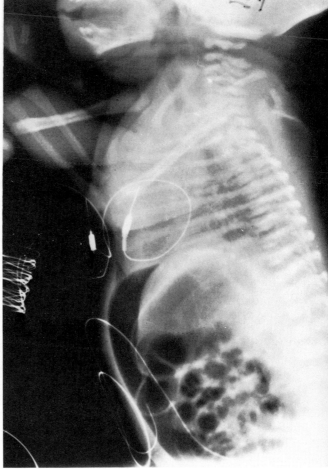

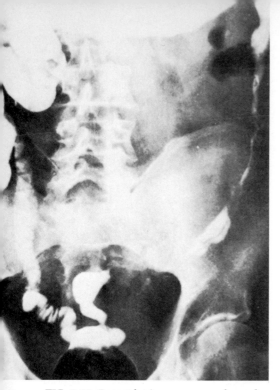

Lumen with a Lumen Sign

Ischemic colitis may cause sloughing of long continuous fragments of colonic mucosa. Radiographs from barium enema examinations may demonstrate filling of the lumen as well as intramural extravasation of barium, creating a "lumen with a lumen" effect (Fig. 1-91). Long segments of bowel may be involved, and the separation between the intraluminal and the intramural barium may be quite wide. Repeat barium studies performed during the healing phase demonstrate a long stenotic segment corresponding in location to the area of mucosal slough shown on the original radiographic examination (Fig. 1-92).

BIBLIOGRAPHY
Chino S, Johnson JC, Keith LM: New clinical and radiographic sign in ischemic colitis. Am J Surg 128:640–643, 1974

FIG. 1-92. Repeat barium enema performed during the healing phase shows a long stenotic segment of the descending colon corresponding in location to the area of mucosal slough shown in Fig. 1-91. (Chino S, Johnson JC, Keith LM: New clinical and radiographic sign in ischemic colitis. Am J Surg 128:640–643, 1974)

FIG. 1-91. (A) Oblique view of a barium enema examination shows areas of mucosal slough with intramural extravasation of barium in the rectal and sigmoid areas. **(B)** Lateral and **(C)** axial views show the "lumen with a lumen" effect in the rectosigmoid. Note that, in some areas, the separation between the intraluminal and intramural barium is quite wide. **(D)** Postevacuation film shows a considerable amount of barium retained on the left side of the colon. This barium is largely intramural rather than intraluminal. The area of mucosal slough extends from the proximal descending colon just beyond the splenic flexure down to the rectum. The remainder of the colon appears relatively normal. (Chino S, Johnson JC, Keith LM: New clinical and radiographic sign in ischemic colitis. Am J Surg 128:640–643, 1974)

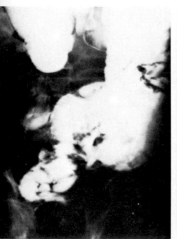
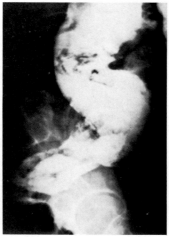
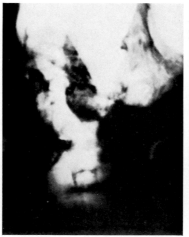
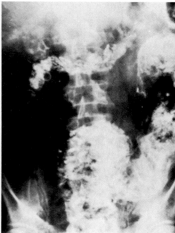

A B   C   D

Medusa Locks Sign ▬▬▬▬

In *Ascaris* infestation, the roundworms may multiply to such an extent that they form conglomerate masses (Fig. 1-93), which may cause intestinal obstruction. Trapping of intestinal gas between the masses of worms may give rise to an appearance suggesting coiled locks of hair (Medusa locks) that is sometimes detectable on plain abdominal radiographs (Fig. 1-94). Other terms to describe this bizarre appearance of a bolus of worms include *whirlpool, breadcrumbs, beehive,* and *tangled thick cord.*

BIBLIOGRAPHY

Bean WJ: Recognition of ascariasis by routine chest or abdomen roentgenograms. AJR 94:379–384, 1965

Ellman BA, Wynne JM, Freeman A: Intestinal ascariasis: New plain film features. AJR 133:37–42, 1980

Isaacs I: Roentgenographic demonstration of intestinal ascariasis in children without using barium. AJR 76:558–561, 1956

Okumura M, Nakashima Y, Curti P et al: Acute intestinal obstruction by ascariasis: Analysis of 455 cases. Rev Inst Med Trop Sao Paulo 16:292–300, 1974

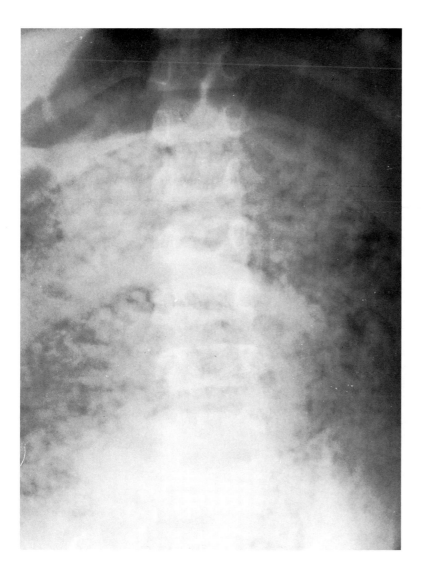

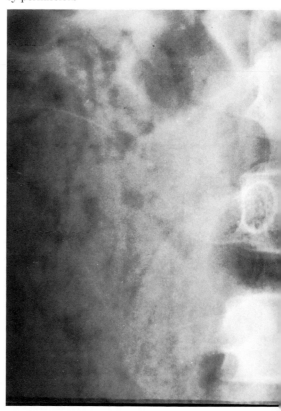

FIG. 1-93. (*Left*) Enormous numbers of impacted worms appear as convoluted masses outlined by gas. (Ellman BA, Wynne JM, Freeman A: Intestinal ascariasis: New plain film features. AJR 133:37–42, 1980. Copyright 1980. Reproduced by permission)

FIG. 1-94. (*Below*) Aggregation of worms contrasts with normal small bowel gas, producing the typical "Medusa locks" appearance. (Ellman BA, Wynne JM, Freeman A: Intestinal ascariasis: New plain film features. AJR 133:37–42, 1980. Copyright 1980. Reproduced by permission)

Mega-Aeroesophagus Sign

FIG. 1-95. (*Upper left*) Frontal chest radiograph demonstrates a markedly distended air-filled esophagus (**arrows**) in this patient with mega-aeroesophagus with gastroesophageal reflux due to cerebral palsy. (*Upper right*) Lateral view demonstrates the same findings (**arrows**). (*Lower left*) Three years later, the same findings are present (**arrows**). (*Lower right*) Barium swallow examination performed at the same time as the third radiograph demonstrates massive reflux (**arrow**) (Swischuk LE, Hayden K, van Caillie BD: Mega-aeroesophagus in children: A sign of gastroesophageal reflux. Radiology 141:73–76, 1981)

A small amount of air in the esophagus of children is a normal radiographic finding. However, distention and filling of the entire esophagus with air, producing the mega-aeroesophagus sign, is almost invariably associated with gastroesophageal reflux (Fig. 1-95). This finding is especially common in children with cerebral palsy or mental retardation. The mega-aeroesophagus sign is occasionally seen transiently in severely ill or moribund patients, also as a result of gastroesophageal reflux. Rare causes of this appearance are distal esophageal obstruction and acute lye burns.

BIBLIOGRAPHY

Swischuk LE, Hayden CK, van Caillie BD: Mega-aeroesophagus in children: A sign of gastroesophageal reflux. Radiology 141:73–76, 1981

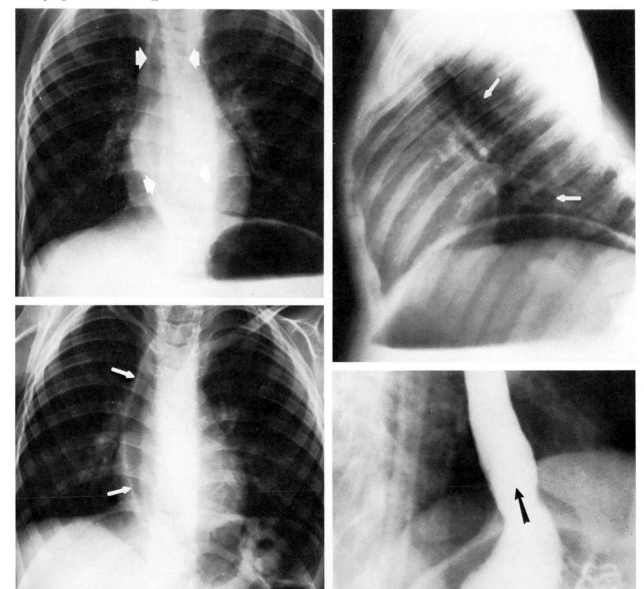

Mercedes-Benz Sign

Noncalcified gallstones are occasionally identified on plain abdominal radiographs because of distinctive stellate lucencies in the right upper quadrant (Fig. 1-96). This phenomenon is called the *Mercedes-Benz sign* because the lucent gas-containing fissures within the gallstones have a triradiate pattern similar to that of the symbol of the German automobile. The mechanism underlying this phenomenon appears to be nitrogen filling of faults that are created by shrinkage of cholesterol crystals composing the gallstones.

BIBLIOGRAPHY
Meyers MA, O'Donohue N: The Mercedes-Benz sign: Insight into the dynamics of formation and disappearance of gallstones. AJR 119:63–70, 1973

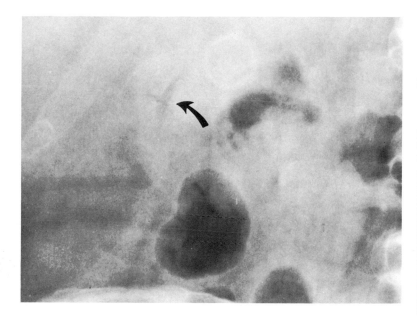

FIG. 1-96. Plain abdominal radiographs demonstrate gas-containing fissures within a gallstone (**arrow**) simulating the triradiate symbol of the Mercedes-Benz automobile. Note the adjacent gallstone with a radiopaque rim. (Eisenberg RL: Gastrointestinal Radiology: A Pattern Approach. Philadelphia, JB Lippincott, 1983)

FIG. 1-97. Barium-filled loops of small bowel in a patient with sprue show smooth contours and unindented, moulded margins.

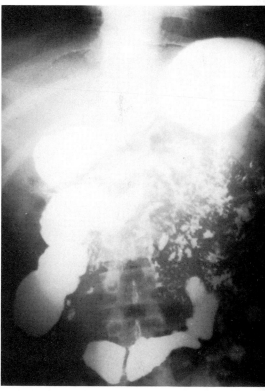

Moulage Sign

The moulage sign is one radiographic appearance of the jejunum in sprue. The French term means *moulding* or *casting* and refers to the smooth contour and unindented margins of barium-filled loops of small bowel. This tubular appearance in sprue is probably due to atrophy and effacement of the jejunal mucosal folds (Fig. 1-97).

BIBLIOGRAPHY
Margulis AR, Burhenne HJ: Alimentary Tract Roentgenology. St. Louis, CV Mosby, 1973

Mucosal Stripe Sign

In a patient with intramural dissection of the esophagus, a sharply defined lucent linear stripe represents the dissected mucosa separating the true and false esophageal lumina (Fig. 1-98). The radiographic appearance is strikingly similar to the typical findings in dissecting aneurysm of the aorta (Fig. 1-99), the esophageal mucosal stripe being the equivalent of the undermined aortic intima. This "double-barrel" appearance of intramural dissection of the esophagus must be differentiated from extraluminal extravasation of contrast medium into the mediastinum.

BIBLIOGRAPHY

Lowman RM, Goldman R, Stern H: The roentgen aspects of intramural dissection of the esophagus: The musocal stripe sign. Radiology 93:1329–1331, 1969

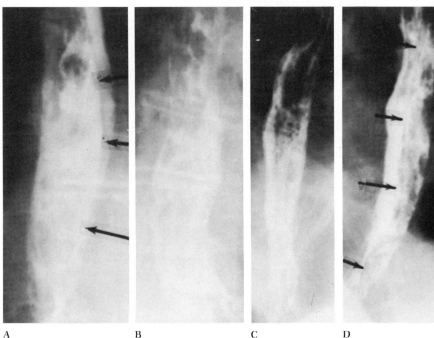

A   B   C   D

FIG. 1-98. **(A)** The sharply defined, lucent linear stripe (**arrows**) represents the dissected mucosa separating the two lumina in this patient with intramural dissection of the esophagus. No extra-esophageal extravasation of barium is present. **(B)** After the barium has been washed out of the central lumen, the retained barium is contained in the outer cylinder. The mucosal stripe sign is now absent. **(C)** During the swallowing of barium, the mucosal stripe sign persists. **(D)** Arrows outline the extent of the mucosal stripe sign. The rent in the mucosa was demonstrated by esophagoscopy. (Lowman RM, Goldman R, Stern H: The roentgen aspects of intramural dissection of the esophagus: The mucosal stripe sign. Radiology 93:1329–1331, 1969)

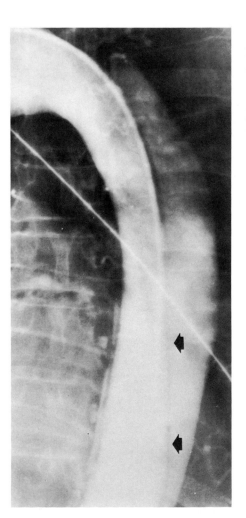

FIG. 1-99. The undermined aortic intima (**arrows**) in a patient with dissection of the aorta mimics the appearance of the esophageal mucosal stripe. (Eisenberg RL: Gastrointestinal Radiology: A Pattern Approach. Philadelphia, JB Lippincott, 1983)

Okra Sign

When seen on end, the pylorus may simulate a discrete mass in the duodenal bulb (Fig. 1-100, *top*). Barium trapped between the mucosal folds produces a stellate pattern that can be fancifully related to the cross section of an okra (Fig. 1-100, *bottom*).

BIBLIOGRAPHY
Eisenberg RL: Gastrointestinal Radiology: A Pattern Approach. Phildelphia, JB Lippincott, 1983

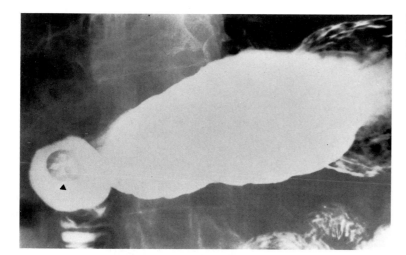

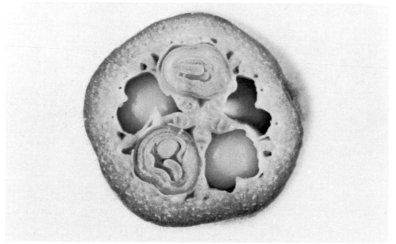

FIG. 1-100. (*Top*) Okra sign (**arrow**). (*Bottom*) Okra in cross section. (Eisenberg RL: Gastrointestinal Radiology: A Pattern Approach. Philadelphia, JB Lippincott, 1983)

Peripheral Bubble Sign

Generalized hydropneumoperitoneum is best diagnosed by demonstration of a gas–fluid level in the abdominal cavity on upright or decubitus radiographs. In critically ill patients in whom only supine radiographs can be obtained, the presence of a large central gas bubble (football sign) is considered diagnostic of pneumoperitoneum (Fig. 1-101). This finding may be enhanced by demonstration of multiple small bubbles ringing the large central collection of gas (peripheral bubble sign; Fig. 1-102).

BIBLIOGRAPHY
Han SY, Shin MS, Tishler JM: Plain film findings of hydropneumoperitoneum. AJR 136:1195–1197, 1981

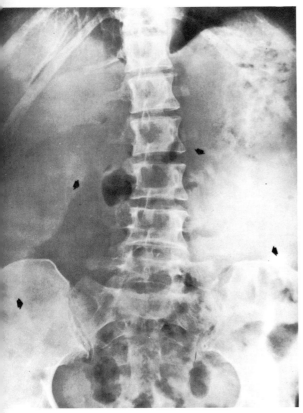

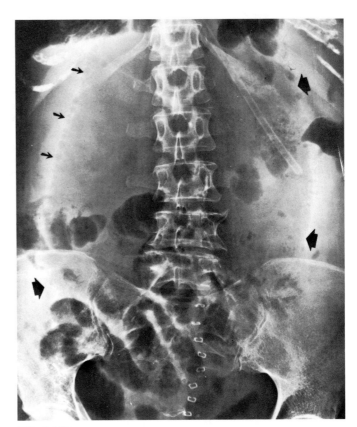

FIG. 1-101.

FIG. 1-102.

FIG. 1-101. Supine abdominal radiograph in a 60-year-old woman with perforation of gangrenous small bowel demonstrates a centrally located gas collection (**arrows**). At surgery, about 3000 ml of serosanguinous fluid were evacuated from the peritoneal cavity. (Han SY, Shin MS, Tishler JM: Plain film findings of hydropneumoperitoneum. AJR 136:1195–1197, 1981. Copyright 1981. Reproduced by permission)

FIG. 1-102. Supine film of the abdomen 1 day after exploratory laparotomy in a 54-year-old woman with ascites due to carcinomatosis. The large collection of gas (**large arrows**) is ringed by smaller bubbles (**small arrows**). (Han SY, Shin MS, Tishler JM: Plain film findings of hydropneumoperitoneum. AJR 136:1195–1197, 1981. Copyright 1981. Reproduced by permission)

Persistent Loop Sign

In a neonate with necrotizing enterocolitis, a loop of bowel that is relatively unchanged in position and configuration over a 24-hr to 36-hr interval has been reported as a sign of advanced bowel necrosis and impending perforation (Fig. 1-103). This persistent loop sign probably reflects mucosal, submucosal, and serosal necrosis, which render the segment aperistaltic. Because of its association with impending perforation, the persistent loop sign has been considered an indication for surgery. In one study, however, almost half of the infants with a persistent loop were managed medically and recovered. This suggests that the persistent loop sign should not be taken as an absolute indication for surgery and that additional clinical data are needed to support operative intervention.

BIBLIOGRAPHY

Leonard T, Johnson JF, Pettett PG: Critical evaluation of the persistent loop sign in necrotizing enterocolitis. Radiology 142:385–386, 1982

Wexler HA: The persistent loop sign in neonatal necrotizing enterocolitis: A new indication for surgical intervention? Radiology 126:201–204, 1978

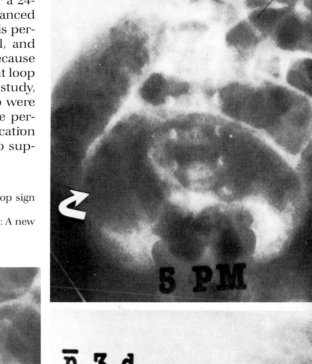

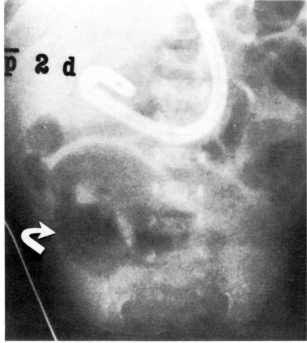

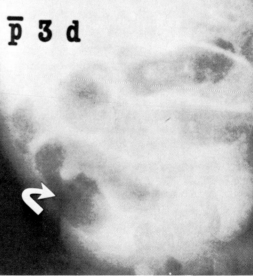

FIG. 1-103. (*Top*) Initial supine abdominal radiograph demonstrates diffuse distention with linear and cystic pneumatosis intestinalis and gas in the portal veins. The **arrow** indicates the position of the future persistent loop. (*Bottom, left*) Repeat examination 2 days later shows decreased distention, probable ascites, and a persistent right lower quadrant bowel loop (**arrow**). (*Bottom, right*) Three days after the onset of symptoms, the ascites has increased and the appearance of other bowel loops has changed, with the exception of the one in the right lower quadrant (**arrow**). (Wexler HA: The persistent loop sign in neonatal necrotizing enterocolitis: A new indication for surgical intervention? Radiology 126:201–204, 1978)

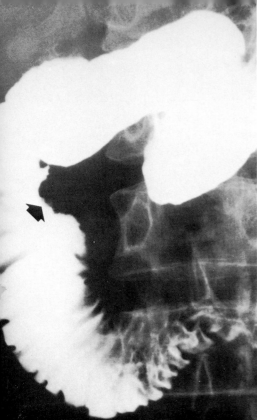

Poppel's Sign

A major cause of enlargement of the papilla of Vater is edematous swelling secondary to acute pancreatitis (Poppel's sign; Fig. 1-104). Although the resulting smooth, elliptical configuration of the edematous papilla was initially described as a manifestation of acute pancreatitis, a similar appearance can be seen in patients with acute duodenal ulcer disease (Fig. 1-105) or an impacted common duct stone (Fig. 1-106).

BIBLIOGRAPHY

Eaton SB, Ferrucci JT, Benedict KT et al: Diagnosis of choledocholithiasis by barium duodenal examination. Radiology 102:267–274, 1972

Jacobson HG, Shapiro JH, Pisano D et al: The Vaterian and peri-Vaterian segments in peptic ulcer. AJR 79:793–798, 1958

Poppel MH: The manifestations of relapsing pancreatitis. Radiology 62:514–521, 1954

FIG. 1-104. Enlargement of the papilla (**arrow**) in acute pancreatitis. (Eisenberg RL: Gastrointestinal Radiology: A Pattern Approach. Philadelphia, JB Lippincott, 1983)

FIG. 1-105. Enlargement of the papilla (**arrows**) in a patient with diffuse peptic ulcer disease. There is generalized thickening of folds throughout the first and second portions of the duodenum. (Eisenberg RL: Gastrointestinal Radiology: A Pattern Approach. Philadelphia, JB Lippincott, 1983)

FIG. 1-106. Enlargement of the papilla caused by an impacted common bile duct stone. (*Left*) Single- and (*right*) double-contrast examinations demonstrate smooth enlargement of the papilla to a diameter several times that of the impacted stone. (Bree RL, Flynn RE: Hypotonic duodenography in the evaluation of choledocholithiasis and obstructive jaundice. AJR 116:309–319, 1972. Copyright 1972. Reproduced by permission)

FIG. 1-105.

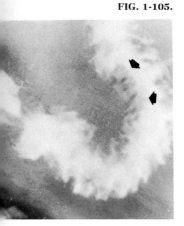

FIG. 1-106.

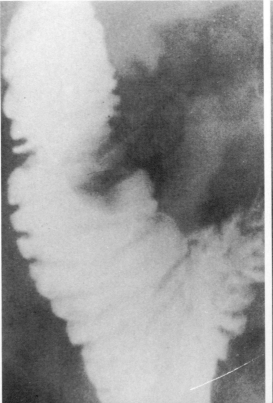
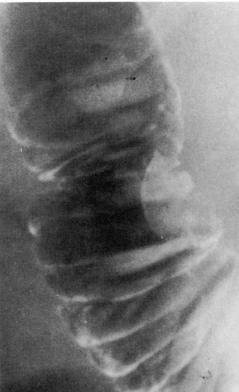

Pseudocalculus Sign

Spasm of the sphincter of Oddi may produce abrupt termination of the distal common bile duct, which has a concave, meniscoid appearance simulating an impacted stone (Fig. 1-107*A*). It is usually seen during operative or postoperative cholangiography but it is occasionally noted on intravenous studies. Serial films are necessary to demonstrate that the defect is transitory and actually due to spasm rather than representing a stone (Fig. 1-107 *B–D*).

BIBLIOGRAPHY

Beneventano TC, Schein CJ: The pseudocalculus sign in cholangiography. Arch Surg 98:731–733, 1969

Martinez LO, Cohen G: The pseudocalculus sign in intravenous cholangiography. South Med J 65:1066–1078, 1972

FIG. 1-107. (*Top, left*) Smooth, slightly lobulated filling defect of the distal common bile duct simulating an impacted stone (**arrow**). Note, however, that some contrast has already flowed into the duodenum. (*Top, right*) and (*bottom, left*) Contrast has encircled the stonelike filling defect (**arrows**) in two projections. (*Bottom, right*) Following relaxation of the sphincter of Oddi, the distal common bile duct appears normal, and contrast flows freely into the duodenum. (Eisenberg RL: Gastrointestinal Radiology: A Pattern Approach. Philadelphia, JB Lippincott, 1983)

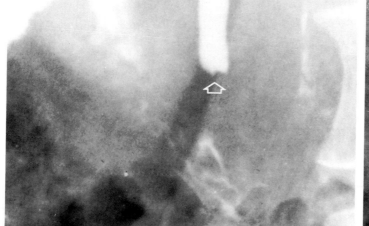
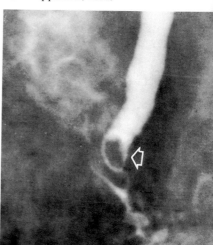
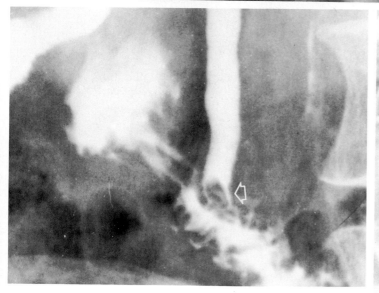
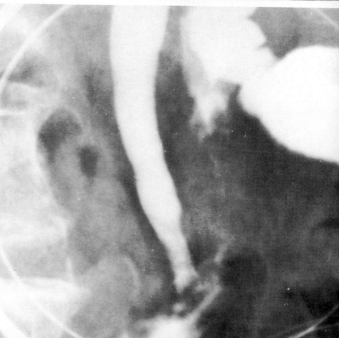

Pseudotumor Sign

The involved segment of bowel in a strangulating closed-loop intestinal obstruction is usually filled with fluid and presents radiographically as a tumor-like mass of water density (Fig. 1-108). The outline of this pseudotumor is easier to detect if there is gas distention of bowel above the obstruction than if there are no gas-distended loops. The pseudotumor sign must be differentiated from fluid-filled loops that are present in simple mechanical obstruction. In closed-loop obstruction, the pseudotumor sign reflects a loop that is fixed and remains in the same position on multiple projections. This is probably due to the combination of fixation of the bowel loop at both ends and vascular compromise, which prevents the normal tendency of bowel to change configuration and position.

BIBLIOGRAPHY

Bryk D: Strangulating obstruction of the bowel: A reevaluation of radiographic criteria. AJR 130:835–843, 1978

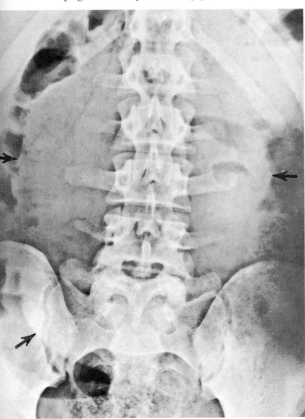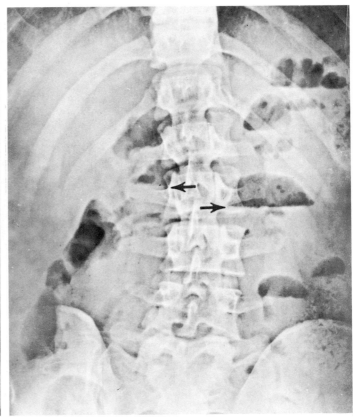

FIG. 1-108. (*Left*) Supine film showing fluid-filled loops as a tumor-like density in the midabdomen with a polycyclic outline indenting adjacent gas-containing loops (**arrows**). (*Right*) Upright film showing fluid levels in the pseudotumor (**arrows**). (Bryk D: Strangulating obstruction of the bowel: A reevaluation of radiographic criteria. AJR 130:835–843, 1978. Copyright 1978. Reproduced by permission)

Psoas Sign

The presence, absence, or attenuation of the psoas muscle outline seen on plain abdominal radiographs, or a difference in appearance between the two psoas shadows, has often been used in the differential diagnosis of intra-abdominal and retroperitoneal pathology. Demonstration of a psoas margin depends on the interface that exists between the cylinder of the mass of muscle itself and the retroperitoneal fat. If there is a large amount of fat, or if the fat is spatially arranged so that it and the margin of muscle are in contact with one another and perpendicular to the beam, the margin of the muscle will be seen. Any process that disturbs the radiolucency of the fat (*e.g.*, infiltration of the fat by blood, edema, fluid, or tumor) obliterates the psoas line (Fig. 1-109). Large amounts of stool or gas in the overlying bowel also make visualization of the muscle shadow difficult. In addition, the right psoas margin may be absent in up to 40% of normal patients. Thus, the psoas sign is not a reliable indication for the differential diagnosis of intraperitoneal and retroperitoneal masses. Conversely, preservation of either or both psoas margins does not exclude the presence of significant extraperitoneal disease.

In patients with abdominal trauma, obliteration of a psoas line suggests retroperitoneal hemorrhage (Fig. 1-110). Laceration of the spleen with intraperitoneal bleeding should not of itself obliterate the left psoas margin; absence of the psoas line in a patient with abdominal trauma is therefore highly suggestive of retroperitoneal hemorrhage, such as some injury to the kidney. In children with right lower quadrant pain, absence of the right psoas margin is often considered an indication of ruptured appendicitis due to edema of the right retroperitoneal tissues secondary to peritonitis.

BIBLIOGRAPHY

Elkin M, Cohen G: Diagnostic value of the psoas shadow. Clin Radiol 13:210–217, 1962

Moskowitz M: The psoas sign, hepatic angle, normal patients, and everyday practice. Gut 14:308–310, 1973

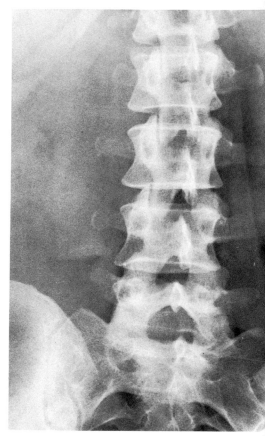

FIG. 1-109. Obliteration of the right psoas margin due to diffuse retroperitoneal inflammation.

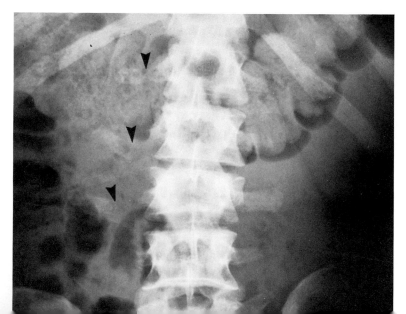

FIG. 1-110. Obliteration of the right psoas shadow due to traumatic right retroperitoneal hematoma and laceration of the psoas muscle. Displaced fractures involve the upper four right lumbar transverse processes (**arrowheads**). (Harris JH, Harris WH: The Radiology of Emergency Medicine. Baltimore, Williams & Wilkins, 1981)

Pyloric String Sign

Pyloric string sign refers to the characteristic elongation and narrowing of the pyloric canal seen as a result of thickened sphincter muscles in patients with hypertrophic pyloric stenosis (Fig. 1-111). Although hypertrophic pyloric stenosis is most commonly seen in children, the term *pyloric string sign* was originally applied to this disorder occurring in adults (Fig. 1-112).

BIBLIOGRAPHY

Kleitsch WP: Diagnosis and treatment of pyloric hypertrophy in the adult. Arch Surg 65:655–664, 1952

FIG. 1-111. Narrowing and elongation of the pyloric canal with characteristic concave, crescentic indentation at the base of the duodenal bulb in an infant with congenital pyloric stenosis. (Eisenberg RL: Gastrointestinal Radiology: A Pattern Approach. Philadelphia, JB Lippincott, 1983)

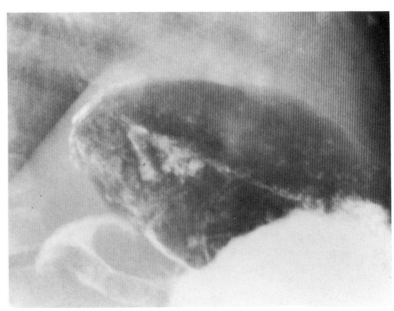

FIG. 1-112. Identical pattern of narrowing and elongation of the pyloric canal with concave, crescentic indentation at the base of the duodenal bulb in an adult with hypertrophic pyloric stenosis. (Eisenberg RL: Gastrointestinal Radiology: A Pattern Approach. Philadelphia, JB Lippincott, 1983)

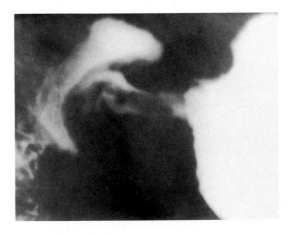

Pyloric Tit Sign

A pyloric tit is a projection from the lesser curvature of the gastric antrum seen in infants with hypertrophic pyloric stenosis (Fig. 1-113). In these patients, the obstructed antrum adjoining the pyloric canal assumes the contour of a breast and nipple when the canal is completely empty of barium. Because pyloric narrowing prevents the peristaltic wave from passing downward, the normal peristaltic pouch is converted into a pyloric tit by persistent peristaltic activity attempting to push past the obstruction (Fig. 1-114). Occasionally, a normal peristaltic pouch may be so prominent that it simulates a pyloric tit. However, this normal finding does not persist or become pointed and diminishes as it passes promptly to the distal end of the pylorus.

BIBLIOGRAPHY

Shopfner CE: The pyloric tit in hypertrophic pyloric stenosis. AJR 91:674–679, 1964

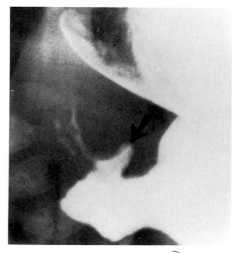

FIG. 1-113. Pyloric tit (**arrow**). (Shopfner CE: The pyloric tit in hypertrophic pyloric stenosis. AJR 91:674–694, 1964. Copyright 1964. Reproduced by permission)

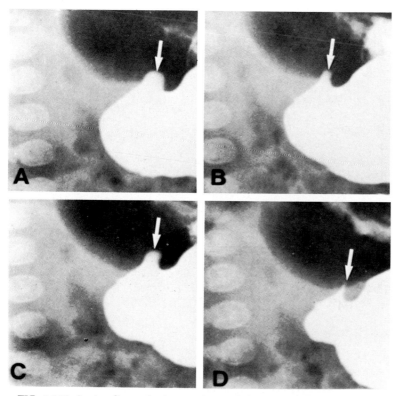

FIG. 1-114. Spot radiographs in a patient with hypertrophic pyloric stenosis demonstrate conversion of a peristaltic pouch into a fully developed pyloric tit (**arrows**). (**A–C**) show intermediate steps and reveal the progressive narrowing and pointing of the pouch. In (**D**), the tit is fully formed. (Shopfner CE: The pyloric tit in hypertrophic pyloric stenosis. AJR 91:674–694, 1964. Copyright 1964. Reproduced by permission)

Ram's Horn Sign

Crohn's disease involving the stomach can result in a smooth, tubular antrum that is poorly distensible and exhibits sluggish peristalsis. The narrowed antrum tends to flare out into a relatively normal gastric body and fundus (Fig. 1-115), giving the appearance of a ram's horn or sacramental "shofar" used to sound the advent of the Jewish New Year (Fig. 1-116). The presence of this deformity, especially in young patients, suggests the need for full radiographic investigation of both large and small bowel to document Crohn's disease in these areas.

BIBLIOGRAPHY

Farman J, Faegenburg D, Dallemand S et al: Crohn's disease of the stomach: The "ram's horn" sign. AJR 123:242–251, 1975

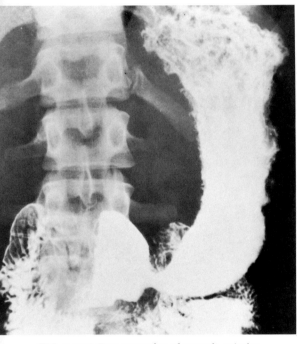

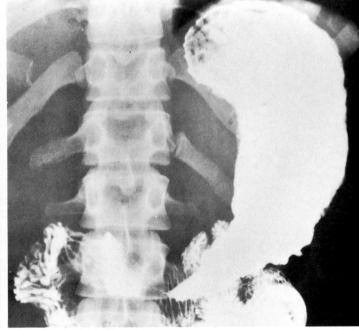

FIG. 1-115. Two examples of smooth, tubular narrowing of the antrum flaring out into a relatively normal gastric body and fundus in patients with Crohn's disease of the stomach. (Farman J, Faegenburg D, Dallemand S et al: Crohn's disease of the stomach: The "ram's horn" sign. AJR 123:242–251, 1975. Copyright 1975. Reproduced by permission)

FIG. 1-116. Ram's horn. (Farman J, Faegenburg D, Dallemand S et al: Crohn's disease of the stomach: The "ram's horn" sign. AJR 123:242–251, 1975. Copyright 1975. Reproduced by permission)

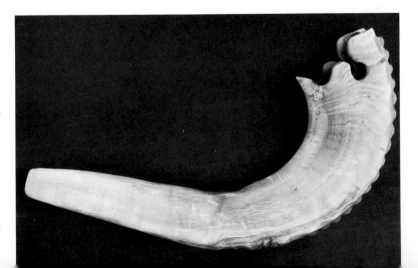

Reverse 3 Sign

In a patient with acute appendicitis, the edematous mesoappendix may cause persistent pressure and indentation of the cecum. This typically presents as a reverse 3 (Fig. 1-117), similar to Frostberg's sign seen in the descending duodenum as a result of enlargement of the head of the pancreas. The center of the 3 is produced by the rigid, inflamed lumen of the appendix, which on occasion shows slight proximal filling with barium (Fig. 1-118). Unlike an infiltrating tumor, the cecal mucosa appears smooth and intact.

BIBLIOGRAPHY
Soter CS: The contribution of the radiologist to the diagnosis of acute appendictis. Semin Roentgenol 8:375–388, 1973

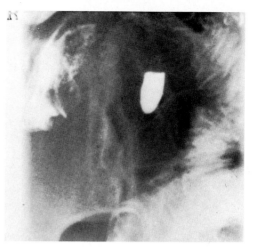

FIG. 1-117. Reverse 3 sign in a patient with acute appendicitis. An appendiceal stone composed of barium caused obstruction of the lumen and acute appendicitis. Note the pressure on the terminal ileum. (Soter CS: The contribution of the radiologist to the diagnosis of acute appendicitis. Semin Roentgenol 8:375–388, 1973. Reproduced by permission)

FIG. 1-118. Reverse 3 indentation on the cecum in a patient with acute appendicitis. A trickle of barium has entered the base of the appendiceal lumen, which is narrow and irregular. The round stone that produced the appendiceal obstruction was not visualized on the plain abdominal radiograph of this 260-lb patient. (Soter CS: The contribution of the radiologist to the diagnosis of acute appendicitis. Semin Roentgenol 8:375–388, 1973. Reproduced by permission)

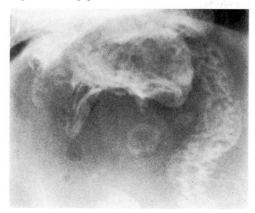

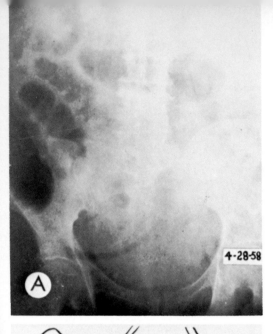

Rigid Loop Sign

Radiographs in patients with mesenteric venous occlusion may demonstrate a rigid, edematous segment of bowel in which a relatively small amount of gas remains in a generally straight or curvilinear lumen and does not change in distribution on upright or decubitus films (rigid loop sign; Figs. 1-119 and 1-120).

BIBLIOGRAPHY

Nelson SW, Eggleston W: Findings on plain roentgenograms of the abdomen associated with mesenteric vascular occlusion with a possible new sign of mesenteric venous thrombosis. AJR 83:886–894, 1960

FIG. 1-119. (A) Supine abdominal radiograph and **(B)** corresponding line drawing demonstrate a narrow, sickle-shaped collection of gas in the right lower abdomen in a patient with mesenteric vascular occlusion. (Nelson SW, Eggleston W: Findings on plain roentgenograms of the abdomen associated with mesenteric vascular occlusion with a possible new sign of mesenteric venous thrombosis. AJR 83:886–894, 1960. Copyright 1960. Reproduced by permission)

FIG. 1-120. (A) Supine abdominal radiograph and **(B)** corresponding line drawing obtained 24 hr after Fig. 1-119 show two sickle-shaped collections of gas in the right lower abdomen. The distance (a) between these collections of gas may be due to intraluminal fluid, extraluminal fluid between the loops, or the markedly edematous walls of two adjacent loops of bowel. Note the distention of several loops of small bowel in the left midabdomen since the original examination made the previous day (Fig. 1-119). (Nelson SW, Eggleston W: Findings on plain roentgenograms of the abdomen associated with mesenteric vascular occlusion with a possible new sign of mesenteric venous thombosis. AJR 83:886–894, 1960. Copyright 1960. Reproduced by permission)

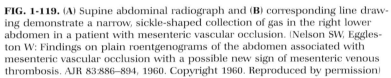

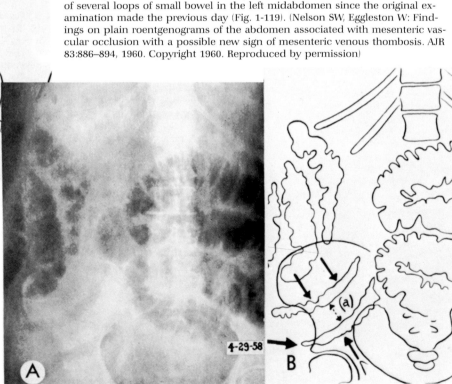

Rim Sign

A choledochal cyst is a congenital localized dilatation of the hepatic or bile duct that presents as a right upper quadrant mass. Although it can be readily diagnosed on ultrasound, a choledochal cyst has always been difficult to opacify by intravenous cholangiography even in patients with normal bilirubin levels. A well-defined opaque rim completely surrounding a lucent cystic mass has been described on high-dose urography (Fig. 1-121) and arteriography (Fig. 1-122) as a sign of choledochal cyst. Opacification of the rim of the cyst is probably due to a delayed diffusion effect related to total body opacification. Demonstration of the rim sign suggests the correct diagnosis by showing that the choledochal cyst is separate from the kidney and liver.

BIBLIOGRAPHY

Rabinowitz JG, Kinkhabwala MN, Rose JS: Rim sign in choledochal cyst: Additional diagnostic feature. J Can Assoc Radiol 24:226–230, 1973

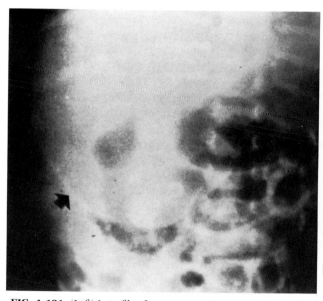
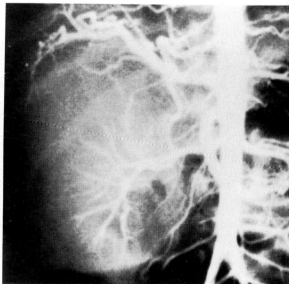
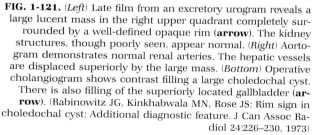
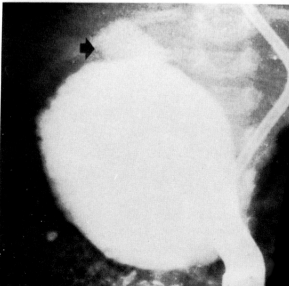

FIG. 1-121. (*Left*) Late film from an excretory urogram reveals a large lucent mass in the right upper quadrant completely surrounded by a well-defined opaque rim (**arrow**). The kidney structures, though poorly seen, appear normal. (*Right*) Aortogram demonstrates normal renal arteries. The hepatic vessels are displaced superiorly by the large mass. (*Bottom*) Operative cholangiogram shows contrast filling a large choledochal cyst. There is also filling of the superiorly located gallbladder (**arrow**). (Rabinowitz JG, Kinkhabwala MN, Rose JS: Rim sign in choledochal cyst: Additional diagnostic feature. J Can Assoc Radiol 24:226–230, 1973)

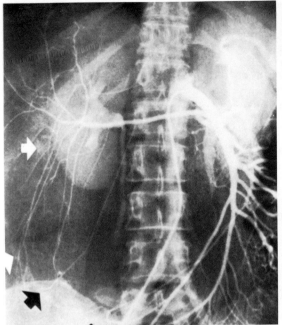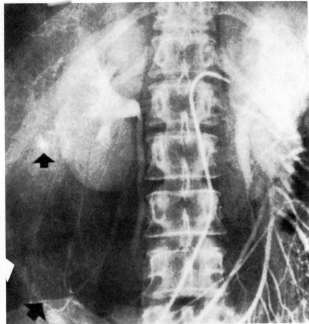

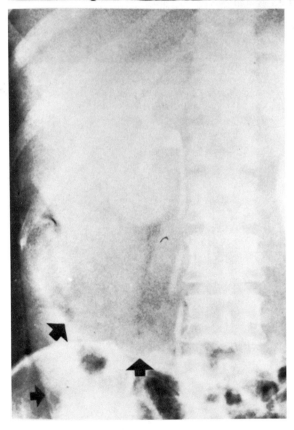

FIG. 1-122. (*Left*) Early and (*right*) late films from a superior mesenteric arteriogram demonstrate an irregular, dense rim of tissue outlining a large mass within the right upper quadrant (**arrows**). The major superior mesenteric artery is displaced to the left and gives rise to a large hepatic vesel. (A previous celiac arteriogram revealed no hepatic artery.) The intrahepatic branches are markedly stretched and elongated. Within the region of the mass, there is a small puddle of contrast (**small arrows**) caused by the presence of granulation tissue. (*Bottom*) Plain abdominal radiograph taken 20 min after the *right* figure again demonstrates the large radiolucent mass and its opacified rim (**large arrows**). The lateral border of the liver extends well below the level of the iliac crest (**lower arrows**). (Rabinowitz JG, Kinkhabwala MN, Rose JS: Rim sign in choledochal cyst: Additional diagnostic features. J Can Assoc Radiol 24:226–230, 1973)

Ring Stricture Sign

A discrete circumferential narrowing of the lumen (ring stricture), almost always situated in the upper descending duodenum, is a sign of chronic postbulbar ulceration (Fig. 1-123). The stricture is usually 2 mm to 3 mm wide and has no visible mucosal pattern. There is usually an abrupt transition to a normal duodenal caliber at both ends. Even if no ulcer crater is visible on barium studies, the ring stricture is indicative of peptic ulcer disease. Ring strictures are not quiescent lesions; rather, they are chronic and progressive. Residual or increasing narrowing of the lumen may cause such severe symptoms as intractable pain, recurrent bleeding, and vomiting.

BIBLIOGRAPHY

Bilbao MK, Frische LH, Rosch J et al: Postbulbar duodenal ulcer and ring-stricture: Cause and effect. Radiology 100:27–35, 1971

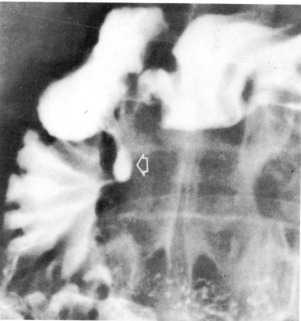

FIG. 1-123. (*Left*) Circumferential narrowing of the lumen of the second portion of the duodenum (**arrow**). (*Right*) Previous postbulbar ulcer in the same patient (**arrow**). (Eisenberg RL: Gastrointestinal Radiology: A Pattern Approach. Philadelphia, JB Lippincott, 1983)

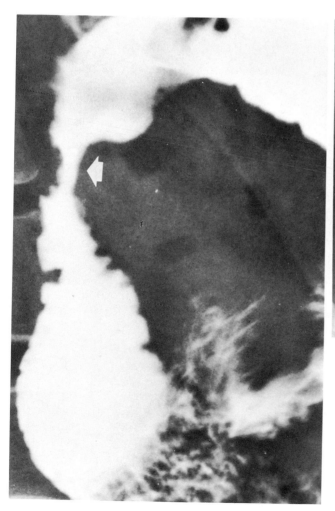

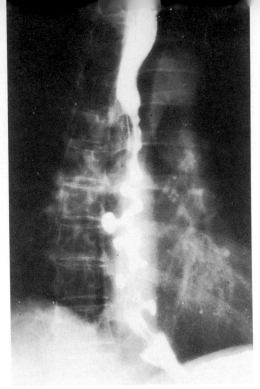

Rosary Bead (Corkscrew) Esophagus Sign

Diffuse esophageal spasm has a classic clinical triad of massive uncoordinated esophageal contractions, chest pain, and increased intraluminal pressure. In the lower two thirds of the esophagus, tertiary contractions of abnormally high amplitude often obliterate the lumen and cause compartmentalization of the barium column (Fig. 1-124). These segmental, nonpropulsive contractions may be accompanied by pain and cause barium to be displaced both proximally and distally from the site of spasm, producing transient sacculations or pseudodiverticula and a corkscrew appearance radiographically (rosary bead or corkscrew esophagus sign; Fig. 1-125).

BIBLIOGRAPHY
Westgaard T, Keats TE: Diffuse spasm and muscular hypertrophy of the lower esophagus. Radiology 90:1001–1005, 1968

FIG. 1-124. High-amplitude contractions cause pseudodiverticula and irregular narrowing of the lumen of the esophagus in a patient with diffuse esophageal spasm. (Eisenberg RL: Gastrointestinal Radiology: A Pattern Approach. Philadelphia, JB Lippincott, 1983)

FIG. 1-125. Corkscrew appearance of the esophagus in a patient with diffuse esophageal spasm.

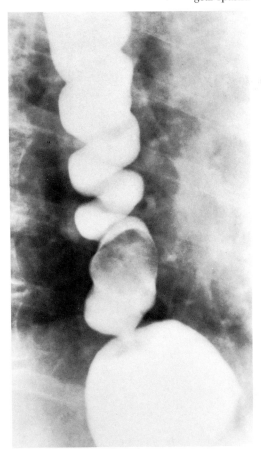

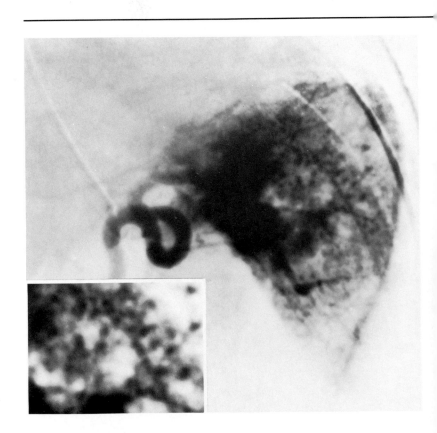

Seurat Spleen Sign

Following publication of an article comparing the arteriographic findings in ruptured spleen to the painting "Starry Night" by Vincent van Gogh, another report suggested that the pattern of extravasation of arteriographic contrast is more reminiscent of the works of Georges Seurat than of those of van Gogh, Seurat's contemporary. Pointillistic paintings, composed of hundreds of tiny dots that merge almost imperceptibly at a distance (Fig. 1-126), often look strikingly similar to the multiple punctate areas of contrast seen in patients with a ruptured spleen (Fig. 1-127).

BIBLIOGRAPHY
Kass JB, Fisher RG: The Seurat spleen. AJR 132:683–684, 1979

FIG. 1-126. Section from "La Parade" by Georges Seurat. Dot patterns from the painting, clearly visible in the magnified *insert*, are strikingly similar to arteriograms of the traumatized spleen. (Kass JB, Fisher RG: The Seurat spleen. AJR 132:683–684, 1979. Reproduced with permission of the Metropolitan Museum of Art, New York)

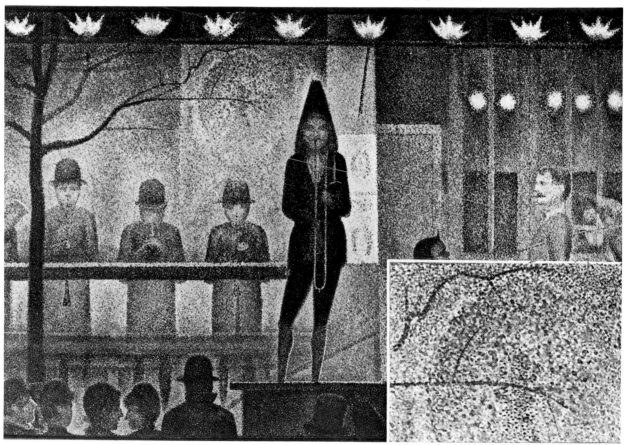

FIG. 1-127. Selective celiac arteriogram in a patient with a ruptured spleen demonstrates multiple punctate areas (magnified in *insert*) most prominent at the midpole of the spleen. (Kass JB, Fisher RG: The Seurat spleen. AJR 132:683–684, 1979. Copyright 1979. Reproduced by permission)

Sigmoid Elevator Sign

The normal colon with a competent ileocecal valve functions as a closed pressure system. Pressure generated during a barium enema examination is distributed throughout the large bowel in all directions. In patients with a redundant sigmoid, the bowel remains in the pelvis until the cecum is filled. Only at this point does the transmitted retrograde pressure cause recoil of the mesenteric sigmoid segment and elevation and displacement of the "pelvic colon" outside of the bony confines. In patients with an intrinsic or extrinsic lesion of the sigmoid colon, the normal pressure distribution is also altered. The pressure of the barium enema is immediately imparted to the mobile portion of the sigmoid, lifting the bowel out of the pelvis at the earliest phase of filling (Fig. 1-128). Presence of this sigmoid elevator sign should lead the radiologist to search the sigmoid colon or adjoining area for a lesion that might otherwise escape detection.

BIBLIOGRAPHY
Rubin S, Lambie R, Davidson KC et al: The sigmoid elevator sign: Its significance. Radiology 93:867–870, 1969

FIG. 1-128. Serial films from a barium enema examination in a patient with carcinoma demonstrate early elevation of the sigmoid at the junction of the descending colon and sigmoid. (Rubin S, Lambie R, Davidson KC et al: The sigmoid elevator sign: Its significance. Radiology 93:867–870, 1969)

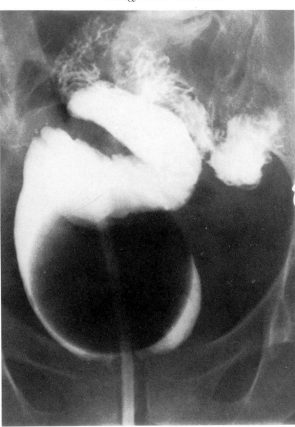
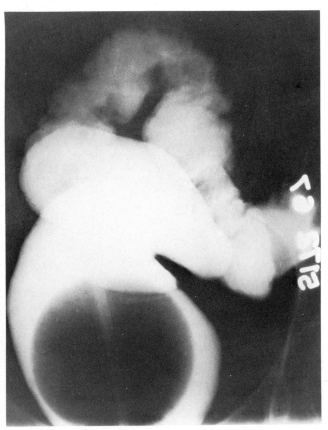

(continued)

Single Bubble Sign

The presence of a single distended, gas-containing viscus in the epigastrium of a newborn infant with little or no distal gas signifies neonatal gastric outlet obstruction (Fig. 1-129). Although the stomach may be distended by gas in normal neonates, some gas is usually seen distally.

BIBLIOGRAPHY
Rabinowitz JG: Pediatric Radiology. Philadelphia, JB Lippincott, 1978

FIG. 1-129. (**A**) A single large gas-containing viscus in a 3-day-old infant with gastric atresia. (The patient also had colonic atresia, for which a colostomy had recently been performed.) (**B**) Oral barium collected and remained within the gastric fundus. Complete gastric atresia was found at surgery. (Rabinowitz JG: Pediatric Radiology. Philadelphia, JB Lippincott, 1978)

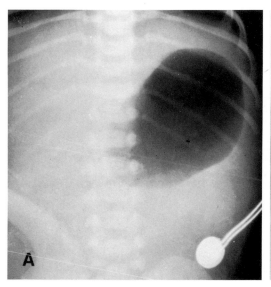

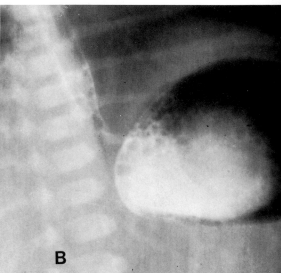

FIG. 1-128. (*continued*)

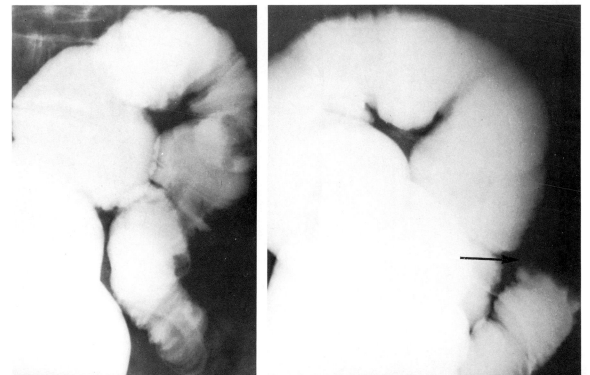

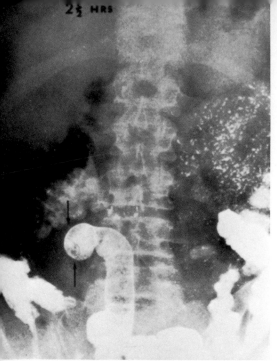

Snake Head Sign

The snake head sign is a radiographic appearance consisting of a short annular constriction (the "neck") immediately proximal to a short dilated segment of small intestine (the "head") adjacent to the site of a nonstrangulating mechanical obstruction (Fig. 1-130). The rounded configuration of the distal end of the obstructed loop is characteristic of an adhesion or other extrinsic nonneoplastic lesion, in contrast to the typical contour of an annular or polypoid intraluminal neoplasm. The snake head sign arises when a strong peristaltic contraction attempting to overcome an obstruction is stopped by the tenacity and tensile strength of the short segment of bowel proximal to the obstruction (the "head"). This contraction persists as the "neck" for several seconds before muscular fatigue and other factors cause its relaxation (Fig. 1-131).

BIBLIOGRAPHY
Nelson SW, Christoforidis AJ, Roenigk WJ: A diagnostic physiologic sign of mechanical obstruction of the small intestine. Radiology 84:881–885, 1965

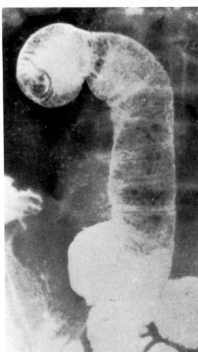

FIG. 1-130. (*Top*) Full and (*bottom*) coned films from a small bowel examination demonstrate a striking snake head configuration (**arrows**) of a loop of ileum just proximal to the site of mechanical obstruction. (Nelson SW, Christoforidis AJ, Roenigk WJ: A diagnostic physiologic sign of mechanical obstruction of the small intestine. Radiology 84:881–885, 1965)

FIG. 1-131. Examples of snake head configurations of the small bowel proximal to the point of obstruction. (Nelson SW, Christoforidis AJ, Roenigk WJ: A diagnostic physiologic sign of mechanical obstruction of the small intestine. Radiology 84:881–885, 1965)

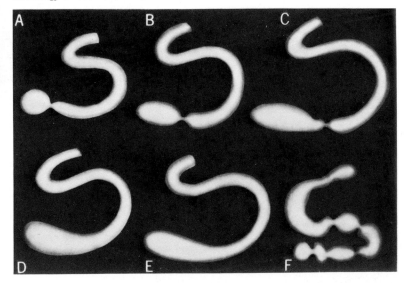

Spheroid Sign

The radiologist must distinguish intramural (mucosal or submucosal) from extramural masses in making a differential diagnosis, because the layer of origin is probably one of the most important factors determing the gross form taken by neoplasms. The distinction can be made according to where the center of the mass lies in relation to the projected luminal contour of the bowel. Defects with estimated centers lying within the projected luminal contour of the bowel are likely to be intramural (Fig. 1-132). Those with estimated centers lying outside the projected luminal contour are likely to be extramural (Fig. 1-133). Those with centers lying along the luminal contour tend to be intramural (Fig. 1-134). When a mass is viewed partially face-on, two defects appear in the barium column. If the estimated center of either of these lies outside the luminal contour of the bowel, the origin of the mass is extramural (Fig. 1-135 A, B); if both lie within the projected luminal contour, the mass arises intramurally (Fig. 1-135 C).

BIBLIOGRAPHY
Stein LA, Margulis AR: The spheroid sign: A new sign for accurate differentiation of intramural from extramural masses. AJR 123:420–426, 1975

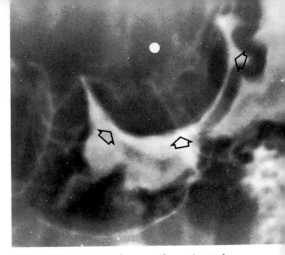

FIG. 1-132. Intramural mass. The estimated center of this leiomyoma lies within the projected luminal contour of the stomach. (Eisenberg RL: Gastrointestinal Radiology: A Pattern Approach. Philadelphia, JB Lippincott, 1983)

FIG. 1-134. Intramural lesion. The center of this duplication cyst lies along the luminal contour of the esophagus. (Eisenberg RL: Gastrointestinal Radiology: A Pattern Approach. Philadelphia, JB Lippincott, 1983)

FIG. 1-133. Extramural lesion. The estimated center of this metastasis to the rectal shelf lies outside the projected luminal contour of the rectosigmoid. (Eisenberg RL: Gastrointestinal Radiology: A Pattern Approach. Philadelphia, JB Lippincott, 1983)

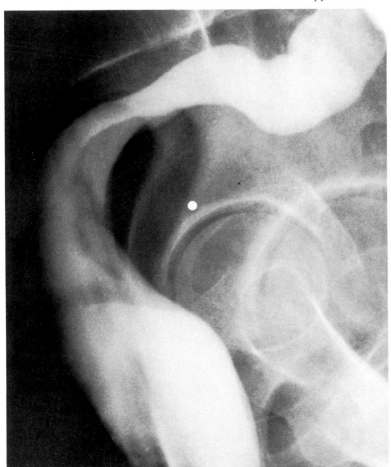

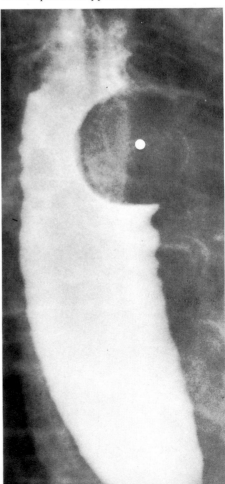

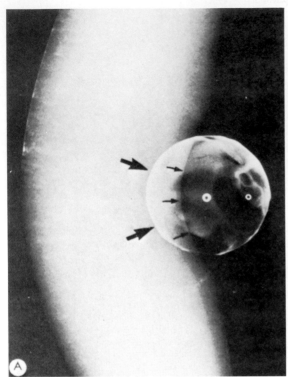

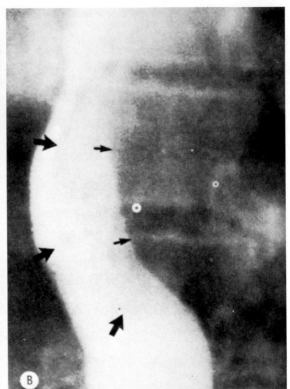

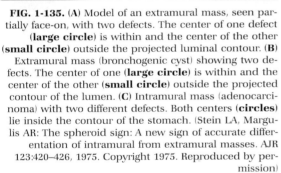

FIG. 1-135. (A) Model of an extramural mass, seen partially face-on, with two defects. The center of one defect **(large circle)** is within and the center of the other **(small circle)** outside the projected luminal contour. **(B)** Extramural mass (bronchogenic cyst) showing two defects. The center of one **(large circle)** is within and the center of the other **(small circle)** outside the projected contour of the lumen. **(C)** Intramural mass (adenocarcinoma) with two different defects. Both centers **(circles)** lie inside the contour of the stomach. (Stein LA, Margulis AR: The spheroid sign: A new sign of accurate differentation of intramural from extramural masses. AJR 123:420–426, 1975. Copyright 1975. Reproduced by permission)

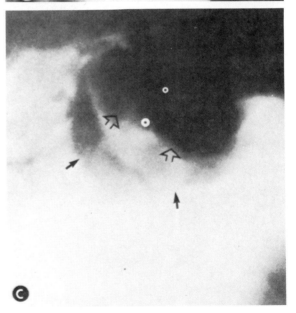

Squeeze Sign

Lipomas are the second most common benign tumors of the colon. These slow-growing lesions are submucosal in origin, usually single, and generally asymptomatic. They are usually found in the right colon, and they are generally found incidentally on barium enema examinations. Because lipomas are extremely soft and pliable, their contours and configurations can be altered by peristalsis and palpation. Thus, a malleable lipoma that appears round or oval on filled films (Fig. 1-136, *left*) characteristically appears sausage or banana-shaped on postevacuation films, when the colon is contracted (Fig. 1-136, *right*).

BIBLIOGRAPHY

Meschan I: Analysis of Roentgen Signs in General Radiology. Philadelphia, WB Saunders, 1973

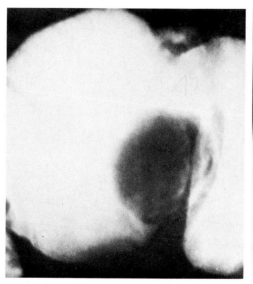 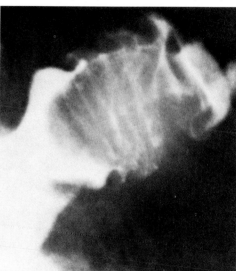

FIG. 1-136. Change in the size and shape of a soft colonic lipoma between the full colon film (*left*) and the postevacuation film (*right*). (Dreyfuss JR, Janower ML: Radiology of the Colon. Baltimore, Williams & Wilkins, 1981)

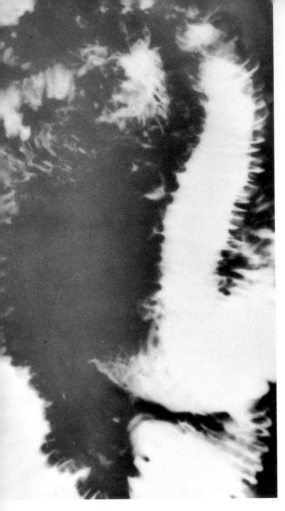

Stack of Coins Sign

Any cause of bleeding into the bowel wall can cause regular thickening of small bowel folds with sharply delineated margins (Fig. 1-137). The parallel arrangement produces a symmetric, spike-like configuration simulating a stack of coins or picket fence (Fig. 1-138). This appearance is more striking in the jejunum than in the distal small bowel because of the better development and normally greater prominence of jejunal folds.

BIBLIOGRAPHY

Eisenberg RL: Gastrointestinal Radiology: A Pattern Approach. Philadelphia, JB Lippincott, 1983

FIG. 1-137. Hemorrhage into the wall of the small bowel produces a symmetric spike-like configuration mimicking a stack of coins. (Eisenberg RL: Gastrointestinal Radiology: A Pattern Approach. Philadelphia, JB Lippincott, 1983)

FIG. 1-138. (*Left*) Regular thickening of small bowel folds in a patient with segmental ischemia produces a picket-fence pattern (**arrows**). (*Right*) The ischemic process completely resolved following conservative therapy. (Eisenberg RL: Gastrointestinal Radiology: A Pattern Approach. Philadelphia, JB Lippincott, 1983)

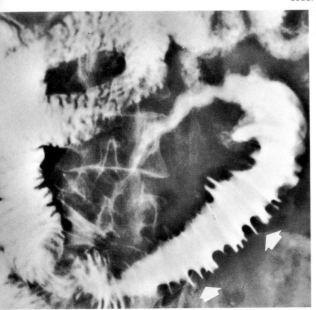

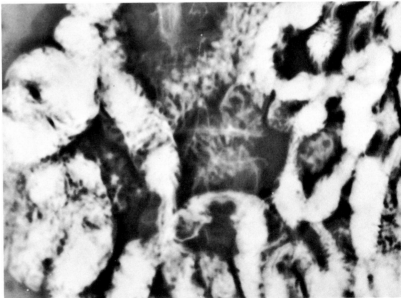

Starry Night Sign

The stasis of contrast material in the malpighian body marginal sinus circulation in a traumatized spleen can appear arteriographically as localized or diffuse, small, rounded shadows (Fig. 1-139, *top*). The capillary phase of the study has been compared to the globular appearance of the stars depicted by van Gogh in his painting "Starry Night" (Fig. 1-139, *bottom*).

BIBLIOGRAPHY

Scatliff JH, Fisher ON, Guilford WB et al: The "Starry Night" splenic angiogram: Contrast material opacification of the malpighian body marginal sinus circulation in spleen trauma. AJR 125:91–98, 1975

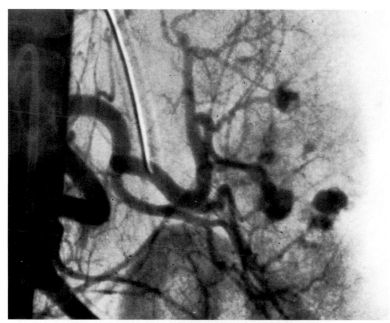

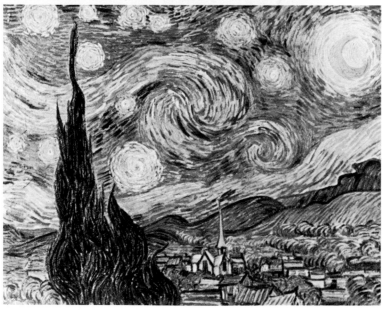

FIG. 1-139. (*Top*) Abdominal aortogram in a patient with a ruptured spleen demonstrates large globular areas of extravasation of contrast reminiscent of (*bottom*) the stars in the painting "Starry Night" by Vincent van Gogh. (Kass JB, Fisher RG: The Seurat spleen. AJR 1232:683–684, 1979. Part B is reproduced with permission of Museum of Modern Art, New York)

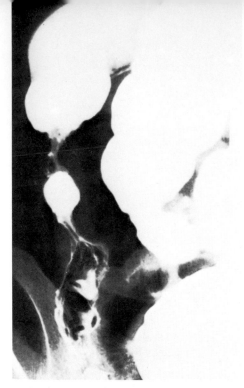

FIG. 1-140. In this patient with ileocecal tuberculosis, the terminal ileum appears to empty directly into the stenotic ascending colon. There is no opacification of the fibrotic, contracted cecum. (Carrera GF, Young S, Lewicki AM: Intestinal tuberculosis. Gastrointest Radiol 1:147–155, 1976)

Stierlin's Sign

Tuberculosis involving the ileocecal region causes edema and irritability with coarsening, irregular nodularity, and ulceration of the mucosa. Subsequent fibrosis results in the classic radiographic appearance of a stiff, severely narrowed terminal ileum emptying directly through a gaping ileocecal valve into a shortened, rigid, or obliterated cecum (Fig. 1-140). Identification of the ileocecal junction is difficult.

BIBLIOGRAPHY
Carrera GF, Young S, Lewicki AM: Intestinal tuberculosis. Gastrointest Radiol 1:147–155, 1976

String Sign

In Crohn's disease involving the small bowel, rigid thickening of the entire bowel wall may produce pipe-like narrowing of the lumen. Continued inflammation and fibrosis may result in a severely narrowed, rigid segment of small bowel in which the mucosal pattern is lost (Fig. 1-141).

BIBLIOGRAPHY
Eisenberg RL: Gastrointestinal Radiology: A Pattern Approach. Philadelphia JB Lippincott, 1983

FIG. 1-141. A severely narrowed, rigid segment of the terminal ileum (**arrows**) reflects the string sign of Crohn's disease. (Eisenberg RL: Gastrointestinal Radiology: A Pattern Approach. Philadelphia, JB Lippincott, 1983)

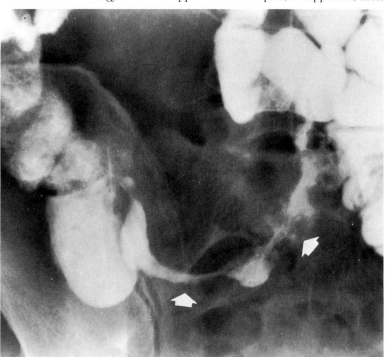

String of Beads Sign

Small amounts of gas in obstructed loops of bowel can produce the characteristic string of beads appearance of small gas bubbles in an oblique line (Fig. 1-142). This sign apparently depends on a combination of fluid-filled bowel and peristaltic hyperactivity. Although often considered diagnostic of mechanical obstruction, the string of beads sign occasionally appears in adynamic ileus secondary to inflammatory disease.

BIBLIOGRAPHY
Levin B: Mechanical small bowel obstruction. Semin Roentgenol 8:281–297, 1973

FIG. 1-142. Two examples of the string of beads appearance (**arrows**) in patients with small bowel obstruction. (Eisenberg RL: Gastrointestinal Radiology: A Pattern Approach. Philadelphia, JB Lippincott, 1983)

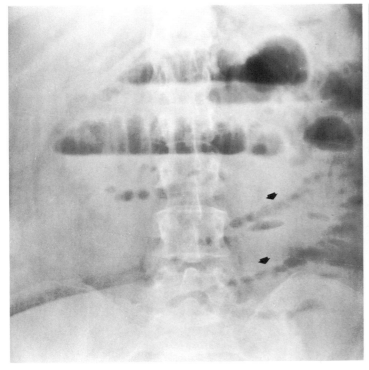

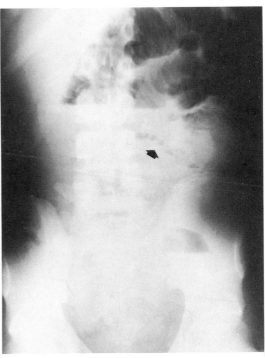

Striped Colon Sign

Metastatic serosal implants incite an intense desmoplastic reaction that appears in profile as characteristic tethering or retraction of folds. When seen *en face* on double-contrast studies, this tethering appears to be projected through the colonic lumen as transverse folds that do not completely traverse the lumen of the colon (Fig. 1-143). This abnormal striped colon pattern must be distinguished from the normal double-contrast appearance, in which transverse folds appear to extend around the entire circumference of the bowel wall.

BIBLIOGRAPHY

Ginaldi S, Lindell MM, Zornoza J: The striped colon: A new radiographic observation in metastatic serosal implants. AJR 134:453–455, 1980

FIG. 1-143. Metastatic serosal implants. A double-contrast barium enema study demonstrates numerous transverse folds in the transverse colon (**arrows**). (Ginaldi S, Lindell MM, Zornoza J: The striped colon: A new radiographic observation in metastatic serosal implants. AJR 134:453–455, 1980. Copyright 1980. Reproduced by permission)

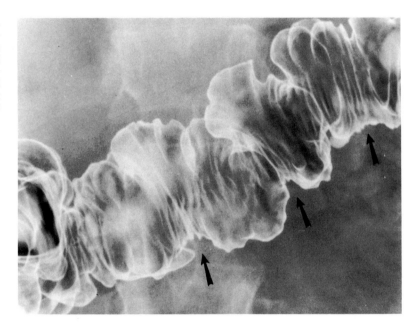

FIG. 1-145.

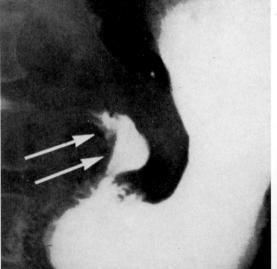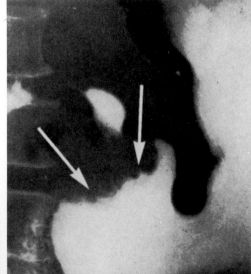

Struggling Antrum Sign

Subtle but definite changes occur in the appearance of the antrum during filling and emptying whenever a portion of the gastric wall is fixed, particularly if it is fixed as a result of infiltration by carcinoma of the pancreas. Abnormalities of antral distensibility and motor activity (struggling antrum), which reflect an attempt by the uninvolved portion of the antrum to maintain adequate mechanical function, may be sufficient to suggest the diagnosis of a perigastric tumor. Abnormal distensibility may appear as pseudoloculation or flattening and ridging of the antrum (Fig. 1-144). Abnormalities of motility include asymmetry and eccentricity (Fig. 1-145), specific alteration of the slopes of the peristaltic waves, fixation, angulation, elevation, and characteristic mucosal changes.

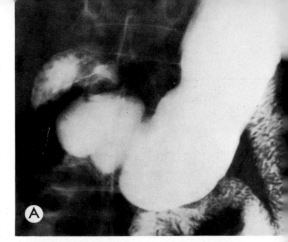

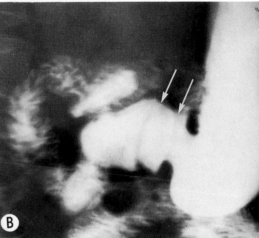

BIBLIOGRAPHY
Keller RJ, Khilnani MT, Wolf BS: The struggling antrum: A new sign of perigastric malignancy. AJR 119:300–310, 1973

FIG. 1-144. Carcinoma of the pancreas. (*Top*) Vertical ridging in the distended antrum simulates two peristaltic contractions. There are no recognizable slopes, and the rings are too narrow to be peristaltic waves. Nodular infiltration of the lesser curvature of the stomach above the incisura angularis is obvious. (*Bottom*) The ridges are accentuated during a phase of partial contraction. Angulation and fixation of the superior aspect of these ridges (**arrows**) may lead to pseudo-diverticulum formation. (Keller RJ, Khilnani MT, Wolf BS: The struggling antrum: A new sign of perigastric malignancy. AJR 119:300–310, 1973. Copyright 1973. Reproduced by permission)

FIG. 1-145. Carcinoma of the pancreas infiltrating the antrum and duodenum. (*Opposite left*) A mass infiltrates the duodenal bulb and indents the pyloric canal primarily along the greater curvature. The mucosal folds in the pyloric canal (**arrows**) are widened, stretched, and fixed in an arcuate configuration by the mass. There is flattening and rigidity of the incisura angularis. (*Opposite right*) The pylorus contracts in an eccentric fashion. The infiltrated folds (**arrows**) in the prepyloric region are distorted and crowded, and there is no draping. (*Lower left*) Nodular infiltration of the region of the incisura is obvious. The distended pyloric canal clearly shows evidence of extrinsic irregular impression of the greater curvature (**arrows**). (*Lower right*) The peristaltic ring (**arrows**) is markedly asymmetric. Indentation of the mass flattens the distal slope along the greater curvature. The folds in the contracted segment are broad and stretched. (Keller RJ, Khilnani MT, Wolf BS: The struggling antrum: A new sign of perigastric malignancy.. AJR 119:300–310, 1973)

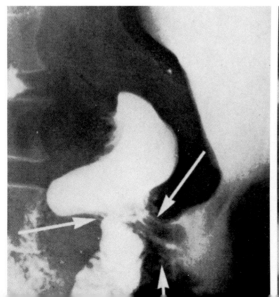

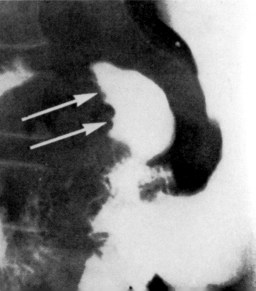

Symmetric Liver Sign

The symmetric liver sign, a soft-tissue density representing the liver that extends from abdominal wall to abdominal wall, was originally reported as a radiographic sign of asplenia (Fig. 1-146). In normal persons, the lower edge of the liver lies obliquely, and the right lobe is markedly larger than the left; in contrast, in persons with hepatic symmetry, the lower edge of the liver lies horizontally. An identical appearance may be seen in patients with polysplenia, in whom multiple accessory spleens can be demonstrated on radionuclide studies.

BIBLIOGRAPHY
Lucas RV, Neufeld HN, Lester RG et al: The symmetrical liver as a roentgen sign of asplenia. Circulation 25:973–975, 1962

FIG. 1-146. Symmetric liver sign in a patient with asplenia. Note the cardiac dextroversion.

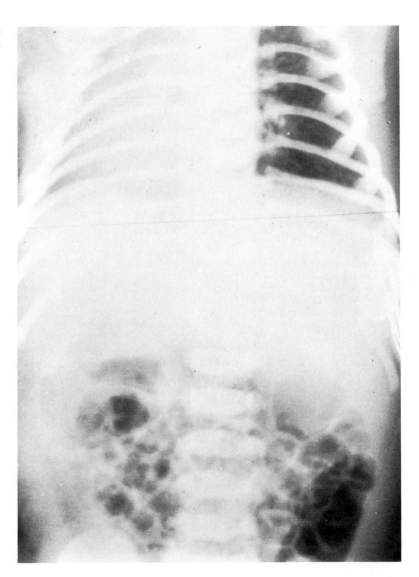

Tacked-Down Sign

Certain desmoplastic tumors involving the mesentery and gut elicit a disproportionate fibrous stromal reaction. Disruption or erosion of the mesothelial covering of bowel serosal surfaces by the tumor also stimulates fibrous peritoneal adhesions. Fibrous adhesions cause fixation and angulation of the bowel as well as stretching and distortion, though usually not destruction, of mucosal folds (Fig. 1-147). Although the tacked-down sign was originally described as typical of diffuse peritoneal carcinomatosis, an identical appearance can be produced by the desmoplastic reaction associated with carcinoid tumors (Fig. 1-148).

BIBLIOGRAPHY

Zboralske FF, Bessolo RJ: Metastatic carcinoma to the mesentery and gut. Radiology 88:302–310, 1967

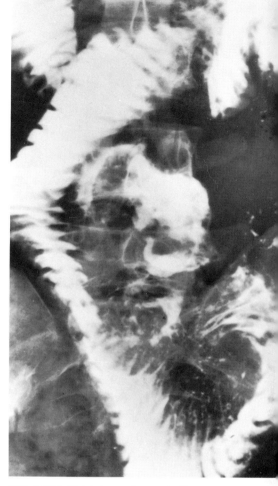

FIG. 1-147. "Tacked-down" sign in a patient with abdominal carcinomatosis (sigmoid primary). (Eisenberg RL: Gastrointestinal Radiology: A Pattern Approach. Philadelphia, JB Lippincott, 1983)

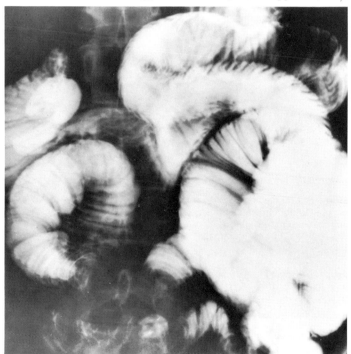

FIG. 1-148. The intense desmoplastic reaction incited by this carcinoid tumor causes kinking and angulation of the bowel and separation of small intestinal loops in the midabdomen. (Eisenberg RL: Gastrointestinal Radiology: A Pattern Approach, Philadelphia, JB Lippincott, 1983)

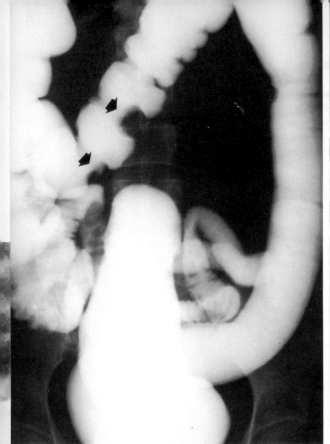

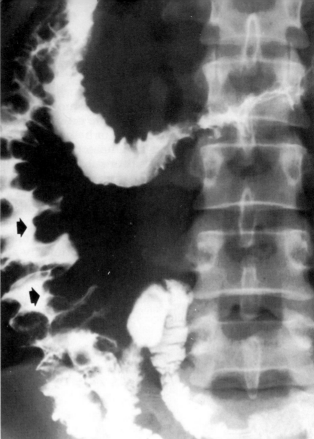

FIG. 1-153. (*Left*) Filled and (*right*) postevacuation films demonstrate marginal filling defects (*arrows*) and overlying mucosal abnormalities in a patient with amebic colitis. (Hardy R, Scullin DR: Thumbprinting in a case of amebiasis. Radiology 98:147–148, 1971)

FIG. 1-154. Thumbprinting in a patient with pneumatosis intestinalis. The polypoid masses indenting the barium column are composed of air rather than soft-tissue density. (Eisenberg RL: Gastrointestinal Radiology: A Pattern Approach. Philadelphia, JB Lippincott, 1983)

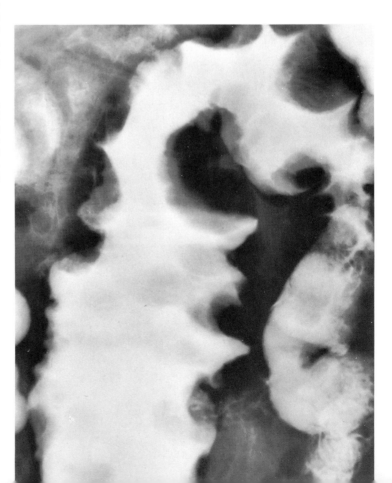

Transverse Stripe Sign

Multiple transverse, narrow, and usually very distinct (though sometimes diffusely outlined) stripes of contrast medium in the colon have been reported as a pathognomonic radiographic sign of Crohn's colitis (Fig. 1-155). These transverse stripes are usually more than 1 cm long and straight, unlike the rest of the haustra, which generally appear somewhat curved. They are sometimes seen as direct continuations of tiny ulcerations extending perpendicularly from the contours of the colon. Transverse stripes result from contrast medium situated in deep grooves between coarse mucosal folds (Fig. 1-156) or within fiord-like fissures or ulcerations. Occasionally, deep grooves between swollen mucosal folds also produce longitudinal stripes of contrast.

BIBLIOGRAPHY

Welin S, Welin B: A pathognomonic roentgenologic sign of regional ileitis (Crohn's disease). Dis Colon Rectum 16:473–478, 1973

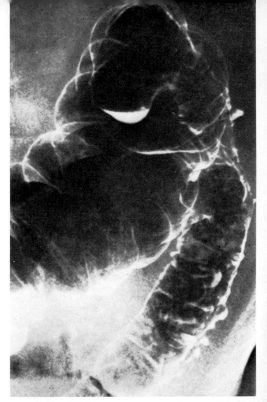
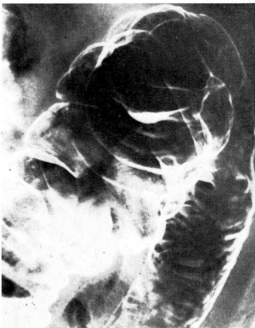

FIG. 1-155. *(Top)* Numerous deep transverse stripes are associated with narrowing and ulcerations in this patient with Crohn's colitis. *(Bottom)* An examination 2 years later shows resolution of the ulcerations but persistence of the stripes. (Welin S, Welin B: A pathognomonic roentgenologic sign of regional ileitis [Crohn's disease]. Dis Colon Rectum 16:473–478, 1973)

FIG. 1-156. Numerous pronounced transverse stripes and longitudinal ulcerations are seen in this patient with Crohn's colitis. (Welin S, Welin B: A pathognomonic roentgenologic sign of regional ileitis [Crohn's disease]. Dis Colon Rectum 16:473–478, 1973)

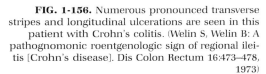
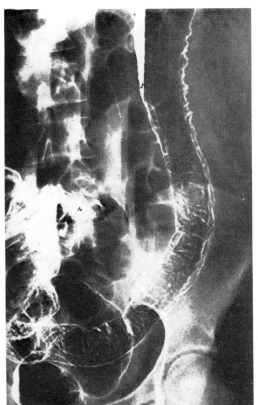

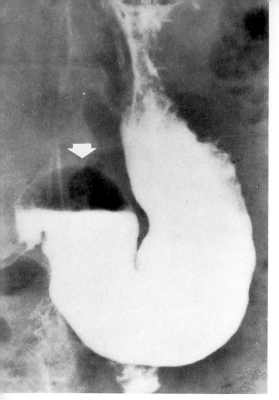

FIG. 1-157. Localized elevation of the gastric antrum with a pocket of gas situated between the elevated portion of the lesser curvature and barium in the stomach (**arrow**) in a patient with benign perigastric adhesions. (Lumsden K, Pexman JHW: The trapped air sign: Its value in the interpretation of antral deformities. Clin Radiol 19:211–220, 1968

Trapped Air Sign

Demonstration of a peculiar pocket of gas along the lesser curvature of the gastric antrum was originally described as an indication of benign perigastric adhesions with elevation and fixation of the gastric antrum to other organs such as the liver and pancreas (Fig. 1-157). Requirements for demonstration of the sign were reported to be the upright position, fixation and elevation of the stomach wall, and a soft, pliable stomach wall to allow tenting. Presence of the sign was thus considered of value in excluding gastric carcinoma. Since then, however, the trapped air sign has been reported in patients with gastric carcinoma (Fig. 1-158). Explanations for this appearance in malignant processes include a cavity within a carcinomatous ulcer on the lesser curvature; gastric fixation due to local spread of gastric carcinoma into an adjacent organ; tumors that irregularly encroach on the antral lumen and permit gas to be trapped in a small, localized elevation along the lesser curvature; development of carcinoma in a stomach that has been deformed by preexisting adhesions; and fibrosis and contraction of the lesser omentum causing antral elevation and trapping of gas in cases of extensive scirrhous carcinoma.

BIBLIOGRAPHY
Lumsden K, Pexman JHW: The trapped air sign: Its value in the interpretation of antral deformities. Clin Radiol 19:211–220, 1968
Shopfner CE: Perigastric adhesions: The "trapped air" sign. AJR 89:810–815, 1963

FIG. 1-158. Two views of a patient with characteristic scirrhous carcinoma involving almost the entire stomach demonstrate a persistent gas bubble in a localized elevation of the antrum (**arrow**). (Lumsden K, Pexman JHW: The trapped air sign: Its value in the interpretation of antral deformities. Clin Radiol 19:211–220, 1968)

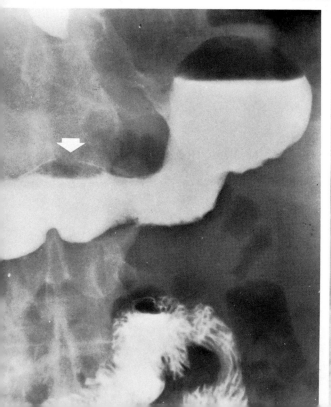

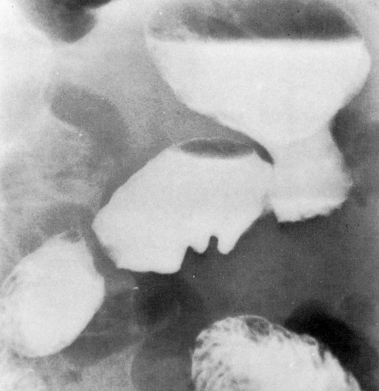

Triangle Sign

Small amounts of free intraperitoneal gas may accumulate in the space in which three loops of bowel adjoin each other to form a radiolucent curvilinear triangle (Fig. 1-159). This triangle sign may also be found in the space between two loops of bowel and other viscera such as the liver or abdominal wall (Fig. 1-160). The triangle is sometimes irregular, but it is always radiolucent. Identification of the triangle sign should lead the observer to search for other evidence of pneumoperitoneum and to obtain confirmatory radiographs.

BIBLIOGRAPHY
Miller RE: The radiological evaluation of intraperitoneal gas (pneumoperitoneum). CRC Crit Rev Diagn Imaging 4:61–85, 1973

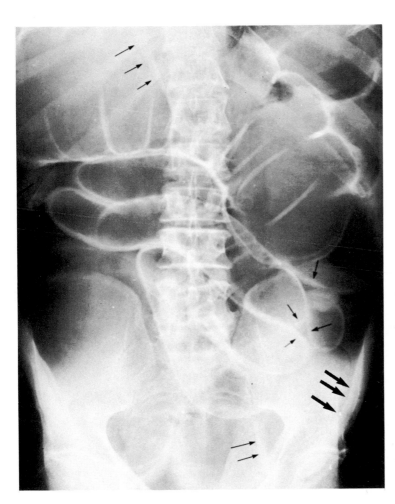

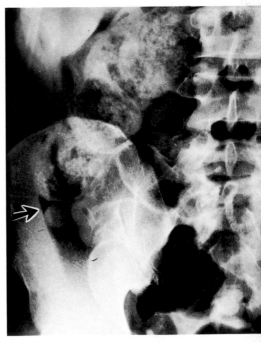

FIG. 1-159. Supine abdominal radiograph demonstrates large amounts of gas both in the small and large bowel and intraperitoneally in a patient with carcinoma of the rectosigmoid and colonic perforation. **Arrows** in the left midabdomen point to two triangle signs between loops of bowel. Other evidence of pneumoperitoneum incudes demonstration of the falciform (**top arrows**) and lateral umbilical ligaments (**lower arrows**), the football signs (**arrows**) in the patient's left lower quadrant, and both the inner and outer walls of the larger and small bowel. (Miller RE: The radiological evaluation of intraperitoneal gas [pneumoperitoneum]. CRC Crit Rev Diagn Imaging 4:61–85, 1973. Copyright Chemical Rubber Co., CRC Press, Inc. Reproduced by permission)

FIG. 1-160. Supine abdominal radiograph in a patient with a perforated duodenal ulcer demonstrates a triangle sign between two fluid-filled loops of large and small bowel and the lateral abdominal wall (**arrow**). A similar sign is seen in the right upper quadrant between the liver edge, colon, and fluid-containing small bowel. (Miller RE: The radiological evaluation of intraperitoneal gas [pneumoperitoneum]. CRC Crit Rev Diagn Imaging 4:61–85, 1973)

Triple Bubble Sign

Congenital jejunal atresia is an important cause of mechanical small bowel obstruction in infants. Plain radiographs of the abdomen demonstrate three large collections of intraluminal gas within the stomach, duodenum, and proximal jejunum. This triple bubble sign is pathognomonic of jejunal atresia (Fig. 1-161).

BIBLIOGRAPHY

Swischuk LE: Radiology of the Newborn and Young Infant. Baltimore, Williams & Wilkins, 1980

FIG. 1-161. Triple bubble sign (stomach, duodenum, proximal jejunum) in an infant with jejunal atresia. (Eisenberg RL: Gastrointestinal Radiology: A Pattern Approach. Philadelphia JB Lippincott, 1983)

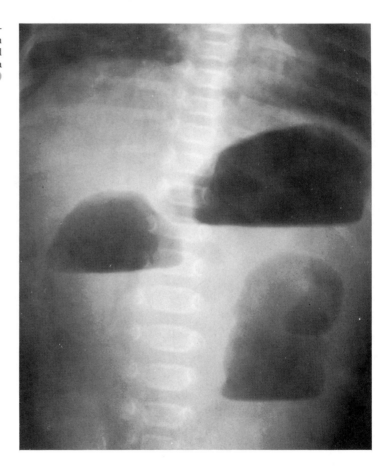

Tumbling Bullet Sign

Abdominal gunshot wounds are surgically managed by immediate laparotomy. If a bullet remains visible on postoperative radiographs, its position is assumed to be retroperitoneal. Given that the retroperitoneal space is only a potential space, a bullet located in this region is embedded in fascia or muscle and does not move. Radiographic demonstration of movement of the bullet on sequential films (Fig. 1-162) indicates that the bullet lies free in a cavity and is therefore diagnostic of the development of a retroperitoneal abscess, even if clinical symptoms are vague and nonspecific.

BIBLIOGRAPHY

Mittelholzer E, Shields JH: The tumbling bullet: A sign of retroperitoneal abscess. Radiology 97:625–627, 1970

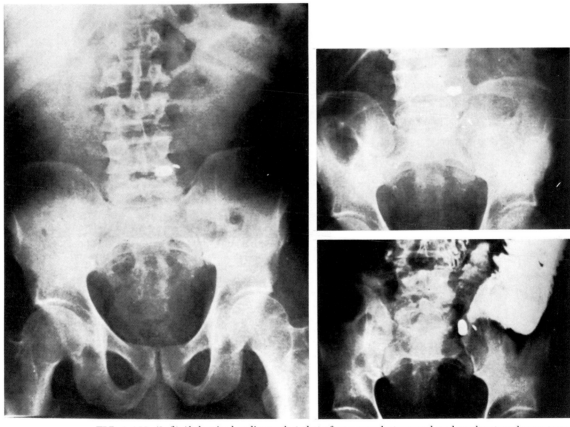

FIG. 1-162. (*Left*) Abdominal radiograph 1 day after a gunshot wound and exploratory laparotomy reveals the bullet and an accompanying small fragment overlying the left side of the L4-L5 intervertebral disk space. (*Top, right*) Abdominal radiograph obtained 3 days later demonstrates a change in the position of the small fragment, which has been substantially displaced caudally. (*Bottom, right*) Seven days after surgery, the bullet itself has changed position. (Mittelholzer E, Shields JB: The tumbling bullet: A sign of retroperitoneal abscess. Radiology 97:625–627, 1970)

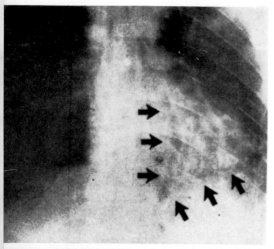

V Sign of Naclerio

Spontaneous rupture of the esophagus is a potentially fatal condition. Early diagnosis gives the best chance of survival. Localized mediastinal emphysema, which can be easily overlooked, is a virtually diagnostic finding that is usually evident before physical signs are present. This characteristically produces a linear lucency in the shape of a V (Fig. 1-166).

BIBLIOGRAPHY

Naclerio NA: The ''V'' sign in the diagnosis of spontaneous rupture of the esophagus (an early roentgen clue). Am J Surg 93:291–298, 1957

FIG. 1-166. Localized mediastinal emphysema in two patients with spontaneous rupture of the esophagus. The linear lucent shadows (**arrows**) correspond to the fascial planes of the mediastinal and diaphragmatic pleurae in the region of the lower esophagus. (Naclerio NA: The ''V'' sign in the diagnosis of spontaneous rupture of the esophagus (an early roentgen clue). Am J Surg 93:291–298, 1957)

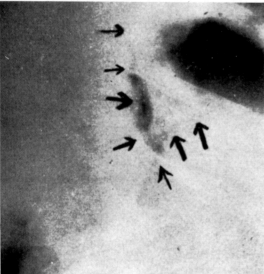

Vallecular Sign

In the normal patient, ingested barium enters the valleculae and is immediately spilled, occasionally leaving small traces that are cleared out by subsequent swallows. The epiglottis, which remains upright during swallowing, divides the barium into equal parts and passes it along the lateral walls into the pyriform sinuses. Prolonged retention of a substantial amount of barium in the valleculae and pyriform sinuses after swallowing is considered the radiographic counterpart of clinical dysphagia (Fig. 1-167). Although first described in association with esophageal malignancy, the vallecular sign may be seen in patients with carcinoma of the hypopharynx or gastric fundus, neurologic and muscular disorders (*e.g.,* bulbar paralysis, multiple sclerosis, myasthenia), and mediastinal neoplastic or inflammatory processes.

BIBLIOGRAPHY
Arendt J, Wolf A: The vallecular sign: Its diagnosis and clinical significance. AJR 57:435–445, 1947

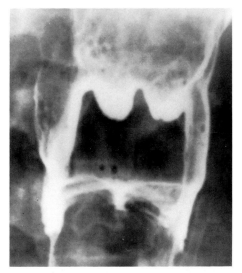

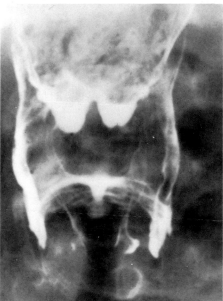

FIG. 1-167. Two examples of the vallecular sign.

Absent Collecting System Sign

An excretory urogram demonstrating a normal nephrogram, good concentration of contrast material in the ureters, but no contrast in the intrarenal collecting systems (absent collecting system sign) has been reported as an indication of severe interstitial edema within the kidney (Fig. 2-1, *top*). Following resolution of the edema, the urographic findings return to normal (Fig. 2-1, *bottom*).

BIBLIOGRAPHY
Murchison RJ, Nicholson TC: Case profile: Absent collecting system sign. Urology 10:343, 1977

FIG. 2-1. (*Top*) Initial excretory urogram demonstrates a normal nephrogram and good concentration of contrast material in the ureters but no contrast in the intrarenal collecting systems. (*Bottom*) The urographic findings have returned to normal 2 weeks later. (Murchison RJ, Nicholson TC: Case profile: Absent collecting system sign. Urology 10:343, 1977)

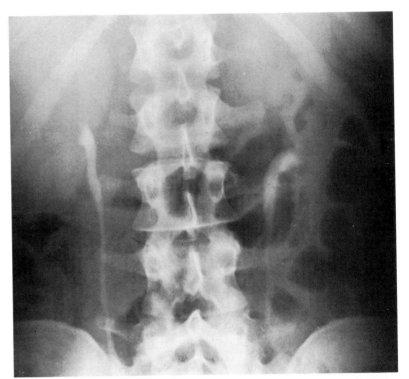

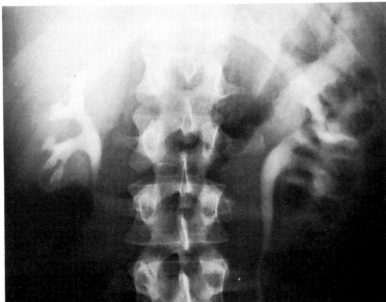

Acorn Deformity
(Spinning-Top Configuration)

In girls with distal urethral stenosis, distinct widening of the urethra above the stenotic ring combined with fixation and narrowing of the bladder neck may produce a characteristic acorn deformity or spinning-top configuration (Fig. 2-2). However, a urethra with this shape can be normal in caliber, and conversely, urethras that appear normal at cystourethrography may have significant stenosis. Variations in the diameter and contour of the urethra probably reflect the volume and rate of urinary flow during voiding. Therefore, the acorn deformities often found in normal children are a result of the forceful passage of a large volume of urine distending the thin-walled urethra (Fig. 2-3).

BIBLIOGRAPHY
Shopfner CE: Analysis of hydronephrosis. Postgrad Sem Unit 6: 1–6, 1967
Witten DM, Myers GH, Utz DC: Emmett's Clinical Urography. Philadelphia, WB Saunders, 1977

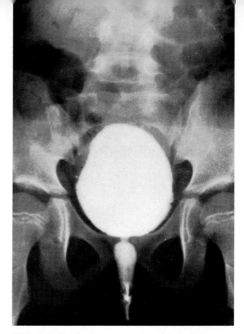

FIG. 2-2. Voiding cystourethrogram demonstrates that the bladder neck and urethra have an acorn or spinning-top contour. This sign is interpreted as representing contracture of the bladder neck and poststenotic dilatation of the urethra. (Gould HR, Peterson CG, Jr: Cystourethrography in children. AJR 98:192–199, 1966. Copyright 1966. Reproduced by permission)

FIG. 2-3. The vesical neck and urethra in this normal child show an acorn or spinning-top deformity. The patient had a negative cystoscopic examination and no residual urine. (Witten DM, Myers GH, Utz DC: Emmett's Clinical Urography. Philadelphia, WB Saunders, 1977)

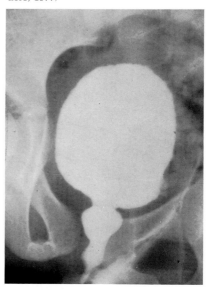

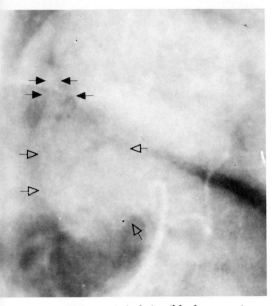

FIG. 2-4. Apical sign (**black arrows**) surmounting a tumor (**open arrows**) of the left adrenal gland indicates a pheochromocytoma in the late phase of this arteriogram. (Ney C, Friedenberg RM: Radiographic Atlas of the Genitourinary System. Philadelphia, JB Lippincott, 1981)

Apical (Dunce-Cap) Sign

Pheochromocytomas are generally spherical tumors that develop within the adrenal medulla and result in mass enlargement of the base of the gland. The superior, or apical, portion of the gland remains intact. The uninvolved apex of the gland, which represents most of the intact glandular cortex, appears radiographically as a small triangular cap at the upper extremity of the bulging mass (Fig. 2-4).

BIBLIOGRAPHY
Meyers MA: Characteristic radiographic shape of pheochromocytomas and adrenocortical adenomas. Radiology 87:889–892, 1966

Beaded (Corkscrew) Ureter Sign

Tuberculosis involving the ureter typically causes multiple ulcerations of short or long segments of the ureter with thickening of the ureteral wall. As the disease heals, a pattern of multiple areas of ureteral strictures alternating with dilated segments of ureter is produced (Fig. 2-5).

BIBLIOGRAPHY
Witten DM, Myers GH, Utz DC: Emmett's Clinical Urography. Philadelphia, WB Saunders, 1977

FIG. 2-5. Two examples of tuberculous ureteritis. Segmental areas of dilatation and constriction produce a corkscrew, or beaded, pattern. (Ney C, Friedenberg RM: Radiographic Atlas of the Genitourinary System. Philadelphia, JB Lippincott, 1981)

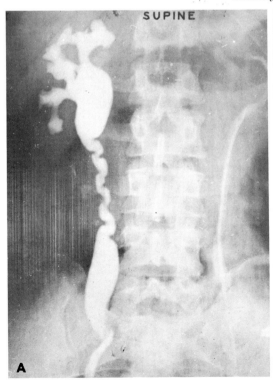

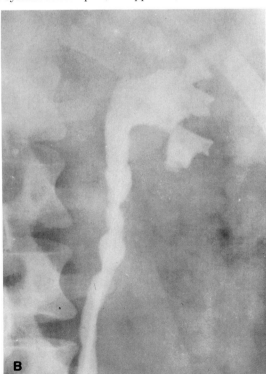

Beak Sign

As a simple renal cyst slowly increases in size, its protruding portion elevates the adjacent edges of the cortex. This cortical margin appears as a very thin, smooth radiopaque rim about the bulging lucent cyst (Fig. 2-6). The beak sign can be demonstrated by nephrotomography, though it is usually better seen on the nephrogram phase of arteriography. Although the beak sign is generally considered to be characteristic of benign renal cysts, it is a reflection of slow expansion of a lesion and thus may occasionally be seen in slow-growing solid lesions, including carcinoma. Thickening of the rim about a lucent mass suggests bleeding into a cyst, a cyst infection, or a malignant lesion.

BIBLIOGRAPHY
Elkin M: Radiology of the Urinary System. Boston, Little, Brown & Co, 1980

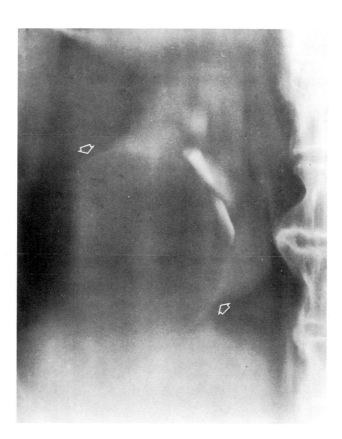

FIG. 2-6. Nephrotomogram demonstrates a thin, smooth radiopaque rim (**arrows**) representing the cortical margin of a large, lucent, benign renal cyst.

Beehive on the Bladder Sign

A distinctively biconvex triangular deformity (beehive) ending in a clearly defined point has been associated with the vesical end of a colovesical fistula (Fig. 2-7). A colovesical fistula develops when involved bowel becomes fixed to the peritoneal surface of the bladder, limiting movement of the bladder wall and impeding efficient contraction. This results in infection due to stasis of urine and may cause the formation of a fistula with triangular elevation of the bladder wall at the vesicular end of the fistulous tract (Fig. 2-8).

BIBLIOGRAPHY

Kaisary AV, Grant RW: "Beehive on the bladder": A sign of colovesical fistula. Ann R Col Surg Eng 63:195–197, 1982

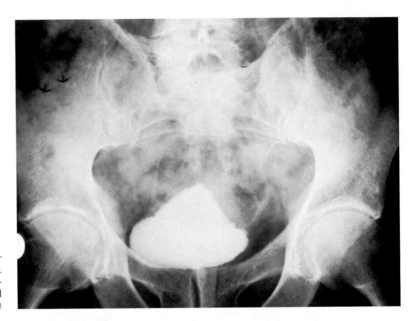

FIG. 2-7. Characteristic biconvex triangular deformity simulates a beehive on the bladder. (Kaisary AV, Grant RW: "Beehive on the bladder": A sign of colovesical fistula. Ann R Col Surg Eng 63:195–197, 1982)

FIG. 2-8. Combined barium enema and cystogram demonstrate a fistulous tract **(arrow)** and "beehive" sign. (Kaisary AV, Grant RW: "Beehive on the bladder": A sign of colovesical fistual. Ann R Col Surg Eng 63:195–197, 1982)

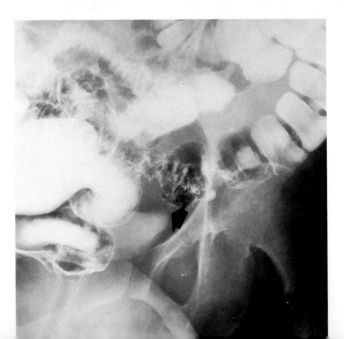

Bell-Shaped Ureter Sign

A bell-shaped configuration with a convex cutoff inferiorly may be produced in the ureter by antegrade intussusception (Fig. 2-9). This rare phenomenon is caused by an underlying sessile or pedunculated neoplasm that is free of submucosal invasion and fixation and is thus able to serve as the lead point of the intussusception.

BIBLIOGRAPHY

Mazer MJ, Lacy SS, Kao L: "Bell-shaped ureter": A radiographic sign of antegrade intussusception. Urol Radiol 1:63–65, 1979

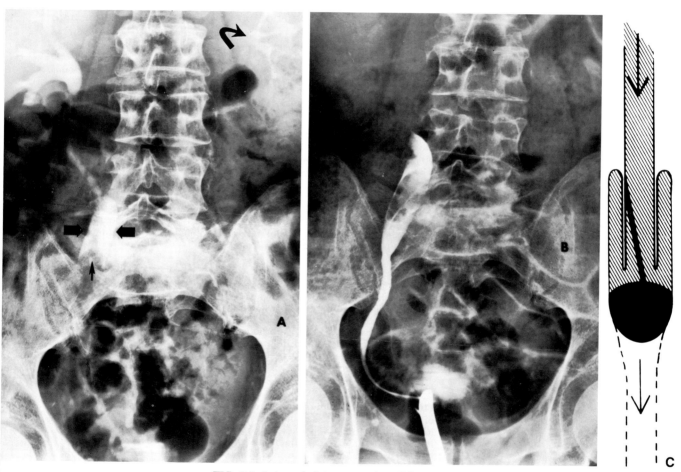

FIG. 2-9. Antegrade intussusception of the ureter secondary to a lead pedunculated polypoid transitional cell tumor. (**A**) The **thick horizontal arrows** delineate the bell-shaped right midureter with a convex cutoff inferiorly. The **thin vertical arrow** shows the lead polypoid tumor. Note the stalk of the tumor mass within the bell and the additional persistent filling defect in the left renal pelvis (**curved arrow**). (**B**) Right retrograde pyelogram better delineates the large polypoid tumor with incomplete filling proximally. (**C**) Schematic drawing of the underlying pathologic process. (Mazer MJ, Lacy SS, Kao L: "Bell-shaped ureter": A radiographic sign of antegrade intussusception. Urol Radiol 1:63–65, 1979)

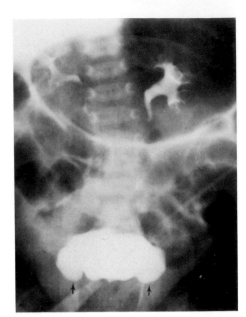

Bladder Ear Sign

So-called bladder ears, which are lateral protrusions of the urinary bladder occurring in infants, represent transitory extraperitoneal herniation of the bladder. Usually bilateral, bladder ears occur in about 10% of all infants under the age of 1 (Fig. 2-16). About 20% of all cases are associated with inguinal hernias. Bladder ears disappear spontaneously and are considered a normal variant.

BIBLIOGRAPHY
Allen RP, Condon VR: Transitory extraperitoneal hernia of the bladder in infants (bladder ears). Radiology 77:979–983, 1961

FIG. 2-16. The lateral walls of the bladder are displaced downward (**arrows**) and project into the inguinal ring. This is a normal occurrence in infants under the age of 1. (Rabinowitz JG: Pediatric Radiology. Philadelphia, JB Lippincott, 1978)

FIG. 2-17 (*Left*).

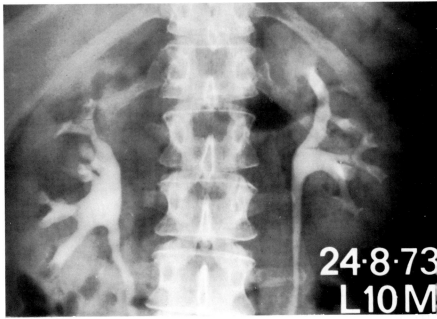

Central Lucency Sign

A renal lobe containing a normal cortex, one pyramid, and a papilla may be displaced deep within the kidney during development (lobar dysmorphism). Excretory urography demonstrates splaying and pressure deformity due to the mass of the misplaced lobe (Fig. 2-17 A); arteriography shows that the interlobar arteries are deviated around the malpositioned lobe but are otherwise normal (Fig. 2-17 B). During the nephrogram phase, there is a well-defined mass with a dense outer rim corresponding to the cortex and a relatively radiolucent center representing the medulla (Fig. 2-17 C). The presence of this central lucency sign distinguishes lobar dysmorphism, containing both cortex and medulla, from prominence of a renal column, which consists only of cortical tissue.

A similar appearance can be seen at angiography when a simple cyst protrudes beyond the cortex of the kidney. When viewed *en face*, the lucent cyst is surrounded by a dense, elevated rim of cortex.

BIBLIOGRAPHY

Dacie JE: The "central lucency" sign of lobar dysmorphism (pseudotumor of the kidney). Br J Radiol 49:39–42, 1976

FIG. 2-17. (*Left*) Ten-minute film from an excretory urogram demonstrates a mass in the center of the right kidney with splaying of the adjacent infundibula. (*Center*) Arterial phase of a right selective renal arteriogram shows slight displacement of the interlobar arteries by the central mass. (The lower pole was supplied by an accessory vessel arising from the aorta just proximal to the bifurcation.) (*Right*) Oblique projection during the nephrogram phase of the right selective renal arteriogram demonstrates a dense blush surrounding a central lucency in this patient with lobar dysmorphism. The diagnosis was confirmed on pathologic examination. (Dacie JE: The "central lucency" sign of lobar dysmorphism [pseudotumor of the kidney]. Br J Radiol 49:39–42, 1976)

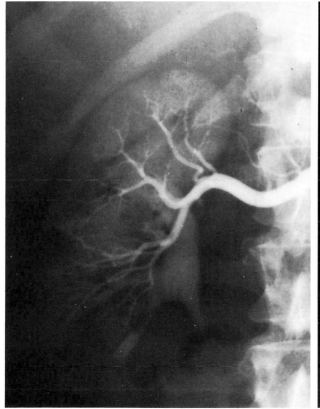

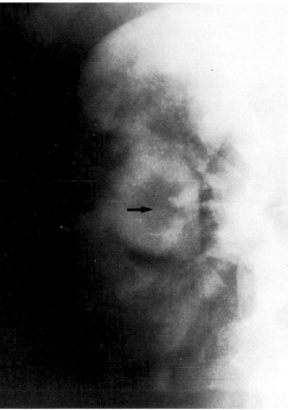

Collateral Vein Sign

Arteriographic visualization of collateral veins draining a kidney that contains a renal carcinoma has been reported as a strong indication of compromise of the renal vein (Fig. 2-21). Since the original description, however, authors have pointed out that collateral or "abnormal" venous communications associated with renal tumors do not necessarily indicate renal vein involvement, and the sign should thus be interpreted with caution. Conversely, although collateral renal veins are seen in most cases of renal carcinoma examined by the high-dosage arteriographic technique, substantial tumor extension into the renal vein can occur with no evidence of collateral vein filling. Therefore, contrast examination of the inferior vena cava or renal vein, ultrasound, or computed tomography may be necessary to establish the status of the renal vein.

BIBLIOGRAPHY

Ahlberg NE, Bartley O, Wahlqvist L: Angiographic diagnosis of tumor thrombus in main trunk of renal vein in renal carcinoma. Acta Chir Scand 132:362–369, 1966

Whitley NO, Kinkhabwala M, Whitley JE: The collateral vein sign: A fallible sign in the staging of renal cancer. AJR 120:660–663, 1974

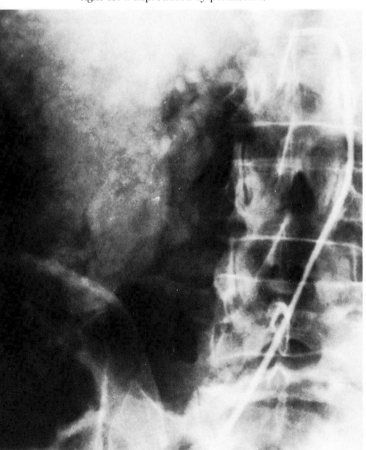

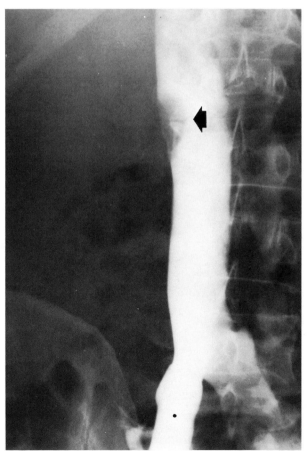

FIG. 2-21. *(Left)* Late phase of a renal arteriogram in a patient with carcinoma of the kidney demonstrates collateral veins but no renal vein. *(Right)* Inferior vena cavogram demonstrates the rounded filling defect of a tumor thrombus (**arrow**) protruding into the inferior vena cava from the renal vein. (Whitley NO, Kinkhabwala M, Whitley JE: The collateral vein sign: A fallible sign in the staging of renal cancer. AJR 120:660–663, 1974. Copyright 1974. Reproduced by permission)

Colon Sign

In patients in whom the kidneys are not visualized on excretory urography, the appearance of the colon can be an aid in differentiation between renal absence (agenesis, ectopia, surgical removal) and extensive renal disease. In renal agenesis or ectopia, lack of development of the perirenal fascia in the renal fossa allows the colon to occupy the renal bed. Thus, on nephrotomography, visualization of sharply outlined gas or fecal material indicates that the colon lies in the plane of the renal fossa where the kidney would normally be located (Fig. 2-22). Conversely, in acquired renal diseases such as renal atrophy, loss of volume is compensated for by adipose deposition between the intact perirenal fascial layers or by fibrotic adhesions, not by the colon. The colon remains in its normal position in acquired renal disease, so that, although nephrotomography may demonstrate gas and fecal material superimposed on the kidneys, it also shows fuzziness and blurring of the colonic margins, indicating that they are outside the plane of the kidneys.

BIBLIOGRAPHY

Dixit JK, Leslie CL, Hagaman FV et al: Value of nephrotomography in evaluating nonvisualized kidney in renal absence: The colon sign. South Med J 72:581–584, 1979

FIG. 2-22. *(Left)* Nephrotomogram does not demonstrate the right kidney. The colonic wall, haustral pattern, and bowel contents, including feces and gas, are sharply outlined **(arrows)**. The left kidney shows changes due to compensatory hypertrophy. *(Right)* Lateral film from a barium enema examination demonstrates characteristic malposition of the colon. The posteromedial location of the hepatic flexure occupying the right renal bed **(arrows)** confirms the diagnosis of renal agenesis. (Dixit JK, Leslie CL, Hagaman FV et al: Value of nephrotomography in evaluating nonvisualized kidney in renal absence: The colon sign. South Med J 72:581–584, 1979)

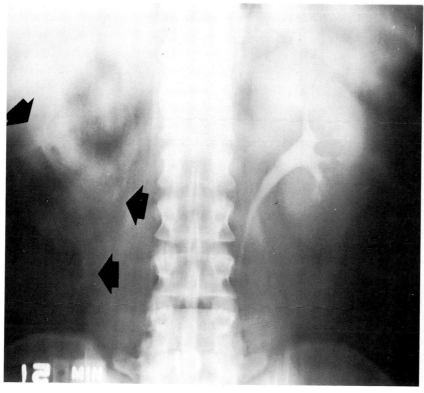

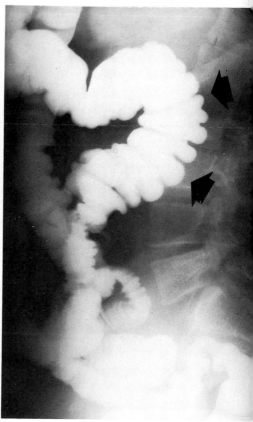

Crescent Sign

In patients with chronic obstructive uropathy with preserved glomerular filtration and tubular reabsorption of water, excretory urography may demonstrate thin curvilinear collections of contrast material in the renal parenchyma overlying nonopacified, dilated calyces (Fig. 2-26 *A* and *B*). This crescent sign is attributed to the accumulation of contrast in collecting tubules that have been flattened and displaced by the hydronephrotic calyces so that they lie parallel to the renal convexity and near its surface. As the calyces slowly opacify, the crescents are no longer visible (Fig. 2-26 *C*). Some remaining excretory function is required for the crescent sign to appear, in contrast to the rim sign of chronic obstructive uropathy (see Fig. 2-78).

BIBLIOGRAPHY
LeVine M, Allen A, Stein JL et al: The crescent sign. Radiology 81:971–973, 1963

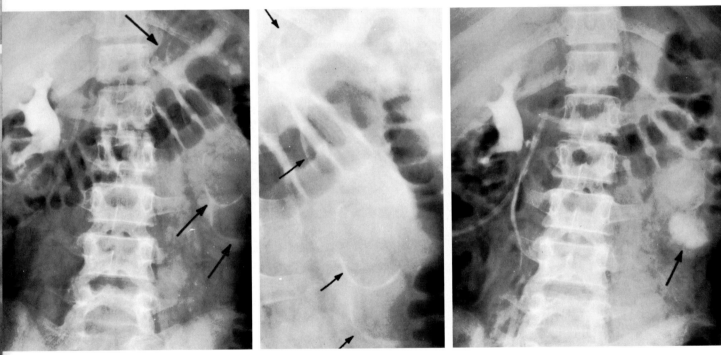

FIG. 2-26. (*Left*) Excretory urogram demonstrates good opacification of the right renal pelvis and calyces. The pelvis and calyces of the left kidney are not opacified, but crescentic collections of contrast (**arrows**) are seen in the renal parenchyma overlying dilated calyces. (*Center*) Enlargement of part of the film shown in (*left*). The crescent sign of hydronephrosis is exaggerated (**arrows**). (*Right*) Delayed film obtained 1 hr later than (*center*). Some contrast has collected in the dilated calyces (**arrow**). The crescent sign has almost completely disappeared. (Witten DM, Myers GH, Utz DC: Emmett's Clinical Urography. Philadelphia, WB Saunders, 1977)

Curlicue Ureter Sign

Herniation of the ureter is very rare, occurring most often in the inguinal region in men and in the femoral region in women. Herniation into the sciatic foramen is even rarer. A virtually diagnostic sign of ureteral herniation is a characteristic looping of the ureter (Fig. 2-27). The position of the loop may be an indication of the type of herniation. In scrotal, inguinal, and preinguinal herniations of the ureter, the curlicue is positioned in a vertical direction. Herniations into the sciatic foramen tend to have a horizontal loop and are more likely to be associated with a hydroureter above the point of herniation.

BIBLIOGRAPHY
Beck WC, Baurys W, Brochu J et al: Herniation of the ureter into the sciatic foramen ("curlicue ureter"). JAMA 149:441–442, 1952
Ney C, Miller HL, Gordimer H: Preinguinal canal herniation of the ureter: Value of the curlicue sign direction. Arch Surg 105:633–634, 1972

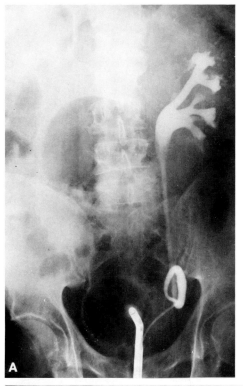

FIG. 2-27. Retrograde pyelogram in a patient with an inguinal hernia. **(A)** Frontal view demonstrates vertical redundancy of the pelvic ureter. **(B)** Oblique view demonstrates angulation of the ureter. (Ney C, Friedenberg RM: Radiographic Atlas of the Genitourinary System. Philadelphia, JB Lippincott, 1981)

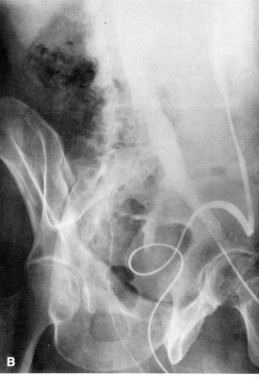

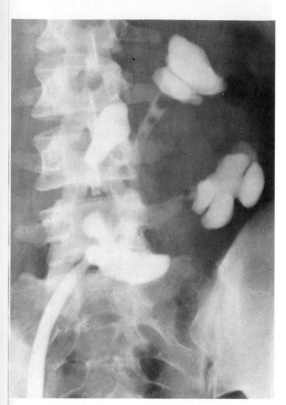

Disk, Cake, Lump, or Doughnut Kidney

Fusion of the kidneys can result in a horseshoe kidney, with an isthmus connecting the lower poles of the two kidneys. Complete fusion may produce a single irregular mass that has no resemblance to a renal structure. The resulting bizarre appearance has been given such varied terms as *disk, cake, lump,* and *doughnut kidney* (Fig. 2-31). The single renal mass has two ureters, each arising from an anteriorly positioned ureteropelvic junction and opening into the bladder at its normal site. The fused kidney usually fails to ascend during development and therefore appears as a single mass of tissue within the bony pelvis. Poor emptying of the pelvocalyceal systems, caused by the abdominal position of the ureteropelvic junction and the ureteral deviation, often results in infection and calculus formation.

BIBLIOGRAPHY
Elkin M: Radiology of the Urinary System. Boston, Little, Brown & Co, 1980

FIG. 2-31. Disk kidney. At cystoscopy, only one ureteral orifice was found in the bladder. Injection of contrast into this orifice demonstrates a centrally placed, irregularly defined single renal mass with four calyceal systems extending out from a small, central renal pelvis. Severe hydronephrosis and pyelonephritis were present. (Ney C, Friedenberg RM: Radiographic Atlas of the Genitourinary System. Philadelphia, JB Lippincott, 1981)

Drooping Lily Sign

Obstruction and subsequent hydronephrosis of the upper segment of a renal duplication causes a mass effect in the kidney that can simulate an upper pole tumor. The mass of the markedly dilated, nonopacified upper calyceal system displaces the visualized lower pelvocalyceal system downward and laterally (Fig. 2-32). Normally, a line connecting the most superior and most inferior calyces runs obliquely downward and laterally in the direction of the psoas line. With obstructive hydronephrosis of the upper segment of a duplicated pelvis, this line tends to run either vertically or, more commonly, obliquely downward and medially (Fig. 2-33).

BIBLIOGRAPHY
Witten DM, Myers GH, Utz DC: Emmett's Clinical Urography. Philadelphia, WB Saunders, 1977

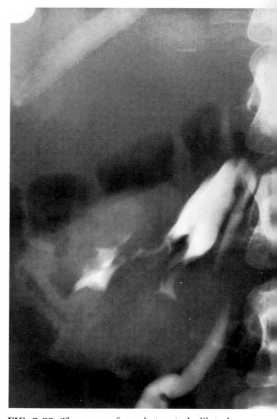

FIG. 2-32. The mass of an obstructed, dilated upper calyceal system displaces the lower pelvocalyceal system downward and laterally, producing a "drooping lily" appearance.

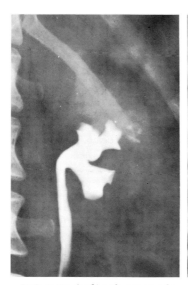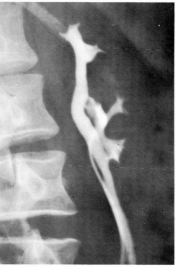

FIG. 2-33. *(Left)* Left retrograde pyelogram demonstrates the drooping lily sign in the lower pelvis of a duplicated collecting system and ureter. Although there are three major calyces, the upper half of the elongated renal outline is not drained by the visualized pelvis, evidence that there must be a duplication. *(Right)* With a catheter in each ureter, the left retrograde pyelogram demonstrates both the upper and lower pelves of the complete duplication. (Witten DM, Myers GH, Utz DC: Emmett's Clinical Urography. Philadelphia, WB Saunders, 1977)

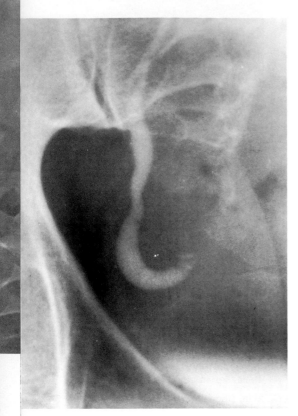

FIG. 2-38. Upward curve of the distal ureter producing a characteristic fishhook appearance in a patient with prostatic hypertrophy.

Fishhook (J-Shaped) Ureter

In patients with prostatic hypertrophy, the prostate gland may elevate the trigone and base of the bladder to such a degree as to cause the terminal portions of the ureter to have an upward curved configuration. This fishhook or J-shaped appearance is pathognomonic of the disease (Fig. 2-38).

BIBLIOGRAPHY
Witten DM, Myers GH, Utz DC: Emmett's Clinical Urography. Philadelphia, WB Saunders, 1977

Goblet (Wine Glass) Sign

In a patient with a ureteral tumor, a contrast examination may demonstrate either the upper or the lower margin of the lucent filling defect of the tumor. It is usually difficult to show both borders on a single film. On retrograde pyelography, there is a characteristic meniscus appearance to the superior border of the contrast, producing a goblet or wine-glass sign outlining the lower margin of the tumor (Fig. 2-39).

BIBLIOGRAPHY
Wood LG, Howe GE: Primary tumors of the ureter: Case reports. J Urol 79:418–430, 1958

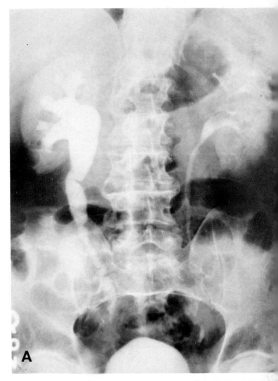

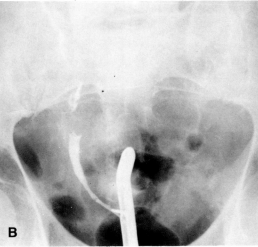

FIG. 2-39. (A) Excretory urogram shows right pyelocaliectasis and proximal ureterectasis from distal ureteral obstruction due to transitional cell carcinoma. The lesion is not well defined. **(B)** Retrograde pyelogram clearly shows the characteristic cupped appearance of the obstructing neoplasm. (Ney C, Friedenberg RM: Radiographic Atlas of the Genitourinary System. Philadelphia, JB Lippincott, 1981)

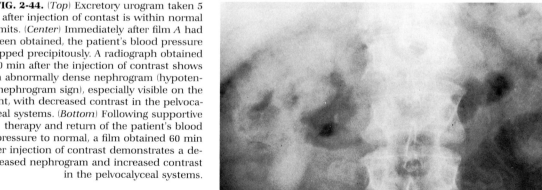

FIG. 2-43. Prolonged and intensified "obstructive" nephrogram of the right kidney in a patient with urinary tract obstruction. Although the left pelvocalyceal system is dilated, the obstruction has been relieved, so that there is no persistent nephrogram on that side.

Hypotensive Nephrogram Sign

During a normal excretory urogram, the nephrogram phase is most intense during the first minute after intravenous injection of contrast and diminishes markedly over the next 10 min. A prolonged and intensified nephrogram involving one kidney is a characteristic finding in patients with urinary tract obstruction (Fig. 2-43). The appearance of prolonged bilateral nephrograms (Fig. 2-44), however, suggests arterial hypotension and indicates the need for immediate blood pressure determination.

BIBLIOGRAPHY
Korobkin MT, Kirkwood R, Minagi H: The nephrogram of hypotension. Radiology 98:129–133, 1971

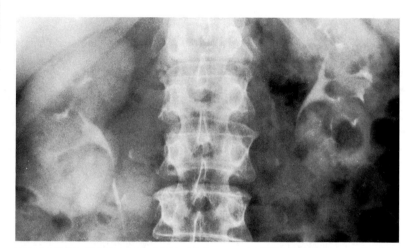

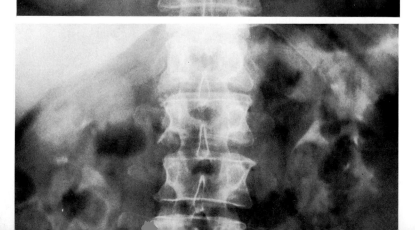

FIG. 2-44. (*Top*) Excretory urogram taken 5 min after injection of contast is within normal limits. (*Center*) Immediately after film *A* had been obtained, the patient's blood pressure dropped precipitously. A radiograph obtained 20 min after the injection of contrast shows an abnormally dense nephrogram (hypotensive nephrogram sign), especially visible on the right, with decreased contrast in the pelvocalyceal systems. (*Bottom*) Following supportive therapy and return of the patient's blood pressure to normal, a film obtained 60 min after injection of contrast demonstrates a decreased nephrogram and increased contrast in the pelvocalyceal systems.

Hysterogram Sign

Persistent uterine opacification can be observed during excretory urography in women with normal renal function and metabolic status (Fig. 2-45). Demonstration of this hysterogram sign suggests the presence of an underlying uterine leiomyoma (Fig. 2-46), though a similar appearance, possibly related to physiologic premenstrual uterine hyperemia, has also been noted in apparently normal uteri.

BIBLIOGRAPHY
Birnholz JC: Uterine opacification during excretory urography: Definition of a previously unreported sign. Radiology 105:303–307, 1972

FIG. 2-45. (*Left*) Preliminary and (*center and right*) postinfusion films from an excretory urogram demonstrate the development of persistent opacificaton (**arrows**) in a pelvic mass above the bladder. The mass was found at surgery to be a large uterine leiomyoma. (Birnholz JC: Uterine opacification during excretory urography: Definition of a previously unreported sign. Radiology 105:303–307, 1972)

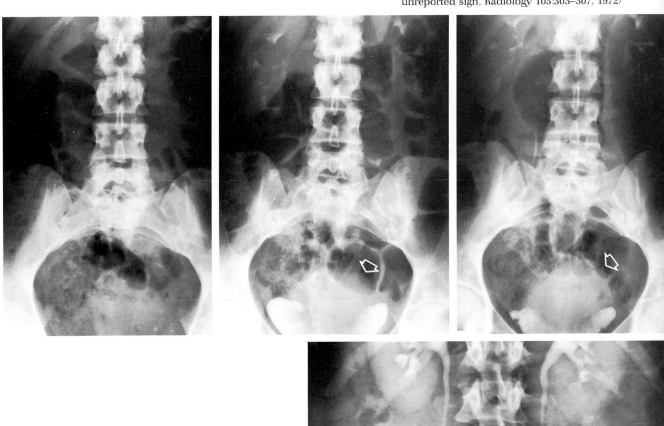

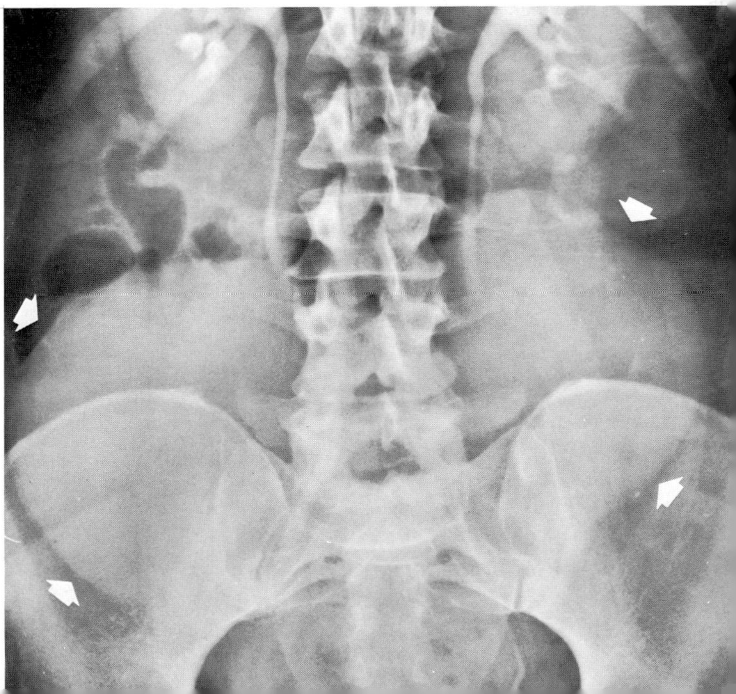

FIG. 2-46. Excretory urogram demonstrates persistent dense opacification of a huge uterine leiomyoma (**arrows**).

Lateral Displaced Ureter Sign

Diagnosis of ureteral duplication is often easy but may be extremely difficult if the ureter to the upper renal segment has an extravesical orifice or if there is distal obstruction causing dilatation of the ureter and failure of the affected renal segment to excrete intravenously injected contrast. If the ureter to an upper renal segment is dilated as a result of a distal obstruction, it is usually displaced laterally. The ipsilateral ureter to the lower segment, which in its distal portion near the bladder shares a common sheath and is closely adherent to the ureter of the upper segment, is ordinarily displaced with it. The ureter to the lower segment may be dilated if it is obstructed by pressure from the nonvisualized dilated ureter to the upper segment. Thus, complete ureteral duplication should be suspected in cases of lateral displacement and dilatation of an apparently single ureter even if no other sign of duplication is visible on the excretory urogram (Fig. 2-50). Lateral displacement of the ureter can also occur in other conditions, including malignant neoplasm. However, ureteral duplication is usually diagnosed during childhood or young adulthood, an age at which cancer causing ureteral displacement is uncommon.

BIBLIOGRAPHY

Amar AD: Lateral ureteral displacement: Sign of nonvisualized duplication. J Urol 105:638–641, 1971

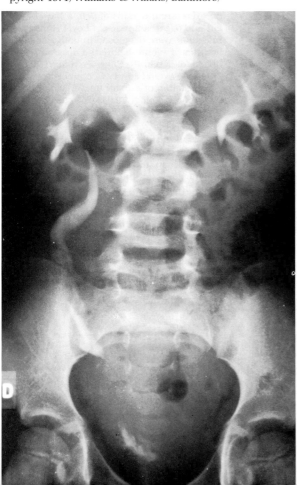
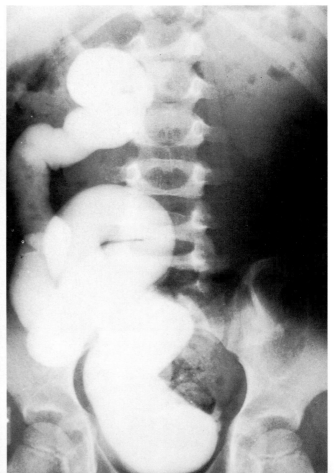

FIG. 2-50. *(Left)* Excretory urogram demonstrates dilatation and lateral displacement of the right ureter. Ureteral duplication was not suspected in this patient. *(Right)* Delayed film following a voiding cystogram demonstrates contrast filling a markedly dilated and tortuous ureter to the upper segment. This ureter, which was not seen on the excretory urogram, has caused lateral displacement of the ureter to the lower segment. (Amar AD: Lateral ureteral displacement: Sign of nonvisualized duplication. J Urol 105:638–641, 1971. Copyright 1971, Williams & Wilkins, Baltimore)

Mickey Mouse Sign

Bilateral hydronephrosis in children, the result of obstruction involving both sides of the urinary tract, may be manifested on excretory urography as the Mickey Mouse sign (Fig. 2-51).

BIBLIOGRAPHY
Rabinowitz JG: Pediatric Radiology. Philadelphia, JB Lippincott, 1978

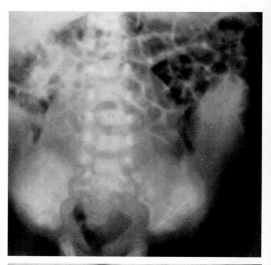

FIG. 2-51. *(Top)* Plain abdominal radiograph reveals soft-tissue masses presenting a Mickey Mouse appearance in a child with bilateral hydronephrosis and posterior urethral valves. The central oval mass represents the dilated bladder; the two lateral "ears" represent the distended and tortuous ureters. *(Bottom)* Retrograde examination demonstrates massive dilatation of the ureters, which occupy almost the entire lateral abdominal flanks. The bladder is now decompressed. (Rabinowitz JG: Pediatric Radiology. Philadelphia, JB Lippincott, 1978)

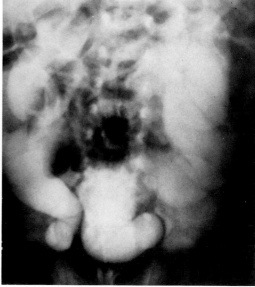

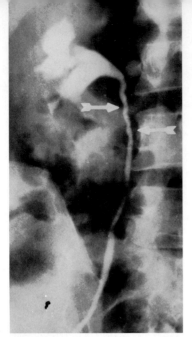

Notched Ureter Sign

The notched ureter sign is the radiographic appearance of numerous sharply defined, scalloped contour deformities of the opacified ureter (Fig. 2-52). This sign is most frequently caused by extrinsic pressure from enlarged and tortuous collateral ureteral arteries, which develop in response to chronic renal artery stenosis. A similar pattern may be due to dilated collateral venous channels resulting from obstruction of the renal vein, splenic vein, or inferior vena cava, varices of the ureteral veins (Fig. 2-53), or compression by enlarged periureteric lymph nodes.

BIBLIOGRAPHY

Beckmann CF, Abrams HL: Idiopathic renal vein varices: Incidence and significance. Radiology 143:649–652, 1982

Halpern M, Evans JA: Coarctation of the renal artery with "notching" of the ureter: A roentgenologic sign of unilateral renal disease as a cause of hypertension. AJR 88:159–164, 1962

Woodward JR: Vascular imprints on the upper ureter. J Urol 87:666–668, 1962

FIG. 2-53. *(Left)* Excretory urogram in elderly woman who presented with left flank pain without hematuria demonstrates notching of the left proximal ureter (**arrows**). *(Right)* Left renal venogram shows massive periureteral varices that extend up to the renal pelvis. (Beckmann CF, Abrams HL: Idiopathic renal vein varices: Incidence and significance. Radiology 143:649–652, 1982)

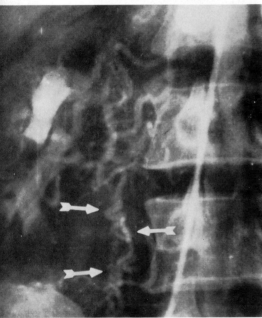

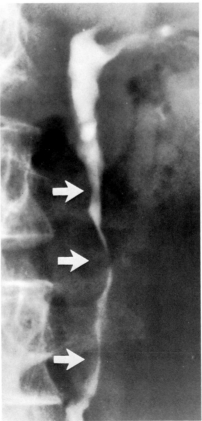

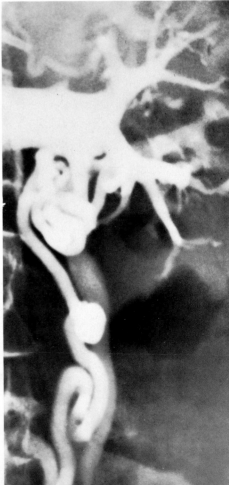

FIG. 2-52. *(Top)* Right retrograde pyelogram demonstrates notching of the proximal ureter (**arrows**). *(Bottom)* Aortogram shows that the ureteral defects were caused by extrinsic pressure from enlarged collateral arteries (**arrows**) surrounding the ureter in this patient with chronic renal artery stenosis. (Witten DM, Myers GH, Utz DC: Emmett's Clinical Urography. Philadelphia, WB Saunders, 1977)

Nubbin Sign

In patients with complete renal duplication, a deficiency of parenchyma may occur in either pole as a result of atrophy secondary to reflux, infection, or obstruction acting singly or in combination, or as a result of congenital hypoplasia. At times, diminution of parenchyma in the lower pole may be so severe that only a small nubbin of tissue remains attached to the inferior border of the healthy upper pole (Fig. 2-54). In such cases, it is essential to search for a faintly visible diminutive collecting system within the nubbin or a paucity of calyces in the upper portion of the kidney (Fig. 2-55) in order to differentiate a lower pole nubbin from a mass protruding from the caudal surface of a small, nonduplicated kidney.

BIBLIOGRAPHY

Curtis JA, Pollack HM: Renal duplication with a diminutive lower pole: The nubbin sign. Radiology 131:327–331, 1979

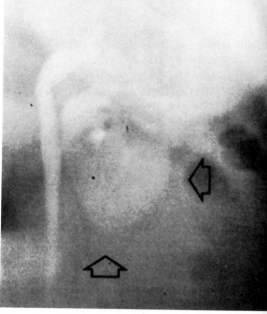

FIG. 2-54. Nephrotomography in a 21-year-old man with unexplained fever demonstrates a marked parenchymal deficiency in the lower half of a duplex left kidney (**arrows**). (Curtis JA, Pollack HM: Renal duplication with a diminutive lower pole The nubbin sign. Radiology 131:327–331, 1979)

FIG. 2-55. (*Left*) Excretory urogram of a 20-year-old woman with a pelvic mass shows a small nubbin of soft tissue arising from the lower pole of the left kidney (**arrows**) and simulating a renal mass. (*Right*) Tomogram obtained after a second injection of contrast material reveals a tiny, faintly opacified collecting system within the nubbin (**arrow**). This finding suggests that the nubbin represents an independent auxiliary renal unit. (Curtis JA, Pollack HM: Renal duplication with a diminutive lower pole: The nubbin sign. Radiology 131:327–331, 1979)

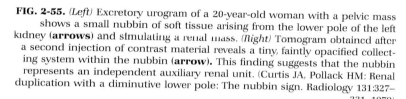

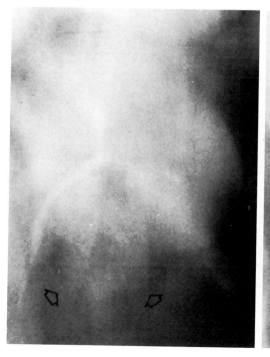

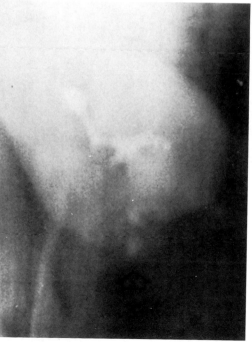

Page Kidney

In his original study, Page reported the production of hypertension in dogs, cats, and rabbits by the wrapping of one or both kidneys in cellophane. The resulting thick, dense perirenal scar did not compromise the main renal vessels but instead altered the intrarenal hemodynamics to produce ischemia and hypertension. Most cases of hypertension due to Page kidney in humans have followed healing of subcapsular or perirenal hematomas in which dense fibrous encasement of the kidney has caused compression of renal parenchyma. Excretory urography demonstrates a functioning, often enlarged kidney with a mass effect and distortion of the collecting system (Fig. 2-56). Arteriography reveals splaying and stretching of the intrarenal arteries (Fig. 2-57) and often irregular staining in the healing portion of the hematoma. Removal of the kidney or evacuation of the offending mass may cause clearing of the hypertension.

BIBLIOGRAPHY

Marshall WH, Castellino RA: Hypertension produced by constricting capsular renal lesions ("Page" kidney). Radiology 101:561–565, 1971

Page IH: A method for producing persistent hypertension by cellophane. Science 89:273–274, 1939

Page IH: The production of persistent arterial hypertension by cellophane and perinephritis. JAMA 113:2046–2048, 1939

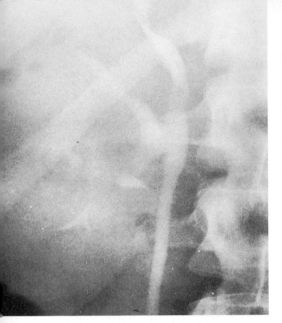

FIG. 2-56. Excretory urogram demonstrates a large intrarenal mass causing splaying and distortion of the collecting system. (Marshall WH, Castellino RA: Hypertension produced by constricting capsular renal lesions ("Page" kidney). Radiology 101:561–565, 1971)

FIG. 2-57. *(Left)* Selective right renal arteriogram demonstrates arterial stretching and medial displacement caused by a large lateral avascular intrarenal mass. *(Right)* The compressed renal parenchyma has an irregular cortical margin. (Marshall WH, Castellino RA: Hypertension produced by constricting capsular renal lesions ("Page" kidney). Radiology 101:561–565, 1971)

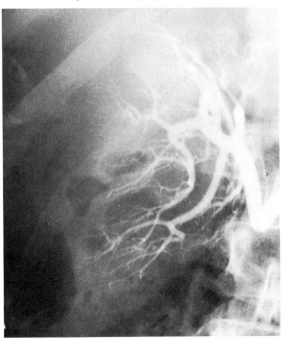
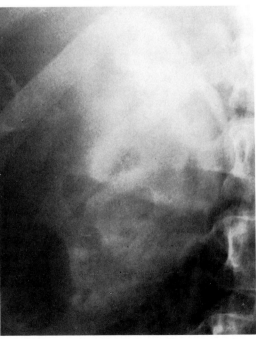

Papillary Ring Sign

Renal medullary necrosis (or papillary necrosis) is a disease characterized by ischemic coagulative necrosis involving a varying amount of the medullary papillae and pyramids. It is most often seen in patients with diabetes, pyelonephritis, urinary tract infection and obstruction, sickle cell disease, or phenacetin abuse. Ischemia leads to a zone of necrosis in the tip of the papilla or in most of the pyramid. When a cleavage plane develops in a zone of ischemia, it usually communicates with the calyx. Different degrees of severity of this process are described by the terms *medullary* (less severe) and *papillary* (more severe). In the medullary type, extravasation may extend from the mid-calyx to the cleavage plane in the papilla, which has an intact fornix. In the papillary type, the cleavage plane is deeper in the pyramid, and the communication usually extends to the fornix. In both cases, a variable amount of papilla becomes a sequestered fragment separated from the pyramid, producing a lucent island surrounded by contrast (Fig. 2-58).

BIBLIOGRAPHY

Ney C, Friedenberg RM: Radiographic Atlas of the Genitourinary System. Philadelphia, JB Lippincott, 1981

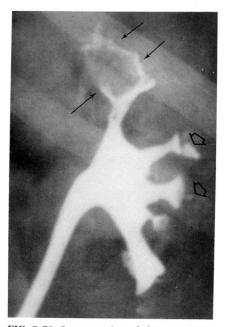

FIG. 2-58. Sequestration of almost a complete papilla with encirclement by contrast produces the papillary ring sign (**long arrows**) in a patient with renal medullary necrosis. The **short arrows** point to a less severe manifestitation of the disease, with contrast extending from the calyces into the papilla. (Ney C, Friedenberg RM: Radiographic Atlas of the Genitourinary System. Philadelphia, JB Lippincott, 1981)

Pear-Shaped (Teardrop) Bladder

The terms *pear-shaped bladder* and *teardrop bladder* were originally used in patients with pelvic hematoma due primarily to trauma (Fig. 2-59). Blood collecting within the pelvis compresses the bladder bilaterally and symmetrically and lifts it up from the pelvic floor, resulting in a pear-shaped configuration. A similar appearance can also be seen with a variety of other conditions, including pelvic lipomatosis (Fig. 2-60), inferior vena cava occlusion, lymphocysts, and enlarged pelvic lymph nodes, as well as in normal persons with iliopsoas muscle hypertrophy and a narrow pelvis (Fig. 2-61).

BIBLIOGRAPHY

Ambos MA, Bosniak MA, Lefleur RS et al: The pear-shaped bladder. Radiology 122:85–88, 1977

Prather GC, Kaiser TF: The bladder in fracture of the bony pelvis. The significance of a "tear-drop bladder" as shown by cystogram. J Urol 63:1019–1030, 1950

Wechsler RJ, Brennan RE: Teardrop bladder: Additional considerations. Radiology 144:281–284, 1982

FIG. 2-59. Pear-shaped bladder in a patient with a large pelvic hematoma resulting from trauma. Note the distraction of the symphysis pubis and the fracture of the right acetabulum (**arrow**).

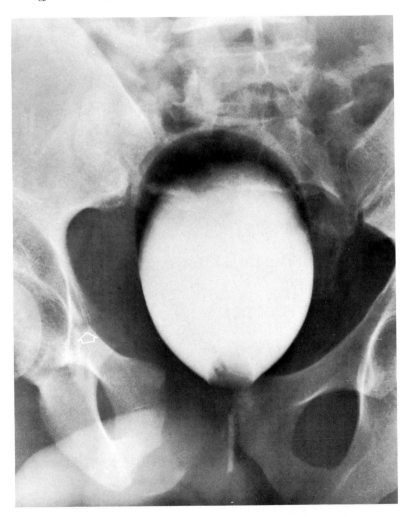

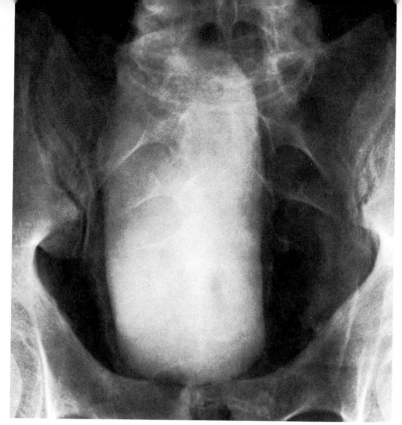

FIG. 2-60. Pear-shaped bladder in a patient with pelvic lipomatosis.

FIG. 2-61. (*Right*) Excretory urogram demonstrates a typical pear-shaped bladder. (*Left*) Computed tomography demonstrates that hypertrophy of the iliopsoas muscle is responsible for the teardrop configuration of the bladder. Note the indentation on the bladder by external iliac vessels as they are displaced medially by the enlarged muscles. (Wechsler RJ, Brennan RE: Teardrop bladder: Additional considerations. Radiology 144:281–284, 1982)

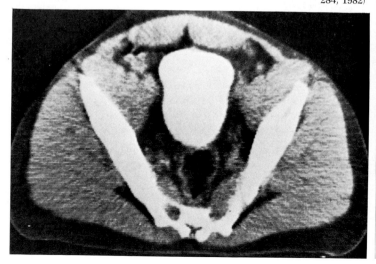

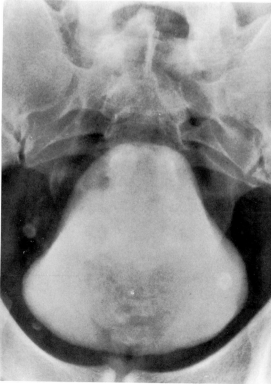

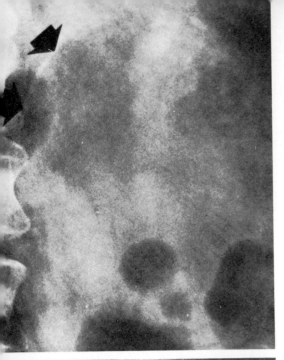

Pelvocalyceal Wall Opacification Sign

A curvilinear density representing opacification of the pelvocalyceal wall during the early stage of an excretory urogram was originally reported as a pathognomonic sign of acute infection in an obstructed urinary tract system (Fig. 2-62). This appearance was attributed to hyperemia of the inflamed wall and equilibration of contrast material between the blood and the interstitial space of the pelvocalyceal wall. However, a pelvocalyceal wall blush was subsequently described in patients with noninfected hydronephrosis (Fig. 2-63), and there has been a report of opacification of the wall of a large pelvic urinoma that mimicked a thickened renal pelvis (Fig. 2-64). Presence of the sign in these cases substantially limits its value as an indication of acute infection.

BIBLIOGRAPHY

Barbaric ZL: Pelvocalyceal wall opacification—A new radiological sign. Radiology 123:587–589, 1977

Older RA, Cleeve DM, McLelland R: The nonspecificity of some radiological signs in excretory urography. Radiology 127:553–554, 1978

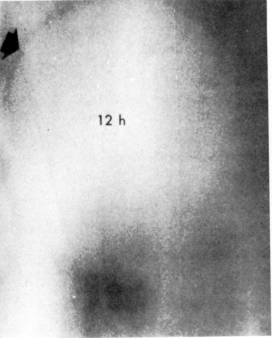

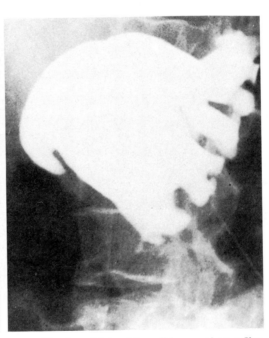

FIG. 2-62. (*Top*) Excretory urogram demonstrates opacification of the pelvic wall (**arrows**) on a film obtained 15 min after the injection of contrast. There is a faint nephrogram present in the laterally displaced kidney. (*Bottom, left*) Twelve hours later, the dilated extrarenal pelvis (**arrow**) is filled with contrast. (*Bottom, right*) Antegrade pyelogram through a temporary nephrostomy shows obstruction at the ureteropelvic junction. (Barbaric ZL: Pelvocalyceal wall opacification—A new radiological sign. Radiology 123:587–589, 1977)

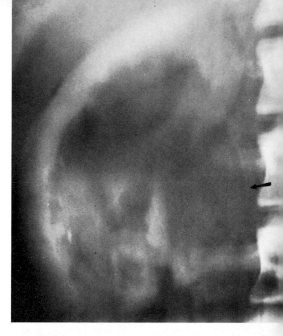

FIG. 2-63. Vascular nephrotomogram obtained immediately after a bolus injection of intravenous contrast demonstrates massive dilatation of the renal pelvis, which is seen as a lucent area within the vascularized kidney. The pelvocalyceal wall (**arrow**) is well visualized. The patient had severe ureteropelvic junction obstruction and hydronephrosis with no evidence of infection clinically, on urinalysis, or at surgery. (Older RA, Cleeve DM, McLelland R: The nonspecificity of some radiological signs in excretory urography. Radiology 127:553–554, 1978)

FIG. 2-64. (*Left*) Vascular nephrotomogram demonstrates the thickened wall of a peripelvic urinoma (**large arrow**) mimicking a thickened renal pelvis. Gerota's fascia can also be seen laterally (**small arrow**). (*Right*) Direct puncture of the peripelvic urinoma shows that it is separate from the dilated renal pelvis (**arrows**). (Older RA, Cleeve DM, McClelland R: The nonspecificity of some radiological signs in excretory urography. Radiology 127:553–554, 1978)

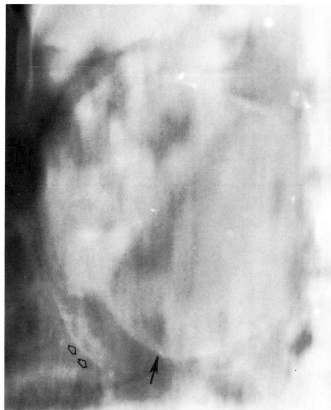

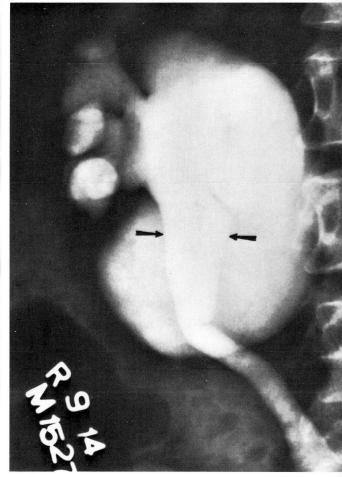

Peripheral Fat Sign

A parapelvic renal cyst appears on excretory or retrograde urography as a parahilar mass that compresses and distorts the pelvis, infundibula, and calyces without invasion. Because of its location in the renal sinus rather than in the renal parenchyma, the usual sharp interface between the contrast-laden parenchyma and the lucent cyst may be absent or incomplete on nephrotomography. As the cyst expands in the renal sinus, it displaces and compresses the normal sinus fat, producing a radiolucent halo that surrounds the parapelvic renal cyst (Fig. 2-65).

BIBLIOGRAPHY

Crummy AB, Madsen PO: Parapelvic renal cyst: The peripheral fat sign. J Urol 96:436–438, 1966

FIG. 2-65. (*Top*) Excretory urogram demonstrates distortion of the superior portion of the left collecting system and pelvis by an extrinsic mass that shows no evidence of invasion or obstruction. (*Bottom*) Nephrotomogram shows that the collecting system is well filled and the cortex normal. The radiolucent halo surrounding the cyst (**arrows**) represents compressed sinus fat. (Crummy AB, Madsen PO: Parapelvic renal cyst: The peripheral fat sign. J Urol 96:436–438, 1966. Copyright 1966, Williams & Wilkins, Baltimore)

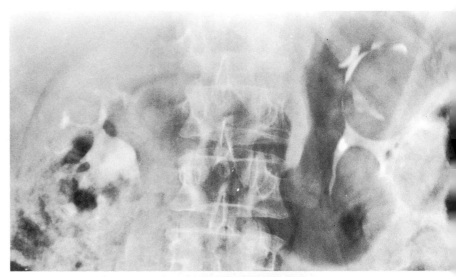

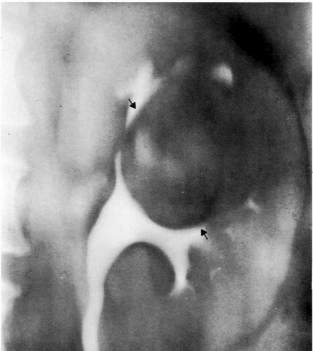

Perirenal P and Subcapsular C Signs

Urinary ascites is an often fatal condition caused by urine filling the abdomen after extravasating through tears in a hydronephrotic collecting system. The radiographic appearance on excretory urography depends on the site of the extrarenal collection of contrast. Extravasation confined to the subcapsular space causes medial and inferior displacement of the kidney with a smooth C-shaped collection of contrast about it (Fig. 2-66). Extracapsular urinary extravasation takes the shape of the letter P (Fig. 2-67). The rounded upper part of the P is roughly formed by urine trapped around the kidney and lying beneath Gerota's fascia (Fig. 2-68). A lucency in the center of the urine pool is produced by the kidney itself; the dilated ureter adds a tortuous leg to the P.

BIBLIOGRAPHY

Barry JM, Anderson JM, Hodges CV: The subcapsular C sign: A rare radiographic finding associated with neonatal urinary ascites. J Urol 112:836–839, 1974

Dockray KT: The perirenal P sign: A new roentgenogram index to the cause and treatment of urinary ascites in babies. Am J Dis Child 119:179–181, 1970

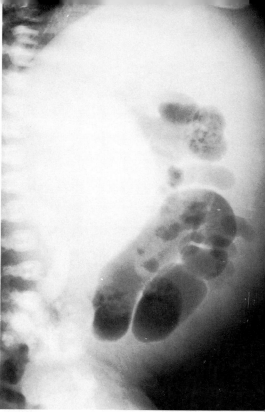

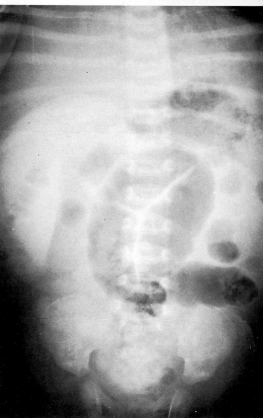

FIG. 2-66. (*Top*) Lateral view from an excretory urogram demonstrates gas-filled loops of bowel floating in ascitic fluid. A smooth, curved collection of contrast material is anterior to the renal outline, forming a reverse C. Dilated calyces and ureter are within the renal parenchymal shadow between the vertebral column and subcapsular C sign. (*Bottom*) Anteroposterior view demonstrates subcapsular contrast material pushing the faintly visible kidney and collecting system medially. (Barry JM, Anderson JM, Hodges CV: The subcapsular C sign: A rare radiographic finding associated with neonatal urinary ascites. J Urol 112:836–839, 1974)

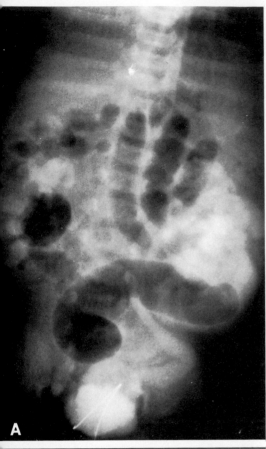

A

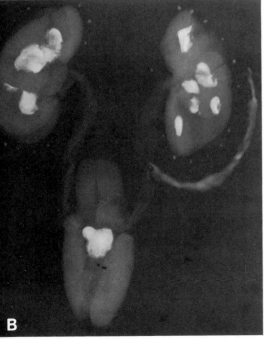

B

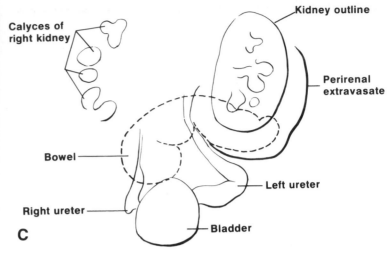

C

FIG. 2-67. (A) Film from an excretory urogram and (B) corresponding line drawing demonstrating the P sign of urine around the left kidney and in the dilated left ureter. (C) Radiograph of autopsy specimen with barium in the calyces of normal-sized kidneys. The opaque arc below and lateral to the left kidney specimen was drawn to parallel the shape of perirenal extravasation as it appeared on the excretory urogram. (Dockray KT: The perirenal P sign: A new roentgenogram index to the cause and treatment of urinary ascites in babies. Am J Dis Child 119:179–181, 1970. Copyright 1970, American Medical Association)

FIG. 2-68. Line drawing demonstrating the subcapsular C sign, formed by contrast under the capsule (right kidney), and the perirenal P sign, produced by extravasated contrast outside the renal capsule and down the ureter inside Gerota's fascia (left kidney). (Barry JM, Anderson JM, Hodges CV: The subcapsular C sign: A rare radiographic finding associated with neonatal urinary ascites. J Urol 112:836–839, 1974. Copyright 1974, Williams & Wilkins, Baltimore)

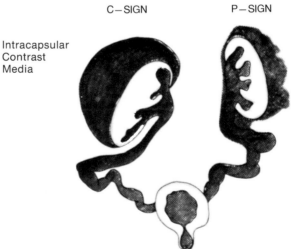

Pine Tree (Christmas Tree) Bladder

A markedly trabeculated bladder with a pointed dome (pine tree or Christmas tree bladder; Fig. 2-69) is usually considered pathognomonic of a spastic neurogenic bladder. However, an identical appearance may also be seen in patients who have no neurologic disease but only simple bladder outlet obstruction, often with superimposed urinary tract infection.

BIBLIOGRAPHY
Elkin M: Radiology of the Urinary System. Boston, Little, Brown & Co, 1980

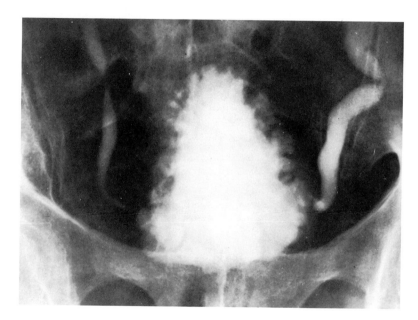

FIG. 2-69. Markedly trabeculated bladder with a pointed dome is seen in a patient with outlet obstruction but no evidence of a neurogenic bladder. (Elkin M: Radiology of the Urinary System. Boston, Little, Brown & Co, 1980)

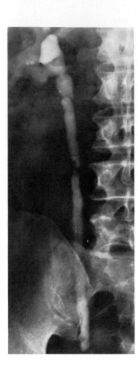

Pipestem Ureter Sign

In advanced cases of tuberculosis of the urinary tract, the wall of the ureter may become thickened and fixed with no peristalsis. This results in a "pipestem" ureter, which runs a course almost as straight as a pencil toward the bladder (Fig. 2-70).

BIBLIOGRAPHY
Witten DM, Myers GH, Utz DC: Emmett's Clinical Urography. Philadelphia, WB Saunders, 1977

FIG. 2-70. Retrograde pyelogram in a patient with advanced tuberculosis demonstrates marked destruction of the kidney and a "pipestem" ureter. (Witten DM, Myers GH, Utz DC: Emmett's Clinical Urography. Philadelphia, WB Saunders, 1977)

FIG. 2-71. The renal (**A**) and calyceal (**B**) axes are parallel to each other and the psoas margin in this normal patient. (Lopez FA, Dalinka M: Renal calyceal axis sign. J Urol 106:639–641, 1971)

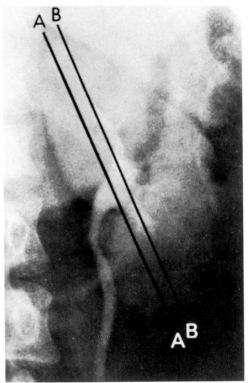

Renal Calyceal Axis Sign

Disproportionate displacement of the calyceal and renal axes on excretory urography has been reported as an aid in the differential diagnosis between intrarenal and extrarenal masses. The calyceal axis is defined as a hypothetical line connecting the most superior and most inferior calyces. Normally, the axis is parallel to the longitudinal axis of the kidney (renal axis) and the psoas margin (Fig. 2-71). An intrarenal mass, such as a cyst, tumor, or hydronephrotic sac of a duplicated collecting system, displaces and distorts the calyceal axis more than the renal axis (Fig. 2-72). In contrast, an extrarenal mass displaces the renal and calyceal axes proportionally (Fig. 2-73).

BIBLIOGRAPHY
Lopez FA, Dalinka M: Renal calyceal axis sign. J Urol 106:639–641, 1971

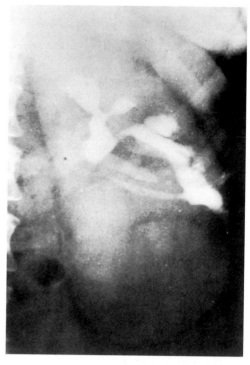

FIG. 2-72. Excretory urogram shows a large mass displacing the lower calyces laterally. Although the calyceal axis is distorted, the renal axis is normal, suggesting an intrarenal lesion. The lesion proved to be a renal cyst. (Lopez FA, Dalinka M: Renal calyceal axis sign. J Urol 106:639–641, 1971)

FIG. 2-73. Excretory urogram shows inferior and lateral displacement of the kidney by a mass. The renal and calyceal axes are displaced proportionately, indicating an extrarenal lesion. The lesion proved to be a retroperitoneal sarcoma. (Lopez FA, Dalinka M: Renal calyceal axis sign. J Urol 106:639–641, 1971)

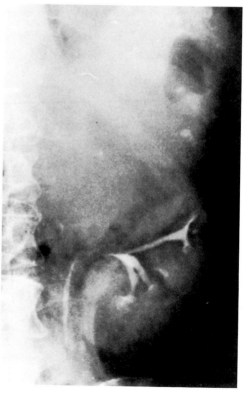

Renal Halo (Perirenal Fat) Sign

Differential absorption between perirenal fat and adjacent inflammatory effusions or diffuse neoplasia in the fatty retroperitoneal space may result in the often striking plain radiographic demonstration of a distinct lucent halo about the left kidney. A renal halo sign on the right has been described in association with such conditions as bacterial inflammation (Figs. 2-74 and 2-75), traumatic hematoma, and disseminated lymphoma and carcinoma in the anterior pararenal space engulfing the perirenal fascia. Although the same pathologic processes may also occur on the left, demonstration of the renal halo sign about the left kidney in a patient with a compatible clinical presentation is strongly suggestive of pancreatitis complicated by an extra-pancreatic fluid collection in the left anterior pararenal space (Fig. 2-76).

BIBLIOGRAPHY

Fritzsche P, Toomey FB, Ta HN: Alteration of perirenal fat secondary to diffuse retroperitoneal infiltration. Radiology 131:27–29, 1979

Susman N, Hammerman AM, Cohen E: The renal halo sign in pancreatitis. Radiology 142:323–327, 1982

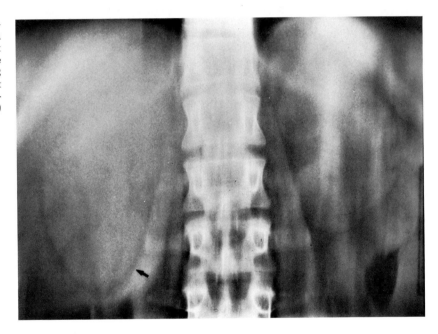

FIG. 2-74. Before the administration of contrast in a patient with acute pyelonephritis, a nephrotomogram demonstrates a thin lucent strip of fat (**arrow**) between the renal capsule and surrounding perirenal fluid. (Fritzsche P, Toomey FB, Ta HN: Alteration of perirenal fat secondary to diffuse retroperitoneal infiltration. Radiology 131:27–29, 1979)

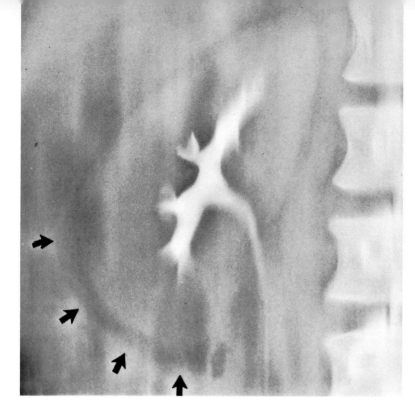

FIG. 2-75. Oblique view from the excretory urogram in a patient with a perirenal abscess shows a lucent band of fat (**arrows**) between the renal capsule and fluid density of the perirenal abscess. (Fritzsche P, Toomey FB, Ta HN: Alteration of perirenal fat secondary to difuse retroperitoneal infiltration. Radiology 131:27–29, 1979)

FIG. 2-76. *(Left)* Plain radiograph and *(right)* corresponding radiograph from an excretory urogram demonstrate a striking lucent perirenal halo on the left in a patient with pancreatitis and pseudocyst formation in the left anterior perirenal space. (Susman N, Hammerman AM, Cohen E: The renal halo sign in pancreatitis. Radiology 142:323–327, 1982)

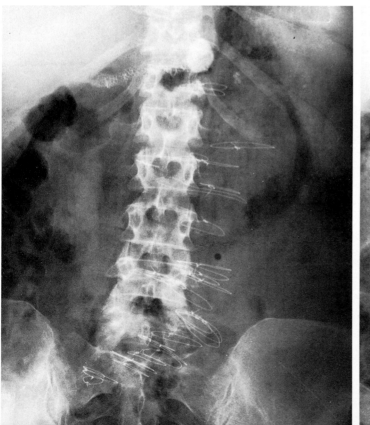 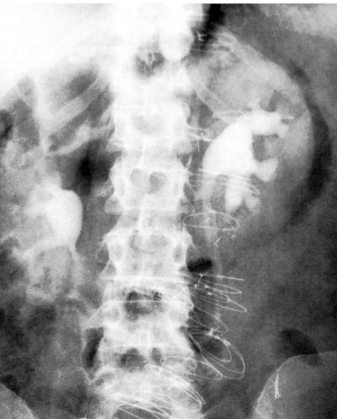

Reversed Appearance Sign

Following surgical relief of significant unilateral main renal artery stenosis, excretory urograms usually show the simultaneous appearance of contrast material in the minor calyces of both kidneys. The reversed appearance sign, in which the contrast appears first in the minor calyces of the operated kidney, where preoperatively it was delayed, suggests significant arterial disease on the unrepaired side (Fig. 2-77).

BIBLIOGRAPHY

Harell GS, Friedland GW, Palmer JM: The reversed appearance sign: An early indication of significant contralateral renal disease following repair of main renal artery stenosis? Radiology 101:305–310, 1971

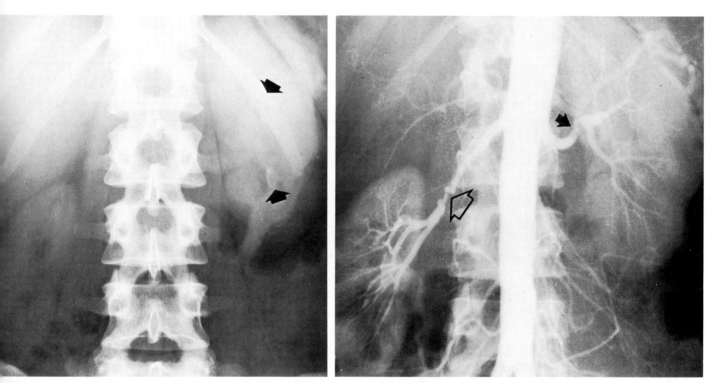

FIG. 2-77. (*Left*) In a preoperative rapid sequence excretory urogram in a patient with hypertension, contrast appears first in the minor calyces of the left kidney (**arrows**) at 3 min. (*Center*) Preoperative abdominal aortogram shows fibromuscular hyperplasia with marked stenosis of the right main renal artery (**open arrow**). There is also stenosis of the left main renal artery (**closed arrow**). (*Right*) Rapid sequence urogram performed on the seventh postoperative day demonstrates contrast in the right pelvocalyceal system at 3 min. No contrast is seen in the minor calyces of the unoperated side. The pre- and postoperative urograms demonstrate the reversed order of the appearance of contrast in patients with significant arterial disease on the unrepaired side. (Harell GS, Friedland GW, Palmer JM: The reversed appearance sign: An early indication of significant contralateral renal disease following repair of main renal artery stenosis? Radiology 101:305–310, 1971)

Rim Sign (Obstructive Uropathy)

In patients with chronic obstructive uropathy, a nephrogram of remaining renal parenchyma can often be seen rimming the dilated lucent calyces (Fig. 2-78). The rim sign is especially well demonstrated during arteriography, and its occurrence, unlike that of the crescent sign, does not require the kidney to have any excretory function.

BIBLIOGRAPHY
Elkin M: Radiology of the Urinary System. Boston, Little, Brown & Co, 1980

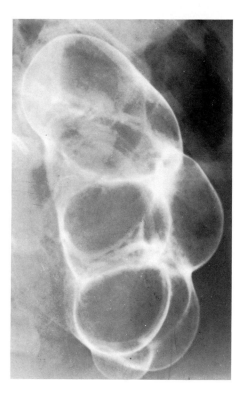

FIG. 2-78. Selective arteriography in a patient with ureteropelvic junction obstruction demonstrates a nephrogram of remaining renal parenchyma rimming the dilated calyces. Urography in this patient showed no excretion of contrast medium from the involved kidney. (Elkin M: Radiology of the Urinary System. Boston, Little, Brown & Co, 1980)

FIG. 2-77 *(Right).*

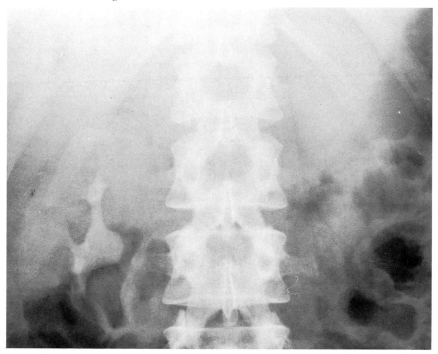

Rim Sign (Adrenal Hemorrhage)

On high-dose excretory urography, neonatal adrenal hemorrhage is occasionally manifested as a dense vascular rim surrounding a lucent avascular suprarenal mass (Fig. 2-79, *top*). This early sign is probably produced by the compression and displacement of adrenal tissue by the central hemorrhage. The vascular rim subsequently calcifies (Fig. 2-79, *bottom*), permitting the condition to be distinguished from a hydronephrotic upper pole renal duplication, which may have a similar urographic appearance.

BIBLIOGRAPHY
Brill PW, Krasna IH, Aaron H: An early rim sign in neonatal adrenal hemorrhage. AJR 127:289–291, 1976

FIG. 2-79. *(Top)* Excretory urogram in a 6-day-old infant demonstrates a lucent mass with dense rim flattening and depressing the right kidney. A study performed 3 days before yielded similar findings. *(Bottom)* Tomographic cut of the right upper quadrant without contrast in the same infant at 23 days of age. Note that the calcific rim is in the identical position as the vascular rim on the previous excretory urogram. (Brill PW, Krasna IH, Aaron H: An early rim sign in neonatal adrenal hemorrhage. AJR 127: 289–291, 1976. Copyright 1976. Reproduced by permission)

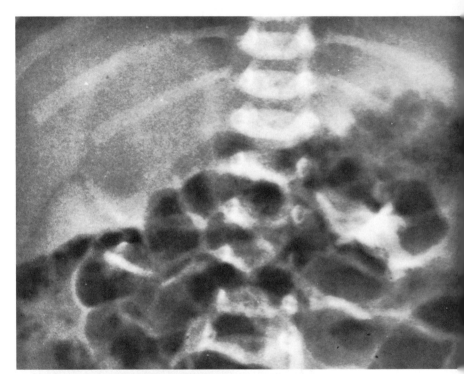

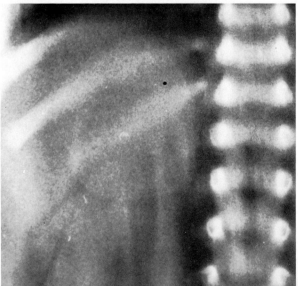

Rim Sign (Pelvic Mass)

A thin curvilinear zone of opacity has been described at the margin of cystic pelvoabdominal masses during infusion urography (Fig. 2-80). This contrast enhancement is reported to be strong evidence for a cystic mass, most likely of ovarian origin (Fig. 2-81), as opposed to the homogeneous contrast enhancement seen with uterine leiomyomata (Fig. 2-82) and the lack of enhancement seen with tubo-ovarian abscesses.

BIBLIOGRAPHY

Phillips JC, Easterly JF, Langston JW: Contrast enhancement of pelvo-abdominal masses: The rim sign. Radiology 112:17–21, 1974

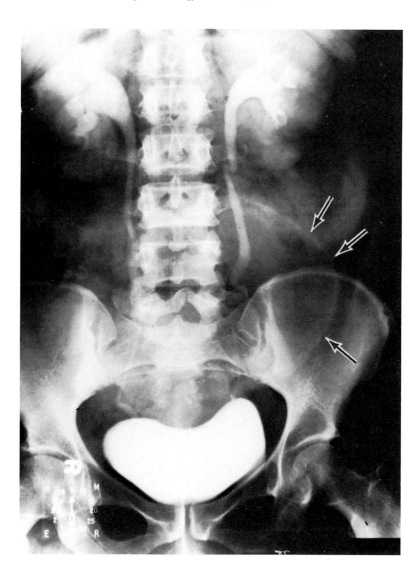

FIG. 2-80. Excretory urogram demonstrates a sharply defined curvilinear zone of opacity in the left lower abdomen (**arrows**) in a patient with cystadenofibroma of the left ovary. (Phillips JC, Easterly JF, Langston JW: Contrast enhancement of pelvo-abdominal masses: The rim sign. Radiology 112:17–21, 1974)

FIGS. 2-81, 82. (continue on overleaf)

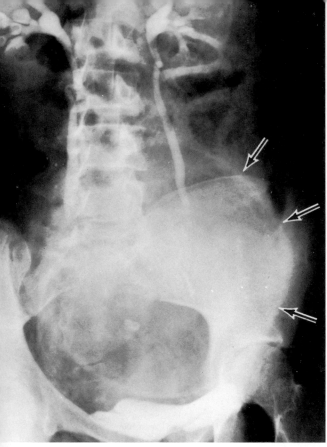

FIG. 2-81. Oblique view from an infusion urogram clearly demonstrates the rim sign (**arrows**) and pelvic calcification in a patient with benign teratoma of the ovary. (Phillips JC, Easterly JF, Langston JW: Contrast enhancement of pelvo-abdominal masses: The rim sign. Radiology 112:17–21, 1974)

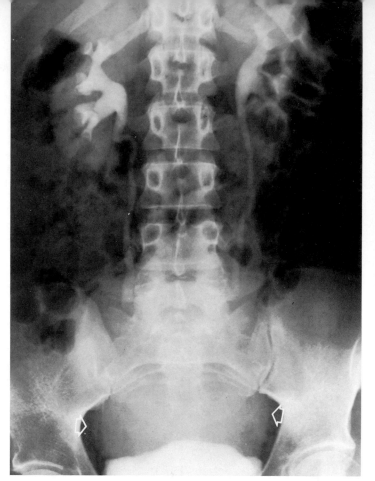

FIG. 2-82. Infusion urography demonstrates diffuse, homogeneous contrast enhancement without a rim sign (**arrows**) in a patient with a uterine leiomyoma. (Phillips JC, Easterly JF, Langston JW: Contrast enhancement of pelvo-abdominal masses: The rim sign. Radiology 112:17–21, 1974)

FIG. 2-83 *(Left)*.

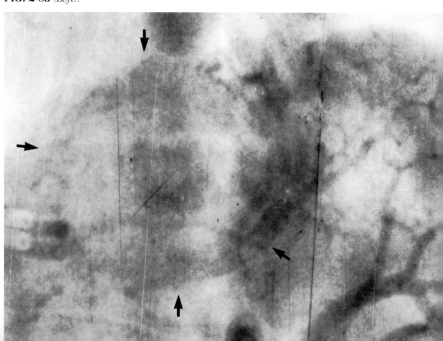

Ring Sign

Pheochromocytomas are usually hypervascular tumors that exhibit a dense stain during arteriography. The cystic nature of the neoplasm or tumor necrosis can result in failure of the mass to opacify or in the presence of a central lucency within an opacified mass. In the latter instance, arteriography demonstrates a central avascular zone surrounded by a dense rim of contrast (Fig. 2-83A). Because this appearance is best seen in the capillary (Fig. 2-83B) and venous (Fig. 2-83C) phases, delayed films are essential.

BIBLIOGRAPHY

Velasquez G, Nath PH, Zollikofer C et al: The "ring sign" of necrotic pheochromocytoma. Radiology 131:69–71, 1979

FIG. 2-83. *(Left)* Oblique view of an abdominal aortogram demonstrates a large avascular pheochromocytoma medial to the upper pole of the left kidney **(arrows).** A fine rim of hypervascular network surrounds the tumor. *(Center)* A frontal projection of the capillary phase in the same patient demonstrates a dense ring of contrast over the upper pole of the left kidney **(arrows).** The rest of the mass is avascular. *(Right)* In the venous phase of the abdominal aortogram, a large tumor **(arrows)** with a dense ring and lucent center is seen lying over the upper pole of the right kidney. (Velasquez G, Nath H, Zollikofer C et al: The "ring sign" of necrotic pheochromocytoma. Radiology 131:69–71, 1979)

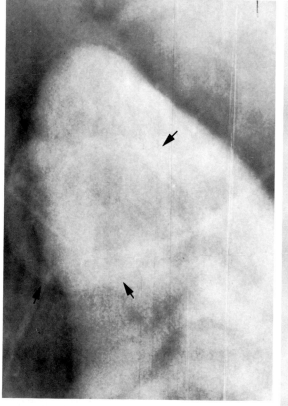
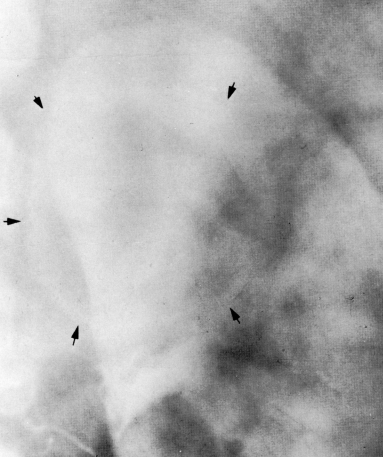

Sinking Pellet Sign

Although numerous metallic pellets may be randomly distributed throughout the pelvis following a shotgun wound, clumping can occur only when the pellets are within the lumen of a hollow viscus such as the bladder (Fig. 2-84). Clumping of pellets that have sunk to the dependent portion of the bladder under the influence of gravity indicates that the bladder has been perforated as a result of penetrating missile injury (Fig. 2-85), even if retrograde cystography fails to show extravasation.

BIBLIOGRAPHY
Conrad MR, Bazan C, Allen T et al: "Sinking pellet" sign of bladder perforation. AJR 132:113–114, 1979

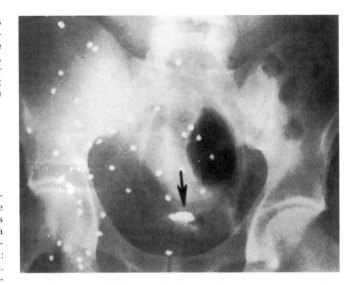

FIG. 2-84. Excretory urogram demonstrates extravasation of contrast material in the pelvis. Note clumping of pellets (**arrow**) in the region of the bladder. (Conrad MR, Bazan C, Allen T et al: "Sinking pellet" sign of bladder perforation. AJR 132:113–114, 1979. Copyright 1979. Reproduced by permission)

FIG. 2-85. (A) Excretory urogram shows scattered metallic pellets in the pelvis. A large clump of pellets is present in the lower pelvis (**arrow**). **(B)** Retrograde cystogram shows a normal bladder without evidence of extravasation. (Conrad MR, Bazan C, Allen T et al: "Sinking pellet" sign of bladder perforation. AJR 132:113–114, 1979. Copyright 1979. Reproduced by permission)

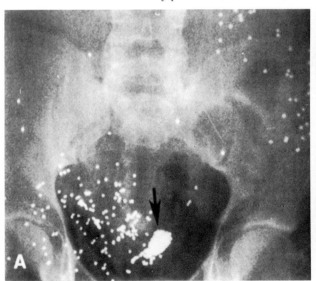

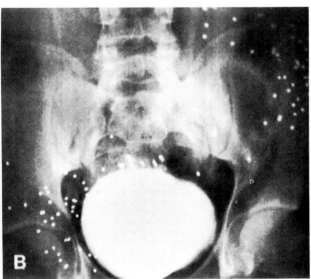

Spaghetti Sign

In patients with hematuria, the presence of filling defects in the bladder on excretory urography suggests that the bleeding arises from the bladder or perivesical structures (*e.g.*, bladder tumor, radiolucent calculi, blood clots, foreign bodies). Worm-like, perfectly tubular filling defects mimicking strands of spaghetti within the opacified bladder represent blood clot casts of the ureter. Their presence implies that the upper urinary tract is the source of the bleeding (Fig. 2-86).

BIBLIOGRAPHY
Komolafe F: The "spaghetti sign": An uncommon radiologic sign of upper urinary tract hemorrhage. AJR 137:1062, 1981

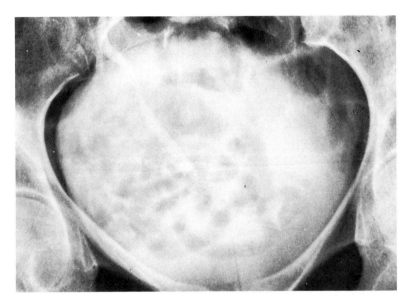

FIG. 2-86. Bladder view from an excretory urogram demonstrates multiple cylindrical filling defects due to blood clots from the left ureter. Contrast material emanates only from the right ureter. (Komolafe F: The "spaghetti sign": An uncommon radiologic sign of upper urinary tract hemorrhage. AJR 137:1062, 1981. Copyright 1981. Reproduced by permission)

Spastic Urinary Tract Sign

In patients with renal artery stenosis, the calyces, pelvis, and ureter are smaller on the affected than on the unaffected side (Fig. 2-87). This "spastic" appearance of the collecting system can be altered by the degree of hydration and therefore is probably a function of the greatly reduced flow of urine in the involved kidney.

BIBLIOGRAPHY
Poutasse EF: Diagnosis and treatment of occlusive renal artery disease and hypertension. JAMA 178:1078–1083, 1961

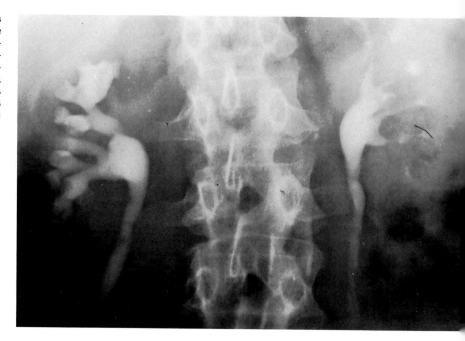

FIG.. 2-87. Excretory urogram demonstrates an ample, well-filled collecting system of the right kidney. A smaller, "spastic" type of collecting system with a small amount of contrast may be seen on the left in the same patient, who had stenosis of the left renal artery. (Witten DM, Myers GH, Utz DC: Emmett's Clinical Urography. Philadelphia, WB Saunders, 1977)

Spiral Sign

In men with spinal cord injury, iatrogenic trauma to the urethra can be caused by an indwelling catheter, intermittent catheterization, cystoscopy, or cystolithoplexy. This can produce a radiographic pattern consisting of two or three rings of contrast medium encircling the membranous urethra at the level of the external sphincter (Fig. 2-88). Because the concentric rings seen radiographically have the appearance of circular muscle fibers of the external sphincter outlined by contrast, the spiral sign probably represents submucosal extravasation of contrast at the level of the external sphincter. Because some small diverticula seen in the same area may retain vague spirals, it is suggested that the spiral sign is a precursor of a diverticulum and results from forceful stretching of the membranous urethra.

BIBLIOGRAPHY

Calenoff L, Foley MJ, Hendrix RW: Evaluation of the urethra in males with spinal cord injury. Radiology 142:71–76, 1982

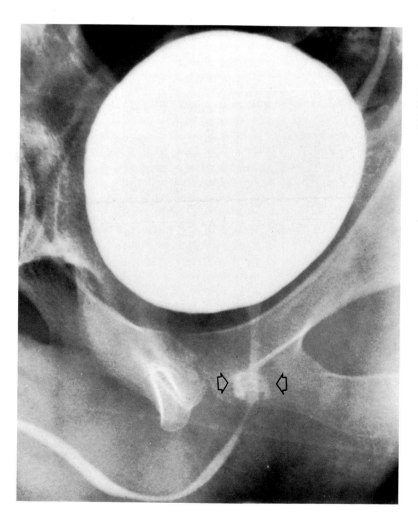

FIG. 2-88. Submucosal undermining of the membranous urethra by contrast material outlining the circular striated muscle fibers of the external sphincter (**arrows**) produces the spiral sign in a quadriplegic with repeated bilateral vesicoureteral reflux. (Calenoff L, Foley MJ, Hendrix RW: Evaluation of the urethra in males with spinal cord injury. Radiology 142:71–76, 1982)

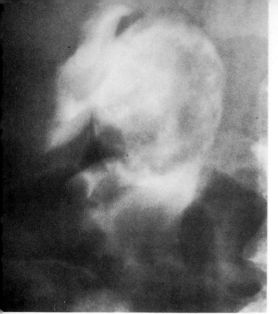

FIG. 2-89. A large oval mass fills the entire renal pelvis. Its smooth margin is suggestive of a radiolucent calculus or clot, but the presence of coarse and fine stipples makes transitional cell carcinoma of the renal pelvis the most likely diagnosis. (McLean GK, Pollack HM, Banner MP: The "stipple sign": Urographic harbinger of transitional cell neoplasms. Urol Radiol 1:77–79, 1979)

FIG. 2-90. A small filling defect occupies an interpolar calyx (**arrows**). Although the defect might at first glance be mistaken for a large but otherwise normal papilla, the numerous small contrast stipples as well as the suggestively irregular border makes its neoplastic nature evident. (McLean GK, Pollack HM, Banner MP: The "stipple sign": Urographic harbinger of transitional cell neoplasms. Urol Radiol 1:77–79, 1979)

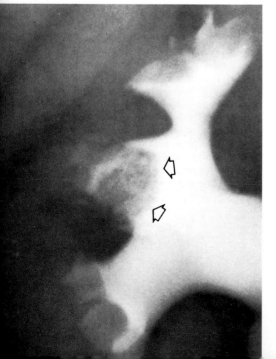

Stipple Sign

The presence on excretory urography of a stippled pattern of contrast within a mass in the urinary tract is highly suggestive of transitional cell carcinoma (Fig. 2-89). This radiographic appearance results from the trapping of small amounts of contrast within the interstices of papillary tumor fronds, which produces a stippled pattern when viewed end on. The stipple sign sometimes aids in identification of the cause of a confusing calyceal or pelvic filling defect (Fig. 2-90). Because urothelial tumors other than transitional cell carcinoma (*i.e.,* squamous cell carcinoma and adenocarcinoma) usually do not grow in papillary fashion, demonstration of the stipple sign is a good indication that the lesion represents a papillary transitional cell tumor (Fig. 2-91).

BIBLIOGRAPHY

McLean GK, Pollack HM, Banner MP: The "stipple sign": Urographic harbinger of transitional cell neoplasms. Urol Radiol 1:77–79, 1979

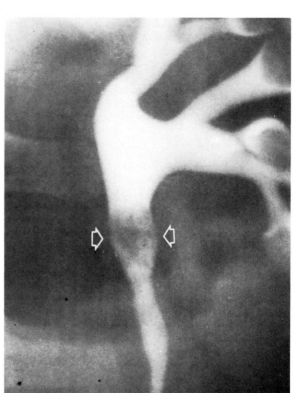

FIG. 2-91. The presence of stippling throughout this proximal ureteral filling defect (**arrows**) and the suggestive papillary contour of its proximal and distal margins allowed the correct diagnosis of transitional cell carcinoma of the ureter to be made preoperatively. (McLean GK, Pollack HM, Banner MP: The "stipple sign": Urographic harbinger of transitional cell neoplasms. Urol Radiol 1:77–79, 1979)

Teat and Udder Sign

Short-stemmed calyces draining small papillae very near the renal pelvis (*i.e.*, deep within the kidney) are often seen in relation to large masses of normal cortical tissue situated within the medullary region (columns of Bertin, or "cloisons"). This appearance has been fancifully described as the *teat and udder sign*, in which the papillae and short-stemmed calyces represent the teats and the large mass of displaced cortical tissue the udder (Fig. 2-92).

BIBLIOGRAPHY
Hodson CJ, Mariani S: Large cloisons. AJR 139:327–332, 1982

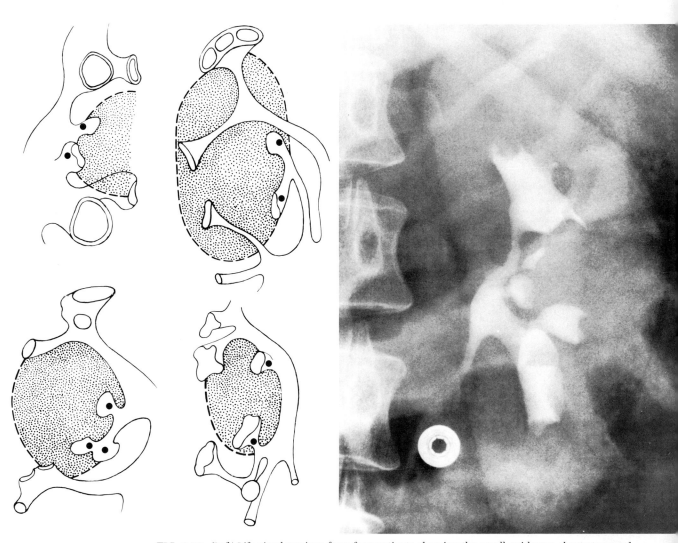

FIG. 2-92. *(Left)* Life-sized tracings from four patients showing the small, midzone, short-stemmed calyces (**black dots**) that make up the teat and udder sign. *(Right)* Film from an excretory urogram demonstrating the teat and udder sign. (Hodson CJ, Mariani S: Large cloisons. AJR 139:327–332, 1982. Copyright 1982. Reproduced by permission)

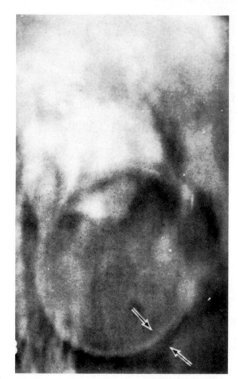

FIG. 2-93. Nephrotomogram demonstrates a lucent, well-demarcated renal mass with a thick wall **(arrows).** A necrotic hypernephroma was found at surgery. (Bosniak MA, Faegenburg D: The thick-wall sign: An important finding in nephrotomography. Radiology 84:692–698, 1965)

Thick Wall Sign

The wall of a true renal cyst resembles the line that a very fine, sharp-pointed pencil would make and can barely be perceived on nephrotomography. If the wall is thicker or simulates the line made by a thick crayon, the lesion cannot be considered a simple benign cyst (Fig. 2-93). Although the thick wall sign often reflects a necrotic avascular carcinoma, a similar appearance can be found in benign tumors, perirenal necrotic abscesses, and infected renal cysts.

BIBLIOGRAPHY
Bosniak MA, Faegenburg D: The thick-wall sign: An important finding in nephrotomography. Radiology 84:692–698, 1965

Toothpaste Sign

Postoperative contracture of the vesical neck can complicate a suprapubic, perineal, or transurethral prostatectomy. If the contrast medium used in retrograde urethrography is more viscid than usual, it retains its shape as it passes through the small opening of the bladder neck and layers out in the bladder, producing a pattern reminiscent of toothpaste being squeezed out of a tube (Fig. 2-94).

BIBLIOGRAPHY
Greene LF, Robinson HP: Postoperative contracture of the vesical neck. V. Clinical findings, symptoms, and diagnosis. J Urol 94:141–147, 1965
Greene LF, Robinson HP: Postoperative contracture of the vesical necks. VI. Prophylaxis and treatment. J Urol 95:520–525, 1966

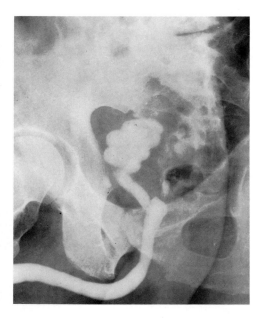

FIG. 2-94. Retrograde urethrogram made with viscid contrast medium in a patient with severe contracture of the vesicle neck demonstrates the toothpaste sign. (Witten DM, Myers GH, Utz DC: Emmett's Clinical Urography. Philadelphia, WB Saunders, 1977)

Wall (Halo) Sign

Ovarian dermoid cysts have a tough fibrous capsule lined internally by squamous epithelium and externally by peritoneum, except at the site of adhesion to abdominal organs. Visualization of the uncalcified wall of a dermoid cyst may be possible because of the contrasting effect of the cyst contents and peritoneal fat on opposite sides of the cyst wall. The fatty contents of the cyst may not be radiolucent enough to be apparent but may be sufficiently radiolucent to enhance a dense fibrous wall seen on edge and surrounded by fatty peritoneal tissues (Fig. 2-95). Depending on the wall thickness and surrounding anatomy, only a segment of an ovarian dermoid capsule may be seen and only in some projections. When a paucity of peritoneal fat causes only the inside surface of the wall to be visible on plain radiographs, it may be possible to outline the outside of the wall indirectly by opacification of adjacent structures such as the ureters, bladder, and bowel (Fig. 2-96).

BIBLIOGRAPHY

Pantoja E, San Pedro CA, Jittivanich U: The radiographic wall—Sign of ovarian dermoids. Rev Interam Radiol 2:33–35, 1977

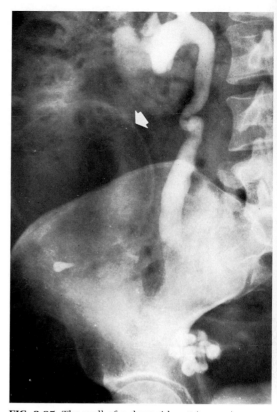

FIG. 2-95. The wall of a dermoid cyst (**arrow**) is almost completely outlined, although the contents are not radiolucent enough to be recognized as such. (Pantoja E, San Pedro CA, Jittivanich U: The radiographic wall—Sign of ovarian dermoids. Rev Interam Radiol 2:33–35, 1977)

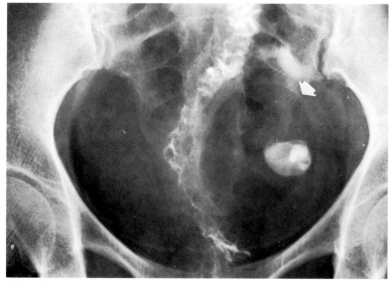

FIG. 2-96. Ovarian dermoid with distinctly radiolucent contents, bone, and a tooth. The **arrow** points to a short-segment wall sign. On the right side, only the inside of the wall is outlined, but the barium in the colon completes visualization of the wall. (Pantoja E, San Pedro CA, Jittivanich U: The radiographic wall—sign of ovarian dermoids. Rev Interam Radiol 2:33–35, 1977)

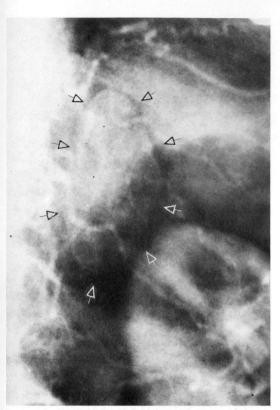

FIG. 2-97. The wedge-shaped contour of an enlarged adrenal gland is visible on the capillary phase of aortography. This sign is diagnostic of cortical adenoma. (Ney C, Friedenberg RM: Radiographic Atlas of the Genitourinary System. Philadelphia, JB Lippincott, 1981)

Wedge Sign

In normal patients, the width of the apex of the adrenal gland is only a fraction of the width of its base. Although cortical adenomas may cause generalized adrenal enlargement, they often result in proportionally much greater enlargement of the upper third of the gland, producing a wedge- or diamond-shaped outline (Fig. 2-97). This radiographic appearance is virtually pathognomonic of cortical adenomas and may be seen in more than half of patients with Cushing's syndrome or the adrenogenital syndrome. The wedge sign has not been reported in cases of adrenocortical carcinoma.

BIBLIOGRAPHY
Meyers MA: Characteristic radiographic shapes of pheochromocytomas and adrenocortical adenomas. Radiology 87:889–892, 1966

White Line Sign

Spurious filling defects caused by gas in overlying loops of bowel, particularly the rectum, can closely simulate true urographic filling defects due to bladder tumors. The white line sign, a thin (2-mm) band of soft-tissue density surrounding a lucent filling defect overlying the bladder, has been reported as evidence of a pseudotumor representing bowel gas (Fig. 2-98). The white line appears to represent the full thickness of the bowel wall lying between gas in the lumen and fat in the surrounding soft tissues. The white line sign is significant only if the bladder is completely opacified, because a similar appearance can be demonstrated about the margin of a tumor when the bladder is incompletely distended with contrast (Fig. 2-99).

BIBLIOGRAPHY
Simpson W, Duncan AW, Clayton CB: A useful sign in the diagnosis of bladder tumours on intravenous urograms. Br J Radiol 47:272–276, 1974

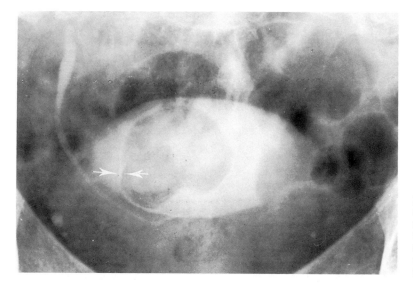

FIG. 2-98. The white line sign (**arrows**) surrounds bowel gas appearing on excretory urography as a filling defect in the bladder. (Simpson W, Duncan AW, Clayton CB: A useful sign in the diagnosis of bladder tumors on intravenous urograms. Br J Radiol 47:272–276, 1974)

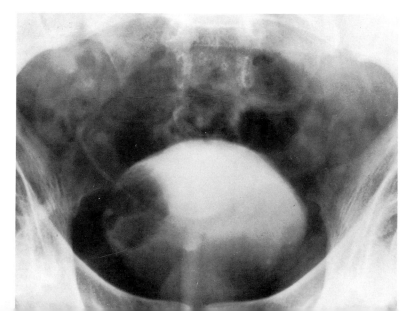

FIG. 2-99. Excretory urogram demonstrates a filling defect in the bladder caused by a transitional cell tumor. An appearance resembling the white line sign is visible around the inferior margin of the tumor where the bladder is incompletely distended with contrast. (Simpson W, Duncan AW, Clayton CB: A useful sign in the diagnosis of bladder tumors on intravenous urograms. Br J Radiol 47:272–276, 1974)

Widened Loop Sign

Perforation of the uterus is an uncommon but serious complication associated with the use of intrauterine contraceptive devices. The space between the loops of a normally placed Lippe's loop is 0.5 cm or less as a result of the relatively small internal cavity of the thick-walled, muscular uterus (Fig. 2-100). In contrast, if partial or complete perforation of the uterus occurs, the intrauterine device widens its natural double-S curve so that the space between the loops becomes approximately 1 cm (Fig. 2-101).

BIBLIOGRAPHY

Eisenberg RL: The widened loop sign of Lippe's loop perforations. AJR 116:847–852, 1972

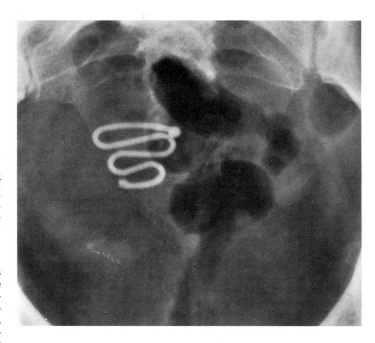

FIG. 2-100. Radiograph showing a well-positioned Lippe's loop. The loop is compact as a result of the relatively small internal cavity of the uterus. (Eisenberg RL: The widened loop sign of Lippe's loop perforations. AJR 116:847–852, 1972. Copyright 1972. Reproduced by permission)

FIG. 2-101. Marked widening of the Lippe's loop in two patients with perforation of the uterus. The contraceptive devices are in extrauterine positions. (Eisenberg RL: The widened loop sign of Lippe's loop perforations. AJR 116:847–852, 1972. Copyright 1972. Reproduced by permission)

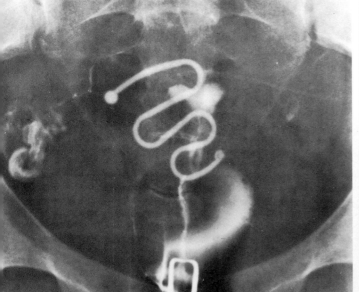

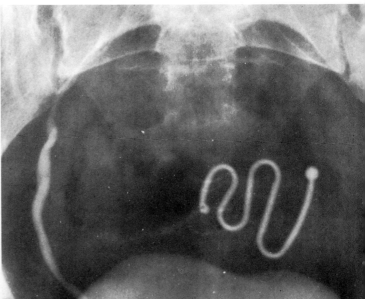

3

Chest

Absent Inferior Vena Cava Sign

Absence of the inferior vena cava shadow on an adequate lateral chest film (Fig. 3-1) is an important clue to the diagnosis of azygos continuation of the inferior vena cava. Absence of the inferior vena cava is commonly associated with complex cardiac anomalies (Fig. 3-2), for which cardiac catheterization is necessary before corrective or palliative surgery. Recognition of the absent inferior vena cava sign is important in patients with the latter condition, since it indicates that an arm vein should be used for cardiac catheterization.

BIBLIOGRAPHY

Heller RM, Dorst JP, James AE et al: A useful sign in the recognition of azygos continuation of the inferior vena cava. Radiology 101:519–522, 1971

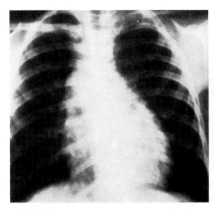
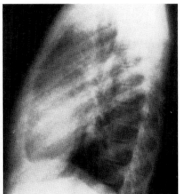

FIG. 3-1. *(Left)* Transposition of the great vessels, other cardiac anomalies, and a right-sided aortic arch in a 2½-year-old boy. *(Right)* The lateral view shows pulmonary vessels in the retrocardiac space but no inferior vena cava. (Heller RM, Dorst JP, James AE et al: A useful sign in the recognition of azygos continuation of the inferior vena cava. Radiology 101:519–522, 1971)

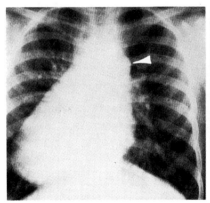
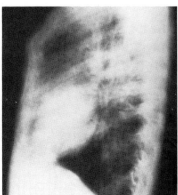

FIG. 3-2. *(Left)* Dextrocardia and complex congenital heart disease in a 10-year-old girl. The left parasternal "mass" (**arrow**) seen on the frontal view is the azygos vein. *(Right)* The lateral view shows no shadow of the inferior vena cava. (Heller RM, Dorst JP, James AE et al: A useful sign in the recognition of azygos continuation of the inferior vena cava. Radiology 101:519–522, 1971)

Air Bronchogram Sign

Air-filled intrapulmonary bronchi have such thin walls that they are not normally seen on chest radiographs. Visualization of air within the intrapulmonary bronchi requires that the surrounding lung parenchyma be airless or contain a markedly reduced amount of air, either as a result of replacement of air by fluid or tissue (consolidation) or as a result of absorption of air, as in atelectasis (Fig. 3-3). The appearance of an air bronchogram also requires the presence of air within the bronchial tree, implying that the bronchus is not completely occluded at its origin. The presence of an air bronchogram excludes a pleural or mediastinal lesion, since there are no bronchi in these regions. An air bronchogram cannot occur within a solid tumor or cyst of the lung, because the bronchi in the region of these lesions are either occluded or displaced. Although the presence of an air bronchogram is an extremely important diagnostic aid, the absence of an air bronchogram is of no value in differential diagnosis.

BIBLIOGRAPHY
Felson, B: Chest Roentgenology. Philadelphia, WB Saunders, 1973
Fleischner FG: The visible bronchial tree: A roentgen sign in pneumonic and other pulmonary consolidations. Radiology 50:184–189, 1948

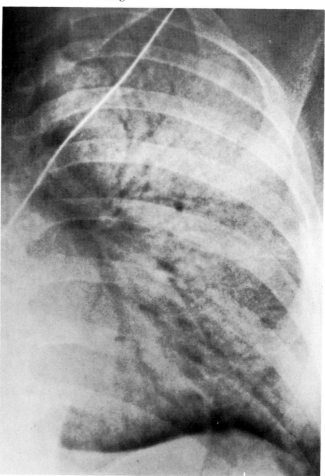

FIG. 3-3. Frontal chest radiograph demonstrates visualization of air within the intrapulmonary bronchi (air bronchogram sign) in a patient with a diffuse pneumonia of the left lung.

Air Crescent (Meniscus) Sign

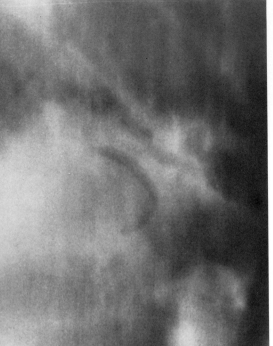

The air crescent or meniscus sign is a crescent-shaped radiolucent shadow at the periphery of a mass lesion of the lung (Fig. 3-4). The sign was originally described in a patient with pulmonary echinococcal cyst and is often considered pathognomonic of hydatid disease. However, it is most commonly produced by an intracavitary fungus ball of *Aspergillus fumigatus* (Fig. 3-5). A similar radiographic appearance has been described in a broad spectrum of disorders, including lung abscess, pulmonary hematoma, benign and malignant lung tumors (Fig. 3-6), granulomatous disease, Rasmussen's aneurysm, and fungus balls due to other causes.

BIBLIOGRAPHY

Bahk YW, Shinn KS, Choi BS: The air meniscus sign in sclerosing hemangioma of the lung. Radiology 128:27–29, 1978

Cubillo-Herguera E, McAlister WH: The pulmonary meniscus sign in a case of bronchogenic carcinoma. Radiology 92:1299–1300, 1969

Curtis AM, Smith GJW, Ravin CE: Air crescent sign of invasive aspergillosis. Radiology 133:17–21, 1979

Watanabe TJ: Mass in a pulmonary cavity (meniscus sign). Semin Roentgenol 14:175–176, 1979

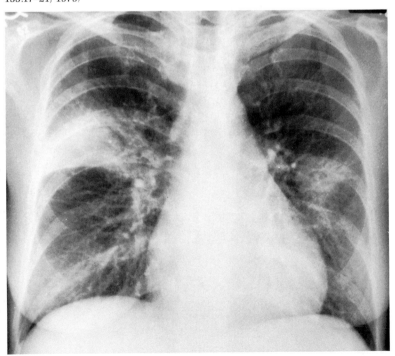

FIG. 3-4. *(Bottom, right)* Frontal chest radiograph demonstrates bilateral upper lobe densities in a patient with invasive aspergillosis. Tomography demonstrates air crescents *(Top, left)* on the right and *(Bottom, left)* on the left. (Curtis AM, Smith GJW, Ravin CE: Air crescent sign of invasive aspergillosis. Radiology 133:17–21, 1979)

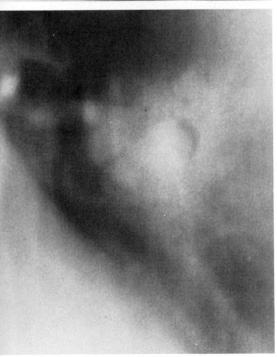

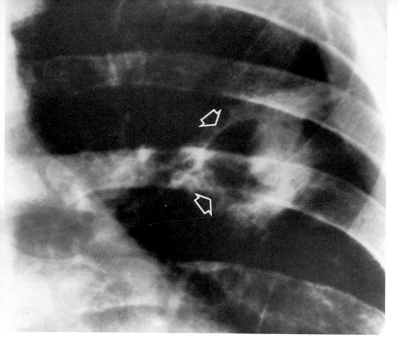

FIG. 3-5. Air crescent sign (**arrows**) associated with an intracavitary fungus ball of aspergillosis in a patient with chronic lymphocytic leukemia.

FIG. 3-6. Air crescent sign (**arrows**) associated with cavitating squamous cell carcinoma of the lung.

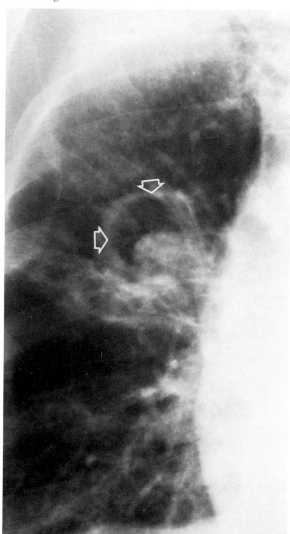

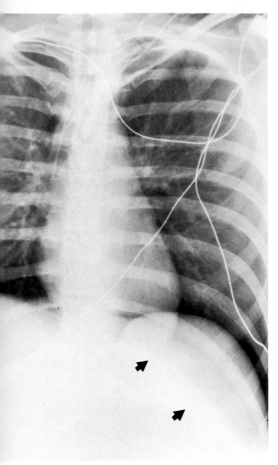

Anterior Sulcus (Double Diaphragm) Sign ▬▬▬▬

In the supine adult, a small pneumothorax may localize anteriorly and inferiorly, the uppermost portion of the thorax in this position. On supine chest radiographs, the pneumothorax may outline the anterior costophrenic sulcus, resulting in an abrupt curvilinear change in density projected over the right or left upper quadrant of the abdomen(Fig. 3-7). The upper quadrant also appears relatively lucent (Fig. 3-8). The anterior sulcus or double diaphragm sign may be the only radiographic finding of a small pneumothorax when the patient is supine; detection of this abnormality should lead to a prompt cross-table lateral or decubitus study to confirm the diagnosis and estimate the size of the pneumothorax.

BIBLIOGRAPHY
Rhea JT, van Sonnenberg E, McCloud TC: Basilar pneumothorax in the supine adult. Radiology 133:583–595, 1979
Ziter FMH, Westcott JL: Supine subpulmonary pneumothorax. AJR 137:699–701, 1981

FIG. 3-7. On a supine chest film, a pneumothorax outlining the anterior costophrenic sulcus results in a double diaphragm sign (**arrows**) and hyperlucency at the left base. Note that the endotracheal tube is abnormally positioned. (Ziter FMH, Westcott JL: Supine subpulmonary pneumothorax. AJR 137:699–701, 1981. Copyright 1981. Reproduced by permission)

FIG. 3-8. Left basilar hyperlucency and double diaphragm sign (**black arrows**) on a supine chest radiograph of a patient with a pneumothorax. The presence of pericardial fat tags (**white arrow**) is another indication of pneumothorax on the supine projection. (Ziter FMH, Westcott JL: Supine subpulmonary pneumothorax. AJR 137:699–701, 1981. Copyright 1981. Reproduced by permission)

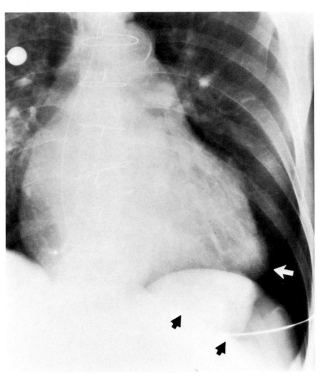

Anterior Tracheal Displacement Sign ━━━━━━━

An obstructed and dilated esophagus in infants and children often causes anterior displacement of the trachea on lateral chest radiographs (Fig. 3-9). The anterior tracheal displacement sign, however, is not pathognomonic of esophageal obstruction; vascular rings, neurenteric cysts, aberrant thyroid tissue, and various malignant tumors may present a similar appearance. The sign must also be distinguished from the anterior buckling of the trachea that may occur in expiration and in flexion of the head.

BIBLIOGRAPHY
Grünebaum M: Tracheal displacement as a sign of esophageal obstruction in infants and children. AJR 104:603–607, 1968

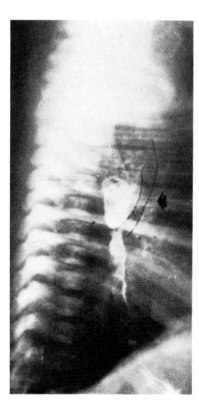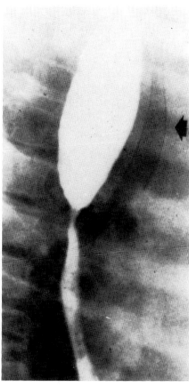

FIG. 3-9. Lateral chest radiographs in two young children demonstrate anterior displacement of the trachea (**arrows**) due to obstruction and dilatation of the esophagus. *(Left)* Congenital stenosis of the esophagus. *(Right)* Chemical (lye) esophagitis with resultant stenosis. (Grünebaum M: Tracheal displacement as a sign of esophageal obstruction in infants and children. AJR 104:603–607, 1968. Copyright 1968. Reproduced by permission.)

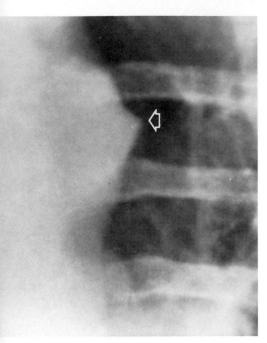

FIG. 3-10. The small, nipple-like mass (**arrow**) adjacent to the lateral aspect of the aortic arch on this frontal radiograph represents the normal left superior intercostal vein.

Aortic Nipple Sign

The appearance on frontal radiographs of a small mass or "nipple" adjacent to the lateral or superior aspect of the aortic arch is indicative of the normal left superior intercostal vein (Fig. 3-10). The aortic nipple may change in size with alterations in intrathoracic pressure, posture, or increased flow when the vein functions as a collateral vein in vena cava obstruction. It is important that this normal vascular shadow not be confused with lymphadenopathy or a small tumor.

BIBLIOGRAPHY
McDonald CJ, Castellino RA, Blank N: The aortic "nipple": The left superior intercostal vein. Radiology 96:533–536, 1970

Aortic Swallowing Sign

There is normally only loose connective tissue between the arch of the aorta and the trachea at the point at which the aorta crosses over the left main stem bronchus. This permits independent movement of these two structures, so that the aortic arch can remain stationary while the trachea rises during swallowing. In fibrous mediastinitis, neoplastic disease, or any other condition producing adhesions between the aortic arch and trachea, the aortic arch is bound to the trachea and must rise with it during swallowing. This is seen at fluoroscopy as the aortic swallowing sign.

BIBLIOGRAPHY
Rabin CB, Baron MG: Radiology of the Chest. Baltimore, Williams & Wilkins, 1980

Apical Cap Sign

In patients with trauma to the chest, the appearance of a collection of blood over the apex of the left lung is an indication of a traumatic aortic aneurysm (Fig. 3-11). The apical pleural cap sign results from the leaking of blood from a ruptured aortic arch into the pleural space over the left lung. There is a normal defect in the pleural covering over the aorta in the region of the transverse arch, so that mediastinal blood can track directly into the left apical pleural space. Presence of this subtle but characteristic sign indicates the need for emergency aortography.

BIBLIOGRAPHY
Swischuk LE: Emergency Radiology of the Acutely Ill or Injured Child. Baltimore, William & Wilkins, 1979

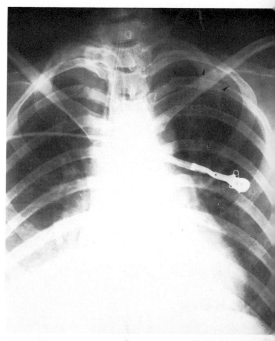

FIG. 3-11. *(Top)* **Arrows** point to the apical cap sign, a collection of fluid over the left lung apex, in a patient with a traumatic aortic aneurysm. The superior mediastinum is widened, and there are fractures of the right upper ribs and left scapula. The endotracheal and esophageal tubes are shifted to the right, substantiating the presence of a mediastinal hematoma. *(Bottom)* Subsequent aortogram demonstrates a traumatic aortic aneurysm **(arrows).** (Swischuk LE: Emergency Radiology of the Acutely Ill or Injured Child. Baltimore, Williams & Wilkins, 1979)

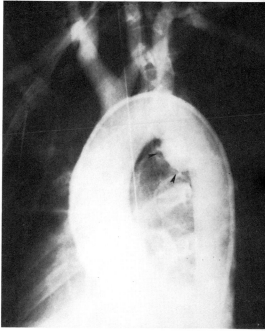

Axillary Mass Sign

Axillary soft-tissue tumor masses may simulate mediastinal tumors on lateral chest radiographs. They usually present in the anterosuperior or middle mediastinum with well-defined curvilinear anterior margins (Fig. 3-12). This axillary mass sign may itself be simulated by heavy anterior axillary folds in obese persons. As a rule, fold lines are straighter in contour and lower in position than the usual axillary mass shadow.

BIBLIOGRAPHY

Bonte FJ, Schonfeld MD: The axillary mass sign on lateral chest roentgenograms. AJR 87:900–907, 1962

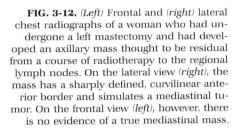

FIG. 3-12. *(Left)* Frontal and *(right)* lateral chest radiographs of a woman who had undergone a left mastectomy and had developed an axillary mass thought to be residual from a course of radiotherapy to the regional lymph nodes. On the lateral view *(right)*, the mass has a sharply defined, curvilinear anterior border and simulates a mediastinal tumor. On the frontal view *(left)*, however, there is no evidence of a true mediastinal mass.

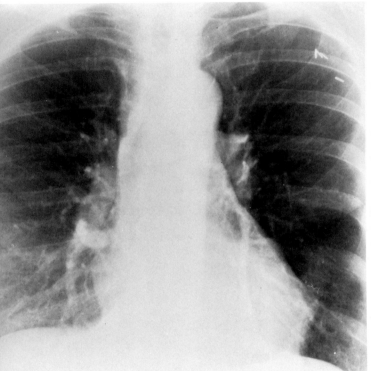
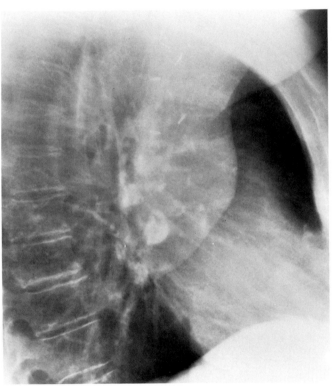

B⁶ Bronchus Sign

The bronchus to the superior segment of the lower lobe has an anteroposterior orientation. In many cases of pneumonia or atelectasis involving this segment, the segmental bronchus remains filled with air and can be recognized on frontal radiographs as an end-on air bronchogram surrounded by the water density of gasless alveoli (Fig. 3-13).

BIBLIOGRAPHY

Friedman PJ: Radiology of the superior segment of the lower lobe: A regional perspective, introducing the B⁶ bronchus sign. Radiology 144:15–25, 1982

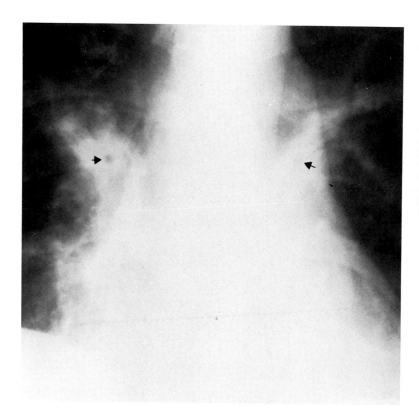

FIG. 3-13. Frontal chest radiograph of a young woman with bilateral B⁶ subsegmental atelectasis as well as posterior basal segmental atelectasis or pneumonia. Note the bilateral B⁶ bronchus sign (air bronchograms; **arrows**), slightly higher on the left side. There is obliteration of part of the descending aorta as well as consolidation in the posterior basal region on the left. On the lateral view, the B⁶ atelectasis was not visible because of superimposed structures and a lack of tangent-forming margins; basal involvement was more evident. (Friedman PJ: Radiology of the superior segment of the lower lobe: A regional perspective, introducing the B⁶ bronchus sign. Radiology 144:15–25, 1982)

Big Rib Sign

Pulmonary disease in the region of the posterior cardiophrenic sulcus may be detectable on lateral radiographs but invisible on standard frontal views. Because such basal pathology usually silhouettes the adjacent hemidiaphragm, it is necessary to devise a way in which to distinguish accurately between the two hemidiaphragms to permit correct localization of disease to the left or right side from the lateral projection alone. The term *big rib sign* is related to the fact that the rib cage farthest from the radiograph is magnified more than the rib cage in contact with the radiograph. Therefore, on well-positioned left lateral radiographs, the ribs that appear larger are those on the right, and the hemidiaphragm related to them is the right hemidiaphragm (Fig. 3-14).

BIBLIOGRAPHY

Naidich JB, Naidich TP, Hyman RA et al: The big rib sign: Localization of basal pulmonary pathology in lateral projection utilizing differential magnification of the two hemithoraces. Radiology 131:1–8, 1979

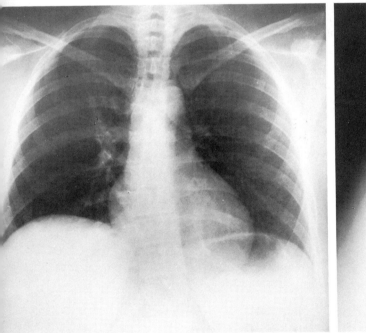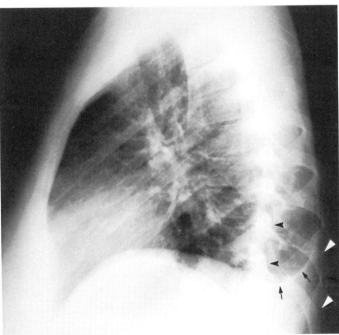

FIG. 3-14. Right pleural effusion, detectable only in lateral projection. Correct lateralization requires use of the big rib sign. *(Left)* Erect posteroanterior chest radiograph shows no evidence of pleural effusion. *(Right)* Left lateral chest radiograph demonstrates a unilateral effusion. Comparable portions of the left ribs **(black arrowheads)** and right ribs **(white arrowheads)** are very different in size. Patient rotation exaggerates the effect of magnification in this radiograph. A meniscus **(black arrows)** in the posterior costophrenic sulcus is easily traced to the magnified, posteriorly projected right ribs. That this meniscus represents a right pleural effusion was confirmed on decubitus views. (Naidich JB, Naidich TP, Hyman RA et al: The big rib sign: Localization of basal pulmonary pathology in lateral projection utilizing differential magnification of the two hemithoraces. Radiology 131:1–8, 1979)

Black Pleura Sign

Extensive alveolar calcification can make the water density pleura appear as a lucent line lying between the calcified pulmonary infiltrate and the adjacent ribs (Fig. 3-15). This black pleura sign was first described in patients with alveolar microlithiasis but has also been seen in a patient with hyperparathyroidism.

BIBLIOGRAPHY

Balikian JP, Fuleihan FJD, Nucho CN: Pulmonary alveolar microlithiasis: Report of five cases with special reference to roentgen manifestations. AJR 103:509–518, 1968

Theros EG: An exercise in radiologic–pathologic correlation. Radiology 91:807–812, 1968

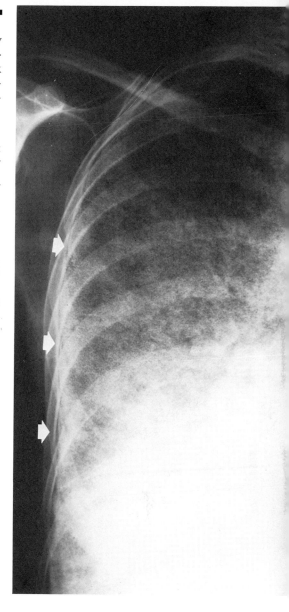

FIG. 3-15. A penetrated coned view of the right upper lung demonstrates nearly uniform distribution of typical fine, fan-like mottling in this patient with alveolar microlithiasis. The tangential shadow of the pleura is displayed along the lateral wall of the chest as a dark, lucent strip **(arrows).** It appears this way because of its relative radiotransparency (water density) when seen between the ribs and the markedly radiopaque lungs that are characteristic of this disease. (Theros EG: An exercise in radiologic–pathologic correlation. Radiology 91:807–812, 1968. Courtesy of the American Registry of Radiologic Pathology at the Armed Forces Institute of Pathology)

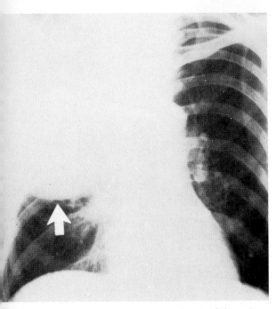

FIG. 3-16. Downward bulging of the minor fissure (**arrow**) in a patient with right upper lobe enlargement caused by Friedlander's pneumonia. (Felson B, Rosenberg LS, Hamburger M: Roentgen findings in acute Friedlander's pneumonia. Radiology 53:559–565, 1949)

FIG. 3-17. Downward bulging of the minor fissure in a patient with an enlarged right upper lobe caused by *Hemophilus influenzae* pneumonia. (Francis JB, Francis PB: Bulging (sagging) fissure sign in *Hemophilus influenzae* lobar pneumonia. South Med J 71:1452–1453 1978)

Bulging Fissure Sign

The bulging fissure sign was first described in patients with acute pneumonia due to Friedlander's bacillus (*Klebsiella*). Infection with this organism causes the involved lobes to be voluminous, heavy, and firmly consolidated. The radiographic appearance of a bulging fissure reflects this lobar enlargement (Fig. 3-16). The bulging fissure sign, especially when combined with the sharp margins of the advancing border of the pneumonic infiltrate and early abscess formation, was reported to be virtually pathognomonic of *Klebsiella* pneumonia. Since the original report was published, a similar appearance of bulging fissure has been described in patients with pneumococcal, plague, and *Hemophilus influenzae* pneumonia (Fig. 3-17), tuberculosis, mass lesions of the lung, and large lung abscesses.

BIBLIOGRAPHY

Felson B, Rosenberg LS, Hamburger M: Roentgen findings in acute Friedlander's pneumonia. Radiology 53:559–565, 1949

Francis JB, Francis PB: Bulging (sagging) fissure sign in *Hemophilus influenzae* lobar pneumonia. South Med J 71:1452–1453, 1978

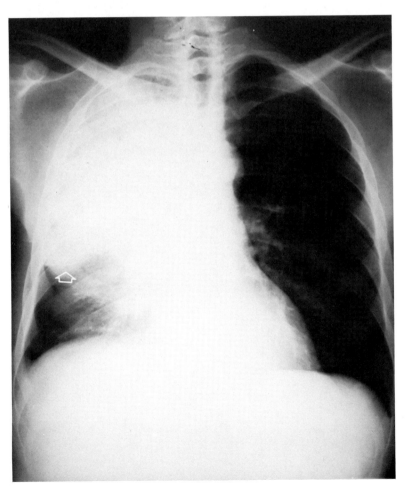

Butterfly (Bat's Wing) Shadow ▬▬▬▬▬▬▬

The butterfly or bat's wing pattern is a diffuse, bilaterally symmetric infiltration that is most prominent in the central portion of the lungs and fades toward the periphery (Fig. 3-18). The apex, base, and lateral portion of each lung are relatively spared. The butterfly shadow was originally described in a patient with uremic pulmonary edema and was considered pathognomonic of this condition. It is now understood that the butterfly shadow implies extensive alveolar disease of any cause, most commonly pulmonary edema. Although usually relatively homogeneous, the butterfly sign can appear as large, ill-defined densities surrounding small areas of normal-appearing lung. Rarely, the sign is unilateral or extends to the periphery of the lung.

BIBLIOGRAPHY
Felson B: Chest Roentgenology. Philadelphia, WB Saunders, 1973
Rendich RA, Levy AH, Cove AM: Pulmonary manifestations of azotemia. AJR 46:802–808, 1941

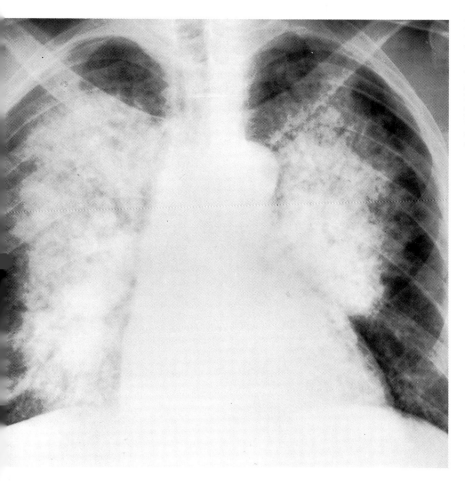

FIG. 3-18. Diffuse, bilaterally symmetric infiltration of the central portion of the lungs with relative sparing of the periphery produces the butterfly, or bat's wing, pattern in this patient with pulmonary edema. The margins of the edematous lung are sharply defined. The consolidation is fairly homogeneous and is associated with a well-defined air bronchogram on both sides. (Fraser RG, Pare JAP: Diagnosis of Diseases of the Chest. Philadelphia, WB Saunders, 1978)

Sign of the Cane

In patients with small hernias through the foramen of Morgagni, the parietal–properitoneal–peritoneal line may be visible well above its normal limits within the thoracic cavity because of the solid or hollow abdominal organs that have migrated through the hiatus of Morgagni. On lateral views, the curvilinear contour assumes the appearance of a cane in profile (Fig. 3-19).

BIBLIOGRAPHY
Lanuza A: The sign of the cane: A new radiological sign for the diagnosis of small Morgagni hernias. Radiology 101:293–296, 1971

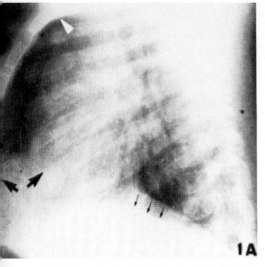

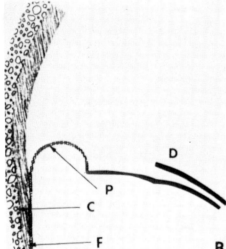

FIG. 3-19. (**A**) Lateral projection demonstrates the sign of the cane (**large arrows**) in a 9-month-old patient with Morgagni hernia. The child also had Down's syndrome. Duplication of the first sternal segment (**arrowhead**) is seen. Only the posterior half of the right hemidiaphragm (**small arrows**) is visible. (**B**) Schematic representation of (**A**). F = fascia; C = cellular tissue; P = properitoneal fat above its normal location; D = diaphragm. (Lanuza A: The sign of the cane: A new radiological sign for the diagnosis of small Morgagni hernias. Radiology 101:293–296, 1971)

Cardiac Blur Sign

The cardiac blur sign is the loss of sharp definition of the left heart border, or a portion of it, on frontal chest films (Fig. 3-20). Although this appearance can be seen in patients with pleuropericardial scarring of inflammatory or surgical origin, pneumonia, some left cardiophrenic angle fat pads, and certain arrythmias, it has been described as highly suggestive of a postinfarction myocardial scar of the anterolateral wall of the left ventricle. Blurring of the left cardiac border cannot be seen with extremely fast exposure times (shorter than 1/20–1/30 sec). Therefore, it is postulated that the sign reflects a variety of rapid irregular and paradoxical movements adjacent to the contracting viable myocardium.

BIBLIOGRAPHY
Sanders I, Woesner ME: The cardiac blur sign of the postinfarction myocardial scar. AJR 113:703–709, 1971

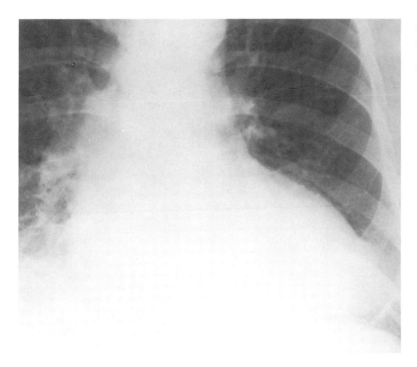

FIG. 3-20. Loss of sharp definition of the left heart border in conjunction with an apical bulge in a patient with postinfarction left ventricular aneurysm. (Sanders I, Woesner ME: The cardiac blur sign of the postinfarction myocardial scar. AJR 113:703–709, 1971. Copyright 1971. Reproduced by permission)

Cervicothoracic Sign

The cephalic border of the anterior mediastinum ends at the level of the clavicle, whereas that of the posterior mediastinum extends much higher. Because any thoracic lesion that is adjacent to the soft tissues of the neck loses its contiguous border, any lesion clearly visible above the clavicles on the frontal view must lie posteriorly and be entirely within the thorax (Fig. 3-21). Conversely, if the upper border of the lesion disappears as it approaches the clavicles, the lesion must lie partly in the anterior portion of the mediastinum and partly in the neck (Fig. 3-22). The trachea is the dividing line: a mediastinal mass anterior to it loses its superolateral margins as it reaches the lower border of the clavicles; a posterior mass remains visible above the clavicles; and a juxtatracheal mass is visible part way above the clavicles (Fig. 3-23).

BIBLIOGRAPHY
Felson B: More chest roentgen signs and how to teach them. Radiology 90:429–441, 1968
Felson B: Chest Roentgenology. Philadelphia, WB Saunders, 1973

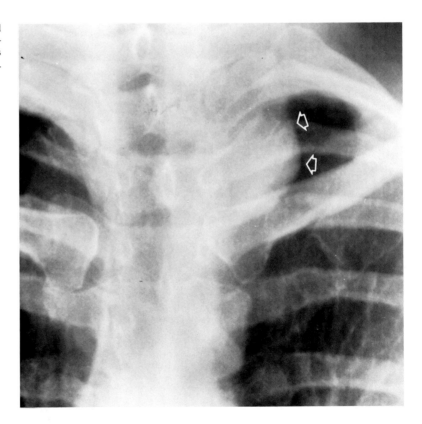

FIG. 3-21. Clear definition of a mediastinal mass above the left clavicle (**arrows**) indicates that the lesion, a neurogenic tumor, lies in a posterior location.

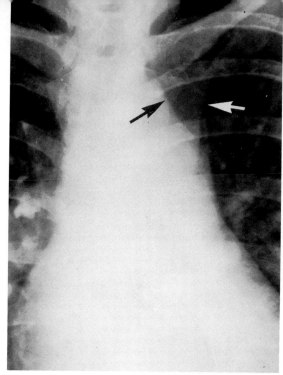

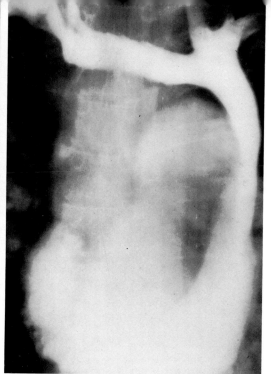

FIG. 3-22. The vertical shadow (**white arrow**) lateral to the aortic knob (**black arrow**) lies anteriorly, as evidenced by the fact that it disappears as it approaches the clavicle. Venous phase of an angiocardiogram in *(top, right)* frontal and *(bottom, left)* lateral views demonstrates that a left superior vena cava en route to the coronary sinus is responsible for the abnormal shadow. *(Bottom, left)* The anomalous vena cava is seen to lie anterior to the trachea in the lateral view. (Felson B: Chest Roentgenology. Philadelphia, WB Saunders, 1973)

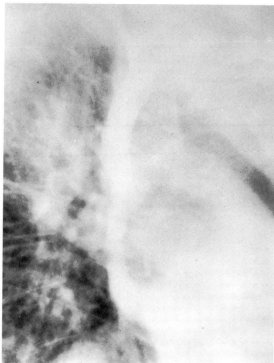

FIG. 3-23. The outer border of this thyroid tumor (**arrows**) is visible part way above the right clavicle, indicating that the tumor is in a juxtatracheal position.

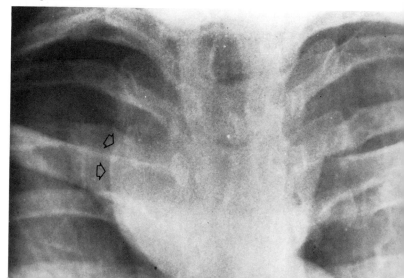

Chest–Abdomen Sign

In children with familial dysautonomia, radiographic changes are seen simultaneously in both the lungs and the gastrointestinal tract. Because of their lack of motor coordination, loss of pain sense, and lack of the swallowing reflex with increased salivation, patients with familial dysautonomia suffer from cyclic vomiting and aspiration pneumonia. Their chest radiographs usually demonstrate evidence of pneumonia, interstitial fibrosis, bronchial wall thickening, and sometimes atelectasis. Chest radiographs that also include the upper part of the abdomen generally demonstrate distended loops of bowel that are not associated with any acute clinical symptoms (Fig. 3-24). In addition to familial dysautonomia, concomitant disease of the chest and abdomen without obvious clinical signs can be found in patients with mucoviscidosis or tracheo-esophageal fistulas, both of which can easily be distinguished from familial dysautonomia.

BIBLIOGRAPHY
Grünebaum M: The "chest–abdomen sign" in familiar dysautonomia. Br J Radiol 48:23–27, 1975

FIG. 3-24. Example of the chest–abdomen sign in a patient with cystic fibrosis. The chest radiograph not only demonstrates the characteristic interstitial fibrosis but also shows distended loops of bowel in the upper abdomen in a patient with no clinical symptoms.

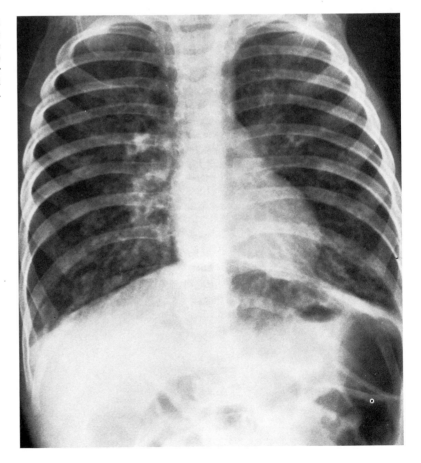

Clear Space Sign

On normal posteroanterior radiographs of the chest is a clear space outlined by the aortic arch and descending aorta, pulmonary outflow tract, and left upper lobe vessels, which form its medial, inferior, and lateral boundaries, respectively (Fig. 3-25). The medial margin of this space has either a vertical orientation or a concave outer border. Lymph nodes of the ligamentum arteriosum and adjoining nodes lie in close proximity to this clear space. In the absence of other processes involving structures of the middle mediastinum, encroachment of the clear space from the medial direction with formation of a convex outer border may be the first radiographic sign of left-sided mediastinal lymph node enlargement (Fig. 3-26) and the earliest indication of neoplastic or granulomatous disease.

BIBLIOGRAPHY
Schwarz MI, Marmorstein BL: A radiographic sign of left sided mediastinal lymph node enlargement. Chest 68:116–118, 1975

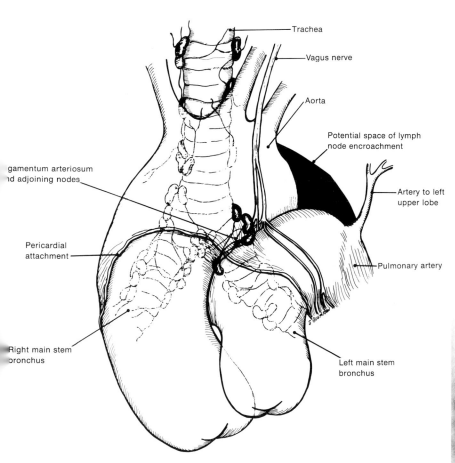

FIG. 3-25. Diagrammatic representation of the normal structures of the middle mediastinum and their anatomic relationships to the space of potential lymph node encroachment. (Schwarz MI, Marmorstein BL: A radiographic sign of left sided mediastinal lymph node enlargement. Chest 68:116–118, 1975)

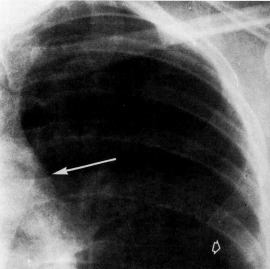

FIG. 3-26. Chest radiograph of a patient with bronchogenic carcinoma and encroachment of the clear space by enlarged mediastinal nodes (**long arrow**). The area of the primary tumor can be identified as an ill-defined density adjacent to the lateral chest wall at the level of the seventh rib posteriorly (**short arrow**). (Swartz MI, Marmorstein BL: A radiographic sign of left sided mediastinal lymph node enlargement. Chest 68:116–118, 1975)

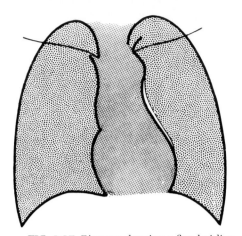

FIG. 3-27. Diagram showing a fine hairline paralleling the left heart border in a patient with a spontaneous pneumothorax and characteristic systolic click. (Wright JT: The radiological sign of "clicking" pneumothorax. Clin Radiol 16:292–294, 1965)

Clicking Pneumothorax Sign

Severe retrosternal pain associated with an unusual systolic click on auscultation (Hamman's sign) was initially described as a manifestation of spontaneous pneumomediastinum with secondary pneumothorax. On frontal radiographs, a sharp and distinct line was often seen running parallel to the border of the heart. In most cases, however, the fine hairline paralleling the left cardiac border is due to a spontaneous pneumothorax in which air becomes trapped in a pocket of the pleural cavity. This pocket is created by the reflection of the pleura from the medial aspect of the left lung onto the pericardium (Fig. 3-27). Its displacement by the forceful action of the left ventricle gives rise to a peculiar noise, which has been variously described as crunching, crackling, bubbling, and grating.

BIBLIOGRAPHY

Hamman L: Spontaneous mediastinal emphysema. Bull Johns Hopkins Hosp 64:1–21, 1939

Wright JT: The radiological sign of "clicking" pneumothorax. Clin Radiol 16:292–294, 1965

Coeur en Sabot Sign

In tetralogy of Fallot, the right ventricular wall is thickened. This displaces the prominent left cardiac apex laterally, sharpens it, and tilts it upward into a contour that resembles the curved toe portion of a wooden shoe (Fig. 3-28).

BIBLIOGRAPHY

Swischuk LE: Plain Film Interpretation in Congenital Heart Disease. Baltimore, Williams & Wilkins, 1979

FIG. 3-28. Lateral displacement and upward tilting of a prominent left cardiac apex producing the *coeur en sabot* appearance in a child with tetralogy of Fallot. (Taken from the Diagnostic Radiological Health Sciences Learning Laboratory, as developed by the Radiological Health Sciences Education Project, University of California at San Francisco, under contract with the Bureau of Radiological Health, Food and Drug Administration, and in cooperation with the American College of Radiology)

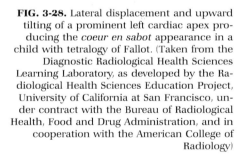

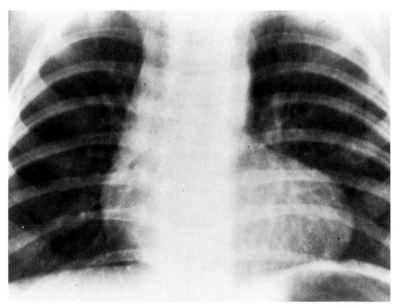

Continuous Diaphragm Sign ▬▬▬▬▬

The silhouette of the two leaves of the diaphragm is normally interrupted in the midline, where the water density of the heart is adjacent to that of the diaphragm and subadjacent viscera. Interposition of gas between the heart and diaphragm in cases of pneumomediastinum permits visualization of the central portion of the diaphragm in continuity with the lateral portions (Fig. 3-29). Although gas in the pericardial sac might cause a similar appearance, patients with pneumopericardium almost always have fluid in the pericardial cavity obliterating the central portion of the diaphragm, at least on radiographs exposed with the patient in the erect position. If uncertainty persists as to whether gas lies in the pericardial sac or mediastinal space, radiographs should be made with the patient in different positions. Demonstration of a change in the appearance of the gas clearly indicates that it lies in the pericardial sac.

BIBLIOGRAPHY
Levin B: The continuous diaphragm sign. A newly-recognized sign of pneumomediastinum. Clin Radiol 24:337–338, 1973

FIG. 3-29. *(Left)* Frontal chest radiograph of a patient with pneumomediastinum demonstrates interposition of gas between the heart and diaphragm permitting visualization of the central portion of the diaphragm in continuity with the lateral portions **(arrows).** *(Right)* The lateral view confirms the diagnosis of pneumomediastinum.

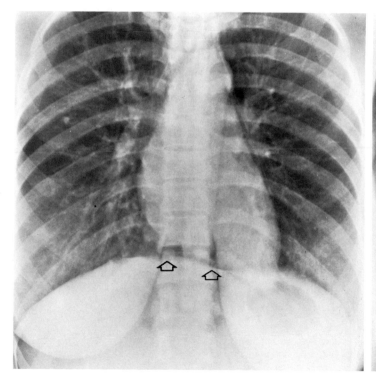
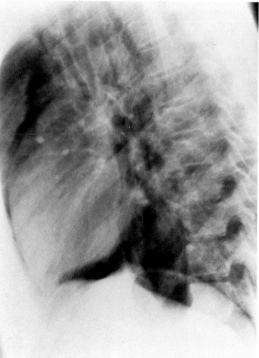

Costal Cartilage Sign

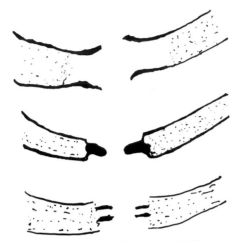

FIG. 3-30. *(Top)* Male type of calcification. *(Center)* Common female type of calcification. *(Bottom)* Uncommon female type of calcification. (Sanders CF: Sexing by costal cartilage calcification. Br J Radiol 39:233–234, 1966)

The pattern of costal cartilage calcification on a chest or upper abdomen radiograph has been shown to be related to the patient's sex. The pattern of calcification in men is constant and quite distinctive. The upper and lower borders of the cartilage become calcified first, extending directly in continuity from the ends of the bony ribs (Fig. 3-30, *top*). Calcification of the central area then follows. In women, two types of calcification are described. The more common is a solid tongue of calcification extending from the rib into the adjacent cartilage (Fig. 3-30, *center*). A less common pattern is two parallel lines of calcification extending from the center of the rib into the adjacent cartilage (Fig. 3-30, *bottom*).

BIBLIOGRAPHY

Sanders CF: Sexing by costal cartilage calcification. Br J Radiol 39:233–234, 1966

FIG. 3-31. Anteroposterior supine radiograph obtained after bilateral attempts at central venous pressure (CVP) line insertion shows subcutaneous emphysema on both sides of the neck. The deep lateral costophrenic angles reflect bilateral pneumothoraces. The small amounts of free air in the apex of each hemithorax are poorly shown. (Gordon R: The deep sulcus sign. Radiology 136:25–27, 1980)

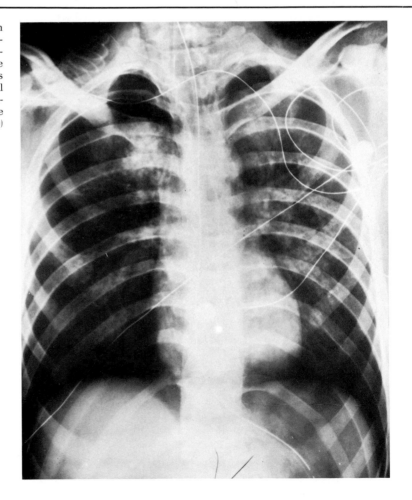

Deep Sulcus Sign

Although upright, expiratory, and decubitus chest radiographs are the best way in which to demonstrate a pneumothorax, a supine radiograph is often all that can be obtained because of the patient's condition. The deep sulcus sign is the appearance of a deep lateral costophrenic angle on the involved side (Fig. 3-31). This appearance may be the only sign of pneumothorax on a supine chest radiograph (Fig. 3-32). It has been suggested that the deep sulcus sign represents a collection of air in a subpulmonary location, which is most likely to be present when the patient is supine. Persons in whom this sign might be interpreted incorrectly include patients with hyperexpansion of the lungs due to chronic obstructive pulmonary disease and large patients in whom one or both costophrenic angles are inadvertently cut off the film.

BIBLIOGRAPHY
Gordon R: The deep sulcus sign. Radiology 136:25–27, 1980

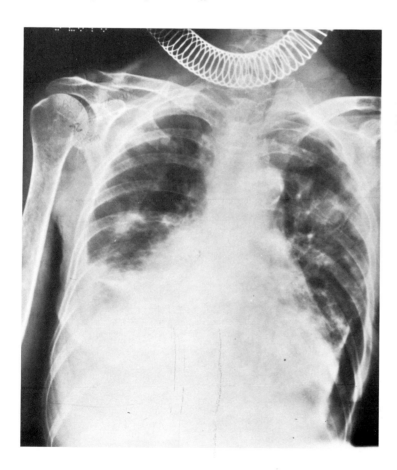

FIG. 3-32. Anteroposterior erect radiograph obtained after a left-sided thoracentesis in an elderly woman with metastatic disease to the chest and no known primary lesion. The radiograph demonstrates a deep left lateral costophrenic angle, indicating a loculated pneumothorax. No other evidence of pneumothorax is seen. (Gordon R: The deep sulcus sign. Radiology 136:25–27, 1980)

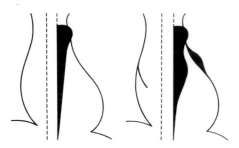

FIG. 3-33. Diagrammatic representation of the contour of *(left)* the normal descending aorta and *(right)* a descending aorta deviated by an enlarged left atrium. (Dee PM: Deviation of the descending thoracic aorta as a sign of left atrial enlargement. Radiology 112:57–59, 1974)

Deviated Descending Thoracic Aorta Sign

On frontal chest radiographs, the contour of the descending aorta normally is a straight line extending inferiorly from the aortic arch and merging with the shadow of the vertebral column. Enlargement of the left atrium encroaching on the retrocardiac mediastinal space may displace the descending aorta posterolaterally tangential to the vertebral bodies (Fig. 3-33). This produces a characteristic deviation of the descending aorta, with the point of maximum convexity of the deviated aorta at the same level as the center of the left atrium (Fig. 3-34). Although not as reliable as the double contour sign, lateral deviation of the descending aorta at the level of the left atrium is a useful subsidiary sign of left atrial enlargement.

BIBLIOGRAPHY
Dee PM: Deviation of the descending thoracic aorta as a sign of left atrial enlargement. Radiology 112:57–59, 1974

FIG. 3-34. Penetrated frontal chest radiograph demonstrates the typical appearance of aortic deviation (**arrows**) by an enlarged left atrium. (Dee PM: Deviation of the descending thoracic aorta as a sign of left atrial enlargement. Radiology 112:57–59, 1974)

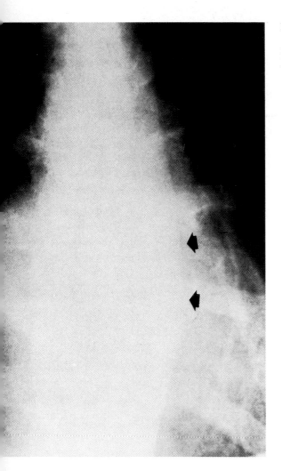

Double Contour Sign

The left atrium lies posteriorly and normally does not form any part of the cardiac contour on radiographs obtained in the frontal projection. Enlargement of the left atrium, such as from rheumatic heart disease, causes the chamber to bulge first posteriorly and then to both the right and left sides. On the right, this enlargement may produce a "double contour" configuration resulting either from the left atrium extending beyond the outer right border of the right atrium and superior vena cava or from the increased density of the enlarged left atrium, which is still projected within the right atrial border (Fig. 3-35).

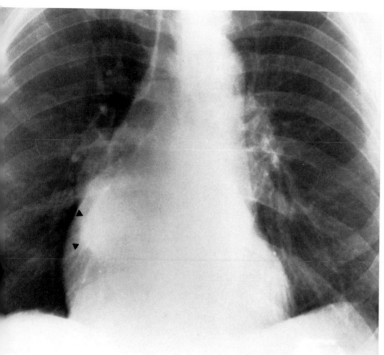
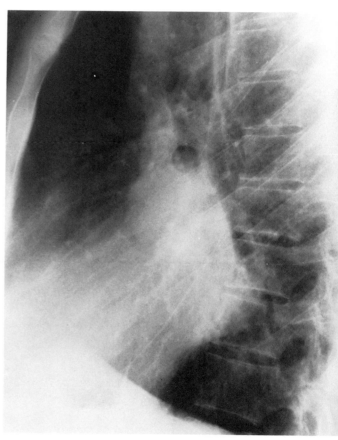

FIG. 3-35. *(Left)* Frontal chest radiograph demonstrates a "double contour" (**arrows**) representing the increased density of an enlarged left atrium. *(Right)* Lateral view confirms the left atrial enlargement in this patient with rheumatic heart disease.

Eggshell Calcification

Eggshell calcification refers to the uncommon appearance of a ring of calcification around the periphery of a lymph node (Fig. 3-36). This appearance is unlike the diffuse or random pattern of calcification typically seen in nodes involved by granulomatous disease (Fig. 3-37). Eggshell calcification is almost pathognomonic of silicosis; however, an identical form of calcification has been infrequently described in conditions not involving industrial dust exposure (sarcoidosis [Fig. 3-38], blastomycosis). Eggshell calcification most commonly affects the bronchopulmonary nodes. Although it has also been found in abdominal, axillary, and cervical lymph nodes in patients with silicosis, its presence in these areas is always accompanied by similar calcifications within intrathoracic nodes.

BIBLIOGRAPHY
Fraser RG, Pare JAP: Diagnosis of Diseases of the Chest. Philadelphia, WB Saunders, 1977
Grayson CE, Blumenfeld H: "Egg shell" calcifications in silicosis. Radiology 53:216–226, 1949

FIG. 3-36. *(Left)* Frontal and *(right)* lateral chest radiographs demonstrate severe chronic pulmonary disease and eggshell calcifications (**arrows**) in a patient with silicosis.

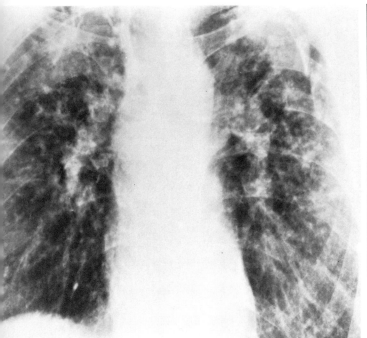
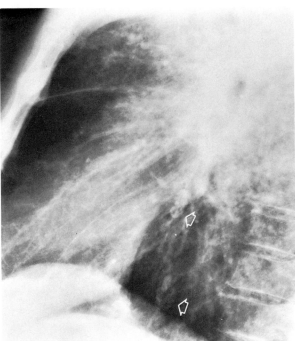

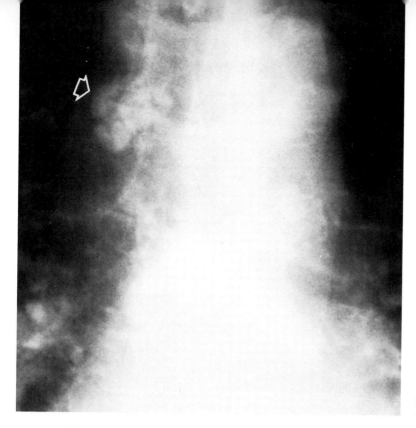

FIG. 3-37. Typical nodal calcification (**arrow**) due to granulomatous disease.

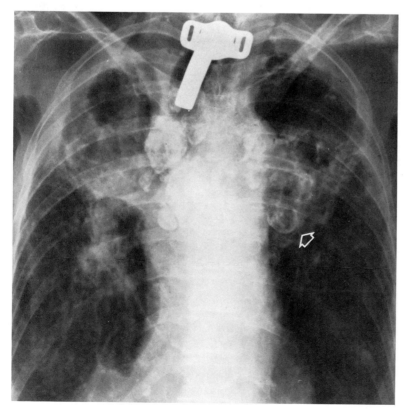

FIG. 3-38. Eggshell lymph node calcification (**arrow**) in a patient with severe chronic sarcoidosis. (Taken from the Diagnostic Radiological Health Sciences Learning Laboratory, as developed by the Radiological Health Sciences Education Project, University of California at San Francisco, under contract with the Bureau of Radiological Health, Food and Drug Administration, and in cooperation with the American College of Radiology)

Empty Mediastinum Sign

Excessive lucency of the anterior mediastinum, giving it an empty appearance (Fig. 3-39), may reflect an abnormally small thymus in infants with combined immune deficiency disease. This is not a pathognomonic finding of dysgenesis of the thymus due to immunologic defect; a similar appearance can be seen in patients with secondary thymic involution due to chronic disease, steroids, or cachexia.

BIBLIOGRAPHY

Presberg HA, Singleton EB: Combined immune deficiency disease: Its radiographic expression. Radiology 91:959–964, 1968

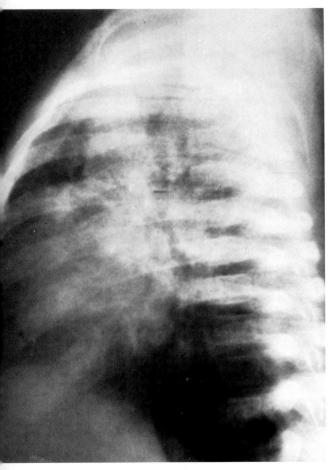

FIG. 3-39. Excessive lucency of the anterior mediastinum in a 9-month-old girl with combined immune deficiency disease and *Pneumocystis* pneumonia. (Presberg HA, Singleton EB: Combined immune deficiency disease: Its radiographic expression. Radiology 91:959–964, 1968)

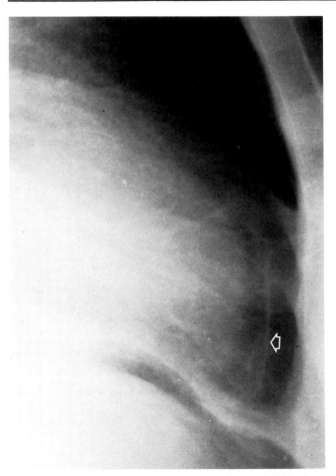

FIG. 3-40. Thin, relatively dense line (**arrow**) representing the normal pericardium lies between the anterior mediastinal and subepicardial fat.

Epicardial Fat Pad Sign

On routine lateral chest films, the anterior mediastinal and subepicardial fat can be visualized on either side of a pencil-thin line representing the normal pericardium (Fig. 3-40). Separation of the subepicardial fat stripe from the anterior mediastinal fat by a soft-tissue density of more than 2 mm is essentially pathognomonic of pericardial effusion or thickening (epicardial fat pad sign; Fig. 3-41). A similar appearance has also been described to be of value in the diagnosis of pericardial effusions on frontal chest radiographs (Fig. 3-42).

BIBLIOGRAPHY

Carsky EW, Mauceri RA, Azimi F: The epicardial fat pad sign: Analysis of frontal and lateral chest radiographs in patients with pericardial effusion. Radiology 137:303–308, 1980

Lane EJ, Carsky EW: Epicardial fat: Lateral plain film analysis in normals and in pericardial effusion. Radiology 91:1–5, 1968

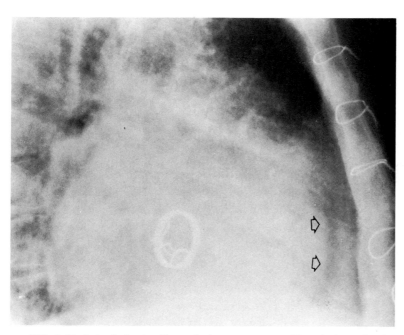

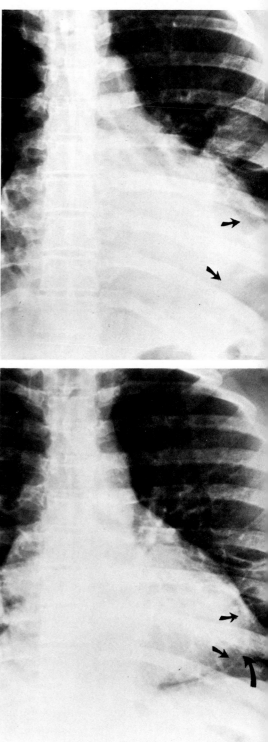

FIG. 3-41. Lateral chest radiograph demonstrates a wide soft-tissue density separating the subepicardial fat stripe (**arrows**) from the anterior mediastinal fat, an essentially pathognomonic sign of pericardial effusion or thickening.

FIG. 3-42. *(Top)* Frontal radiograph demonstrates a positive epicardial fat pad sign (**arrows**) in a patient with myxedema. *(Bottom)* About 10 weeks later, the pericardial fluid has nearly resolved. Epicardial fat (**small arrows**) and mediastinal fat are clearly seen adjacent to the thin pericardial fluid stripe (**large arrow**). (Carsky EW, Mauceri RA, Azimi F: The epicardial fat pad sign: Analysis of frontal and lateral chest radiographs in patients with pericardial effusion. Radiology 137:303–308, 1980)

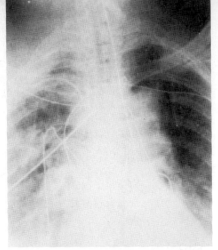

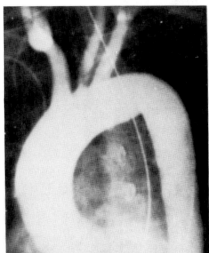

Esophageal Tube Displacement Sign ▰▰▰▰▰▰

Displacement of an opaque nasogastric tube to the right, indicative of esophageal displacement, has been reported as the most reliable plain film sign for the diagnosis of acute traumatic rupture of the thoracic aorta. Blunt trauma to the chest and back produces a hematoma in the anterior and posterior mediastinum, respectively. Although the hematoma may cause widening of the mediastinum visible on frontal chest radiographs, it is not strategically positioned to shift the relationship between the aorta and the esophagus or trachea, both of which are located in the middle mediastinum close to the aortic arch and isthmus (Fig. 3-43). In contrast, a hematoma in the middle mediastinum caused by a traumatic aortic aneurysm does displace the esophagus and trachea (Fig. 3-44). Therefore, demonstration of esophageal tube displacement is considered an indication for emergency aortography.

BIBLIOGRAPHY

Gerlock AJ, Muhletaler CA, Coulam CM et al: Traumatic aortic aneurysm: Validity of esophageal tube displacement sign. AJR 135:713–718, 1980

Tisnado J, Tsai FY, Als A et al: A new radiographic sign of acute traumatic rupture of the thoracic aorta: Displacement of the nasogastric tube to the right. Radiology 125:603–608, 1977

FIG. 3-43. *(Top)* Supine anteroposterior chest radiograph demonstrates multiple right rib fractures and a widened mediastinum but no right displacement of the nasogastric tube. *(Bottom)* Normal thoracic aortogram of the same patient, who had sustained a posttraumatic posterior mediastinal hematoma. (Gerlock AJ, Muhletaler CA, Coulam CM et al: Traumatic aortic aneurysm: Validity of esophageal tube displacement sign. AJR 135:713–718, 1980. Copyright 1980. Reproduced by permission)

FIG. 3-44. *(Left)* Admission chest radiograph demonstrates widening of the mediastinum. The nasogastric tube is in the midline. *(Center)* Chest radiograph obtained 8 hours later demonstrates displacement of the nasogastric tube to the right. *(Right)* Arteriography demonstrates a pseudoaneurysm at the isthmus of the aorta **(arrow).** (Tisnado J, Tsai FY, Als A et al: A new radiographic sign of acute traumatic rupture of the thoracic aorta: Displacement of the nasogastric tube to the right. Radiology 125:603–608, 1977)

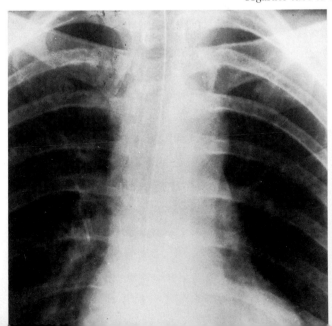

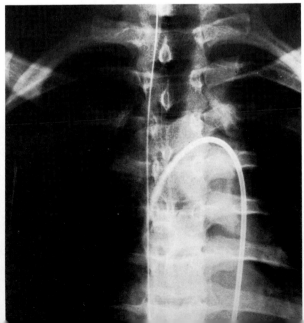

Extrapleural Sign

The extrapleural sign is a combination of radiographic findings caused by mass lesions involving the extrapleural space. Because the overlying intact parietal and visceral pleura tends to smooth out minor surface irregularities of the mass, an extrapleural lesion usually has a very sharp convex contour facing the lung (Fig. 3-45, *left*). An extrapleural mass tends to have tapered superior and inferior edges (Fig. 3-45, *right*) and a horizontal diameter that is often almost as great as the vertical diameter. This sign can generally be used to differentiate extrapleural masses (*e.g.*, those arising from the ribs, mediastinum, and diaphragm) from intrapulmonary lesions (Fig. 3-46).

BIBLIOGRAPHY

Felson B: Chest Roentgenology. Philadelphia, WB Saunders, 1973
Paul LW: Neurogenic tumors at the pulmonary apex. Dis Chest 11:648–661, 1945

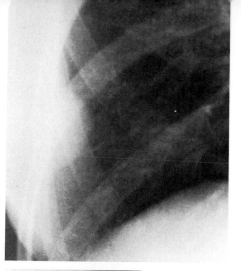
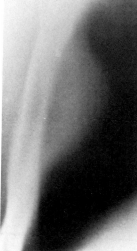

FIG. 3-45. *(Top)* Frontal chest radiograph and *(bottom)* tomographic view demonstrate the extrapleural sign. Note the sharp contour of the mass convex to the lung and the tapered superior and inferior edges.

FIG. 3-46. *(Top)* Rib metastasis from adenocarcinoma of the stomach has produced a large mass with the extrapleural sign. Note the destruction of the left third rib **(arrow).** *(Bottom)* Six months later, the extrapleural sign has disappeared and there is obvious pleural and pulmonary invasion. At autopsy, the tumor was found to have broken through the pleura into the lung. (Felson B: Chest Roentgenology. Philadelphia, WB Saunders, 1973)

. 3-44 *(Right).*

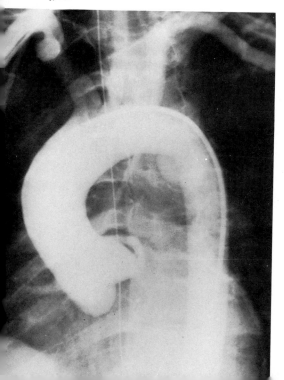

FIG. 3-45.
FIG. 3-46.

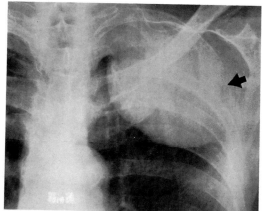

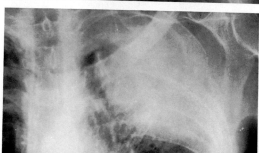

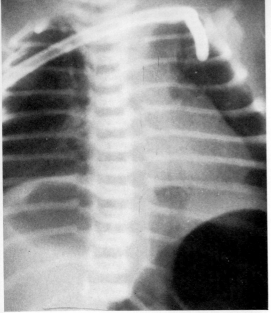

Extrapleural Air Sign

Pneumomediastinum occurs in more than 1% of newborn infants with respiratory distress. Its diagnosis usually requires radiographic demonstration of free air in the various routes of dissection of pulmonary interstitial emphysema. The extrapleural air sign represents a collection of free mediastinal air between the parietal pleura and diaphragm of either hemithorax. It is limited above by a sharp pleural stripe and is located posterior to the domes of the diaphragm (Fig. 3-47). Although the collection of air in pneumomediastinum could be confused with a pneumothorax, it should not shift with change in body position.

BIBLIOGRAPHY

Lillard RL, Allen RP: The extrapleural air sign in pneumomediastinum. Radiology 85:1093–1098, 1965

A

FIG. 3-47. (**A**) Anteroposterior chest film demonstrates a prominent extrapleural air sign on the right that appears to lie below the right hemidiaphragm. A left chest tube is in place. (**B**) Lateral film. The extrapleural air sign is limited above by a well-defined pleural stripe. Barium defines the stomach. (**C**) Frontal view. The gastrointestinal tract is seen to be entirely separate from the extrapleural air. (**D**) Frontal and (**E**) lateral chest films obtained several days later demonstrate spontaneous regression of the free air and the extrapleural air sign. (Lillard RL, Allen RP: The extrapleural air sign in pneumomediastinum. Radiology 85:1093–1098, 1965)

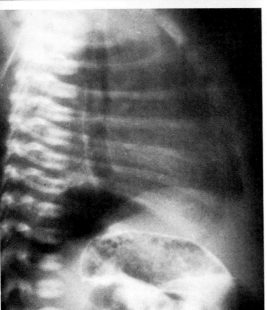

B

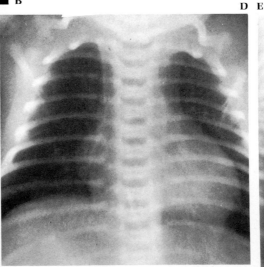

D E

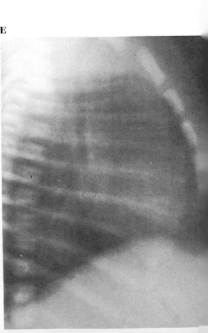

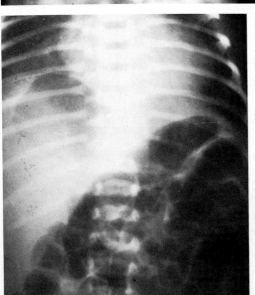

C

Figure 3 and Figure E Signs

Combined prestenotic and poststenotic dilatation of the aorta is present in many cases of postductal coarctation. This is seen as a figure 3 sign on plain chest radiographs (Fig. 3-48, *left*) and as a reverse figure 3, or figure E, sign on a barium esophagram (Fig. 3-48, *right*). The proximal bulge represents dilatation of the proximal aorta and base of the left subclavian artery; the distal bulge represents poststenotic dilatation (Fig. 3-49). When these signs of coarctation of the aorta are noted, the chest radiograph should be evaluated for characteristic rib notching (Fig. 3-50), which usually involves the posterior fourth to eighth ribs and is caused by the progressive dilatation of pulsating intercostal collateral arteries.

BIBLIOGRAPHY

Swischuk LE: Plain Film Interpretation in Congenital Heart Disease. Baltimore, Williams & Wilkins, 1979

FIG. 3-48. *(Left)* Plain chest radiograph in a patient with coarctation of the aorta demonstrates the figure 3 sign (the **arrow** points to the center of the 3). *(Right)* Barium swallow demonstrates the figure E sign (the **arrow** points to the center of the E). (Swischuk LE: Plain Film Interpretation in Congenital Heart Disease. Baltimore, Williams & Wilkins, 1979)

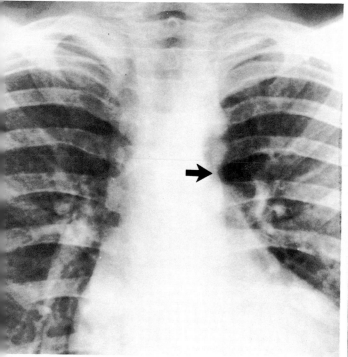
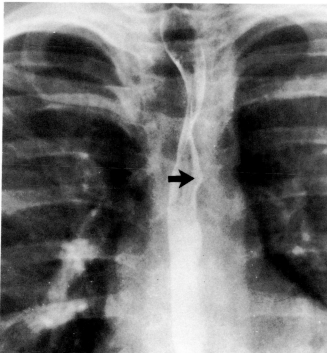

Figure 3 and Figure E Signs——213

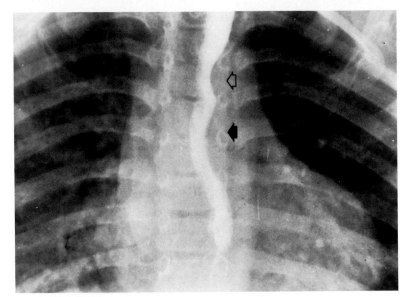

FIG. 3-49. Figure E sign in a patient with coarctation of the aorta. The upper bulge (**open arrow**) represents prestenotic dilatation; the lower bulge (**closed arrow**) represents poststenotic dilatation.

FIG. 3-50. Notching of the posterior fourth through eighth ribs (the **arrows** point to two examples). (Swischuk LE: Plain Film Interpretation in Congenital Heart Disease. Baltimore, Williams & Wilkins, 1979)

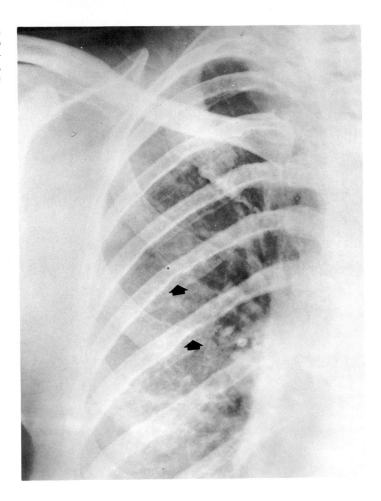

Flat Waist Sign

The *flat waist sign* refers to loss of the concavity of the left heart border on a perfectly symmetric frontal projection (Fig. 3-51). This appearance represents slight right anterior oblique rotation of the heart caused by left lower lobe collapse. The sign can be of value in the differentiation of left lower lobe collapse from compression of the left lower lobe secondary to left upper lobe emphysema, in which the concavity of the left heart border is preserved.

BIBLIOGRAPHY
Kattan KR, Wiot JF: Cardiac rotation in left lower lobe collapse: The "flat waist" sign. Radiology 118:275–276, 1976

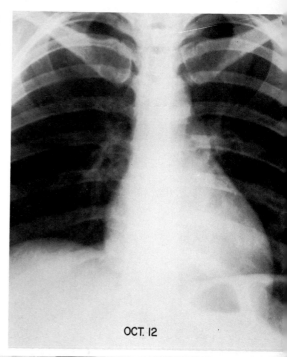

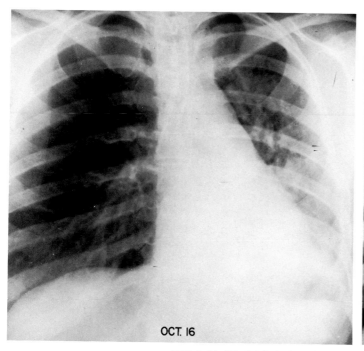

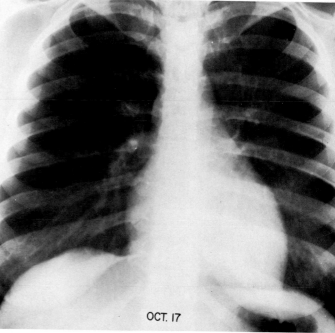

FIG. 3-51. (*Top*) Admission chest radiograph demonstrates normal concavity of the left heart border. (*Bottom, left*) Left lower lobe collapse developed after low insertion of a tracheal tube. In addition to other signs of left lower lobe collapse, the left heart border is straight (flat waist sign). (*Bottom, right*) After adjustment of the tracheal tube, the left lower lobe re-expanded, and the normal concavity of the left heart border is again seen. (Kattan KR, Wiot JF: Cardiac rotation in the lower lobe collapse: The flat waist" sign. Radiology 118:275–276, 1976)

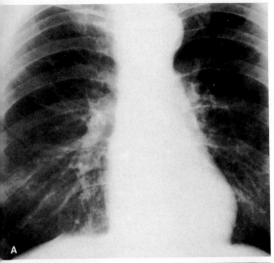

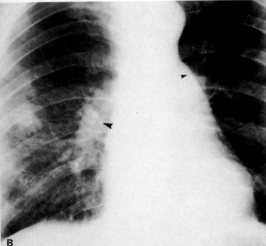

Fleischner (Plump Hilus) Sign

In patients with pulmonary thromboembolism, there is often enlargement of the ipsilateral main pulmonary artery (Fig. 3-52) due to pulmonary hypertension or distention of the vessel by bulk thrombus. In addition to an increase in size, there is usually abrupt distal tapering of the occluded vessel, often with sudden termination. As lysis and fragmentation of clot occurs, the widened pulmonary artery tends to rapidly diminish in size and revert to a normal caliber.

BIBLIOGRAPHY
Fleischner FG: Unilateral pulmonary embolism with increased compensatory circulation through the unoccluded lung. Radiology 73:591–597, 1959

FIG. 3-52. (**A**) Baseline chest radiograph. (**B**) Enlargement of the main pulmonary artery (**small arrow**) and right pulmonary artery (**large arrow**). (**C**) Arteriogram demonstrates multiple bilateral pulmonary emboli with a large right saddle embolus (**arrow**). (Julien P: Pulmonary embolism. In Eisenberg RL, Amberg JR (eds): Critical Diagnostic Pathways in Radiology: An Algorithmic Approach. Philadelphia, JB Lippincott, 1981)

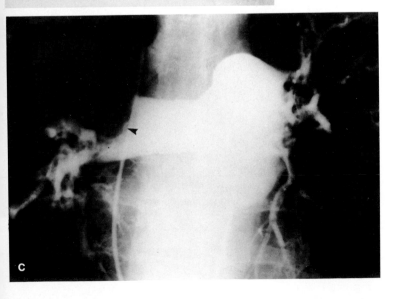

Gloved Finger Shadow Sign

When bronchiectatic segments become filled with retained mucus or pus, their tubular appearance is transformed into homogeneous band-like densities resembling gloved fingers (Fig. 3-53).

BIBLIOGRAPHY

Simon G: Principles of Chest X-Ray Diagnosis. London, Butterworth, 1971

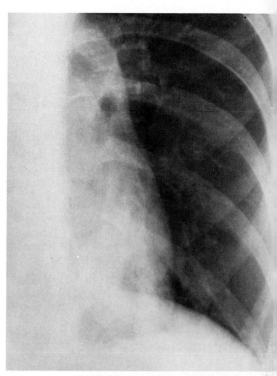

FIG. 3-53. *(Top)* Frontal radiograph of the lower half of the left lung shows several broad, slightly divergent line shadows situated in the bronchovascular distribution of the left lower lobe and producing an appearance resembling gloved fingers. *(Bottom)* A bronchogram shows severe varicose bronchiectasis of several of the basal bronchi of the left lower lobe. The appearance in the *bottom* figure is produced by the filling of these dilated bronchi with mucus and pus. (Fraser RG, Pare JAP: Diagnosis of Diseases of the Chest. Philadelphia, WB Saunders, 1979)

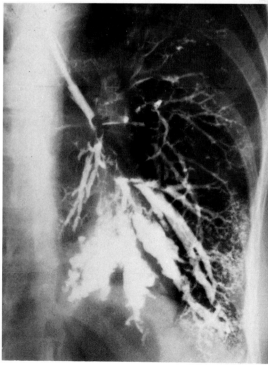

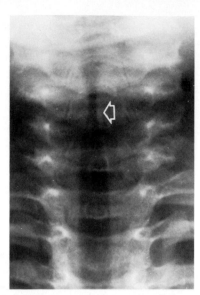

FIG. 3-54. Smooth, tapered narrowing of the subglottic portion of the trachea in a child with croup.

Gothic Arch Sign

In croup, viral or bacterial infection produces inflammatory obstructive swelling localized to the subglottic portion of the trachea. This produces the gothic arch sign (Fig. 3-54), a smooth, tapered narrowing of the airway unlike the broad shouldering seen normally (Fig. 3-55).

BIBLIOGRAPHY
Dunbar JS: Epiglottitis and croup. J Can Assoc Radiol 12:86–95, 1961

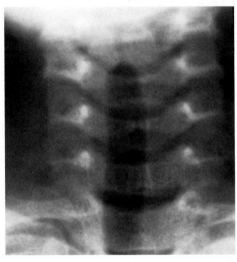

FIG. 3-55. Normal trachea with broad shouldering in the subglottic region.

Gravitational Shift Sign

In intensive care unit patients with diffuse pulmonary infiltrates, it is often difficult to determine whether there is evidence of pulmonary edema. Frontal films obtained before and after prolonged lateral decubitus positioning may demonstrate excess lung water manifested by a shift in infiltrate to the dependent lung with clearing or no change on the opposite side (gravitational shift sign; Fig. 3-56). A positive gravitational shift sign is a strong indication for a trial of diuretic therapy aimed at mobilizing excess lung water.

BIBLIOGRAPHY

Zimmerman JE, Goodman LR, St. Andre AC et al: Radiographic detection of mobilizable lung water: The gravitational shift test. AJR 138:59–64, 1982

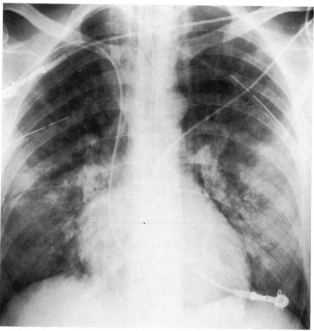

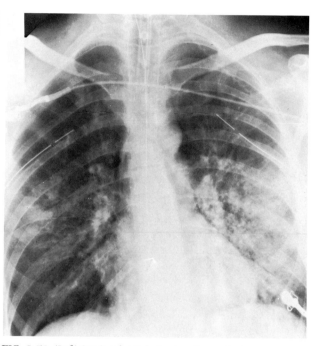

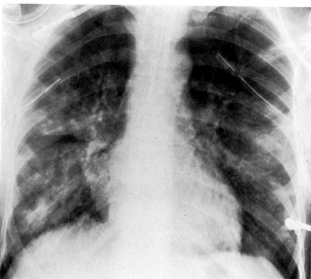

FIG. 3-56. (*Left*) Supine frontal chest radiograph demonstrates bilateral alveolar infiltrates. (*Right*) Shift radiograph exposed by a similar technique after 2 hr of left lateral decubitus positioning. The amount of infiltrate has increased in the dependent left lung; the right lung remains stable. (*Bottom*) Shift radiograph exposed using similar technique after 2.5 liter diuresis and 2 hr of right lateral decubitus positioning. The infiltrate has shifted to the dependent right lung with partial clearing on the left side. Additional diuresis resulted in complete clearing. (Zimmerman JE, Goodman LR, St. Andre AC et al: Radiographic detection of mobilizable lung water: The gravitational shift test. AJR 138:59–64, 1982. Copyright 1982. Reproduced by permission)

Halo Sign

A continuous radiolucent band of gas that conforms to the cardiac outline and does not extend beyond the level of the great vessels is a classic finding in neonatal pneumopericardium (Fig. 3-57). If the pneumopericardium is small, however, the pericardial gas may be present only along a single border. In such cases, pneumopericardium can be distinguished from other forms of extraventilatory gas in that gas in the pericardial space may extend inferior to the heart but not above the level of the great vessels, whereas gas in the pleural or mediastinal space may extend above the great vessels (Fig. 3-58) but does not collect beneath the heart, except in the case of bilateral tension or central pneumothoraces.

BIBLIOGRAPHY
Burt TB, Lester PD: Neonatal pneumopericardium. Radiology 142:81–84, 1982

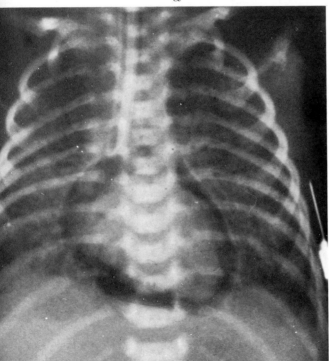

FIG. 3-57. Classic halo appearance of pneumopericardium. The endotracheal tube is in the right main stem bronchus. (Burt TB, Lester PD: Neonatal pneumopericardium. Radiology 142:81–84, 1982)

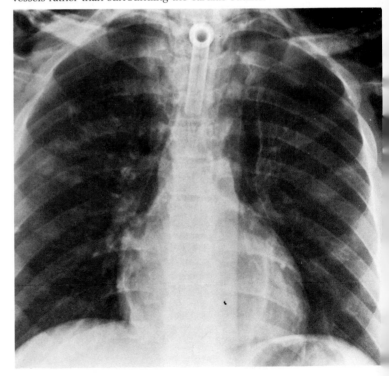

FIG. 3-58. In this patient with pneumomediastinum secondary to a tracheal tear, gas extends well above the level of the great vessels rather than surrounding the cardiac outline.

Hampton's Hump Sign

Hampton's hump sign is an aid in the differentiation of pulmonary infarction from pleural thickening or free pleural fluid in the costophrenic angle. A pulmonary infarct in this common site has a border that is usually convex toward the hilum (Fig. 3-59), in contrast to pleural thickening and free pleural fluid, which tend to have a concave margin toward the hilum (Fig. 3-60).

BIBLIOGRAPHY

Hampton AO, Castleman B: Correlation of postmortem chest teleroentgenograms with autopsy findings: With special reference to pulmonary embolism and infarction. AJR 43:305–326, 1940

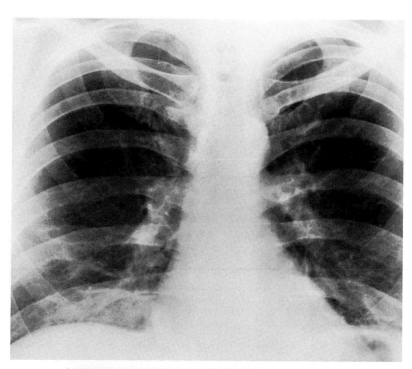

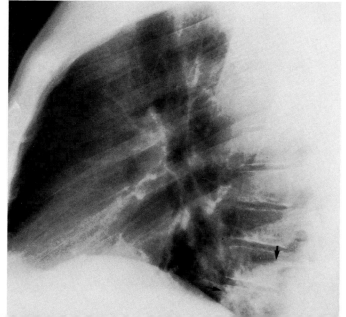

FIG. 3-59. *(Top)* Posteroanterior and *(bottom)* lateral radiographs of a 40-year-old man demonstrate a fairly well circumscribed shadow of homogeneous density occupying the posterior basal segment of the right lower lobe. On lateral projection, the shadow has the shape of a truncated cone and is convex toward the hilum (Hampton's hump; **arrows**). A small effusion can be identified on lateral projection. This combination of changes is highly suggestive of pulmonary infarction; the history and biochemical findings were compatible with the diagnosis. (Fraser RG, Pare JAP: Diagnosis of Diseases of the Chest. Philadelphia, WB Saunders, 1978)

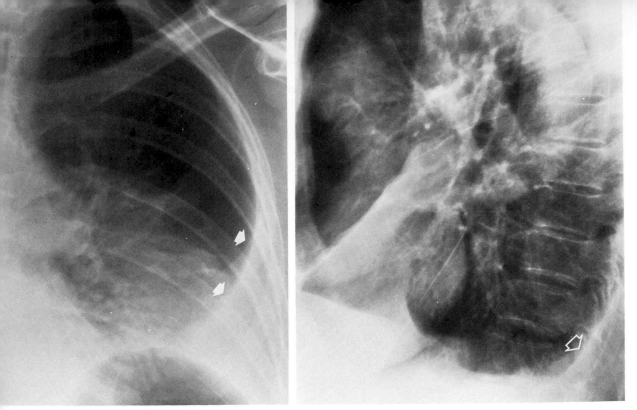

FIG. 3-60. Two patients with free pleural fluid in which the radiographic shadow has a concave margin toward the hilum on *(left)* frontal and *(right)* lateral views.

FIG. 3-61 *(Far, left).*

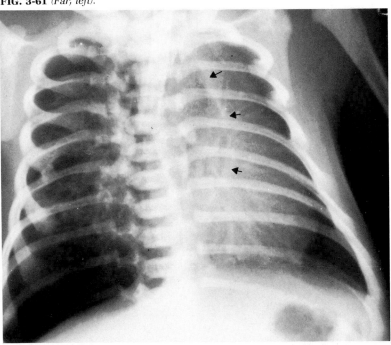

Herniated Mediastinal Pleural Sac Sign ▬▬▬▬▬

In the supine patient, gas in the pleural space tends to collect medial to the lung, producing a medial pneumothorax. In the newborn, pneumothorax is most frequently associated with respiratory distress syndrome, in which there is usually a large amount of intrapleural gas, often under tension. Extension of the medial pneumothorax with herniation of the pleura anteriorly across the midline into the contralateral hemithorax is a common occurrence. On anteroposterior supine radiographs, the gas-containing hernia sac appears as a characteristic crescent-shaped lucency of variable length limited by the curvilinear distended pleura and in contact with the relatively opaque, partially collapsed contralateral lung (Fig. 3-61, *top*). This herniated mediastinal pleural sac sign is often associated with mediastinal shift to the side opposite the pneumothorax, and the overall radiographic appearance is similar to that described in elderly patients with tension pneumothorax. The herniated pleural sac may superficially resemble a pneumomediastinum, though the latter usually demonstrates a spinnaker sail sign without mediastinal shift.

In some patients treated with a chest tube, gas disappears more slowly from the herniated portion of the pleural sac than from elsewhere in the pleural sac (Fig. 3-61, *bottom*), presumably as a result of the rather remote position of the intrathoracic end of the chest tube relative to that of the sac. Therefore, in addition to being a useful confirmatory sign of pneumothorax, the herniated mediastinal pleural sac sign is also important in assessing the completeness of pleural drainage.

BIBLIOGRAPHY

Fletcher BD: Medial herniation of the parietal pleura: A useful sign of pneumothorax in supine neonates. AJR 130:469–472, 1978

Moskowitz PS, Griscom NT: The medial pneumothorax. Radiology 120:143–147, 1976

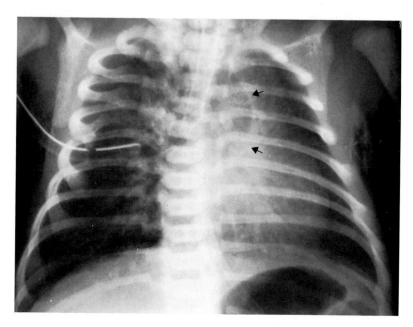

FIG. 3-61. *(Far left)* A large tension pneumothorax causes expansion of the right hemithorax, depression of the ipsilateral diaphragm, mediastinal shift, and bulging of the mediastinal pleura to the left of the midline **(arrows)**. *(Right)* After chest tube drainage, the pneumothorax is less obvious, although herniation of the mediastinal pleural sac into the left hemithorax remains **(arrows)**. Note that gas in the herniated pleural sac has disappeared more slowly than gas elsewhere in the pleural space. (Fletcher BD: Medial herniation of the parietal pleura: A useful sign of pneumothorax in supine neonates. AJR 130:469–472, 1978. Copyright 1978. Reproduced by permission)

Hilum Convergence Sign

The hilum convergence sign is of value in differentiating juxta-hilar mediastinal masses from vascular structures in patients with radiographic evidence of hilar enlargement. Convergence of pulmonary artery branches toward the mass rather than toward the heart implies that the mass represents an enlarged pulmonary artery (Fig. 3-62). The reverse appearance indicates the presence of an extravascular mediastinal mass (Fig. 3-63).

BIBLIOGRAPHY
Felson B: Chest Roentgenology. Philadelphia, WB Saunders, 1973

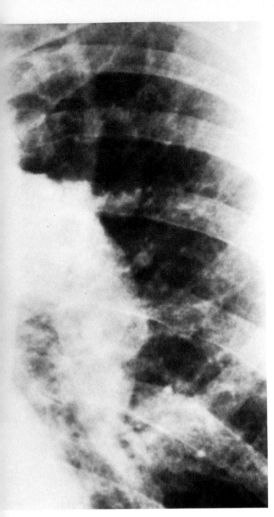

FIG. 3-62. Pulmonary artery branches converge toward a left hilar mass rather than toward the heart, implying that the mass represents an enlarged pulmonary artery in this patient with valvular pulmonary stenosis and poststenotic dilatation of the left pulmonary artery.

FIG. 3-63. Pulmonary artery branches converge toward the heart rather than toward the right infrahilar mass, which represented a bronchogenic carcinoma.

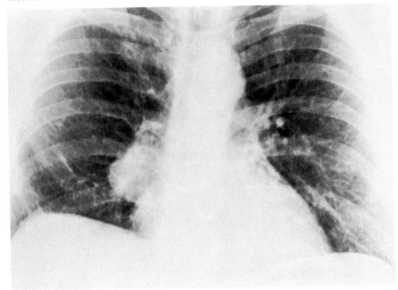

Hilum Overlay Sign

The hilum overlay sign is an aid in the differentiation of true cardiomegaly from a large anterior mediastinal mass mimicking cardiac enlargement. In normal patients, the main pulmonary arteries almost always lie lateral to the cardiac shadow or just within its outer edge. As the heart enlarges, the hilum is displaced laterally, though the normal apposition of the main arteries to the lateral edges of the cardiac margin is preserved. In contrast, an anterior mediastinal mass often overlaps a main pulmonary artery, which is then clearly visible within the margins of the mass (Fig. 3-64). Therefore, an anterior mediastinal mass is indicated on a posteroanterior chest film whenever more than 1 cm of the right or left pulmonary artery is visualized within the lateral edge of what appears to be the cardiac silhouette (Fig. 3-65).

BIBLIOGRAPHY
Felson B: Chest Roentgenology. Philadelphia, WB Saunders, 1973

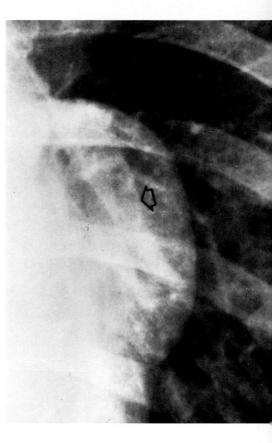

FIG. 3-64. An anterior mediastinal mass (thymic cyst) overlaps the major proximal left pulmonary arteries, which are clearly visible within the margins of the mass (**arrow**).

FIG. 3-65. *(Left)* Hilum overlay sign on a frontal chest radiograph. *(Right)* The lateral view clearly demonstrates the anterior position of the mass.

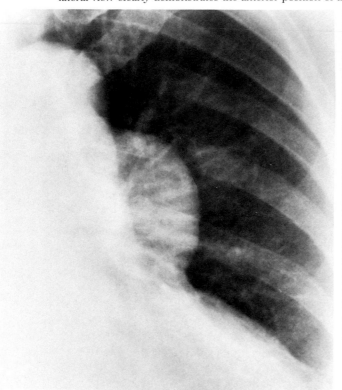
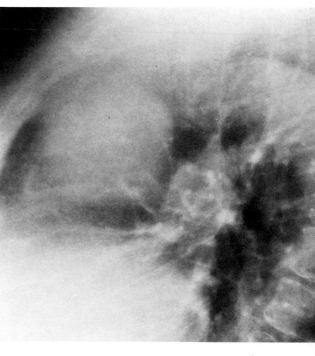

Hyperlucent Hemithorax Sign

On frontal radiographs in infants examined in the supine position, increased lucency of one hemithorax is a sign of free air accumulating over the anterior aspect of the lung (Fig. 3-66). With small volumes of air, the hyperlucent hemithorax can be overlooked, especially since the mediastinum is usually not grossly displaced and the involved hemidiaphragm is only slightly depressed. A valuable concomitant sign is unusual sharpness of the ipsilateral mediastinal edge due to free air, rather than aerated lung, located next to the mediastinal structures. When normal aerated lung abuts these structures, pulmonary bronchovascular markings cause a slight blurring of the mediastinal–pulmonary interface, decreasing the sharpness of the mediastinal edge. When free air is present, the lung and its bronchovascular markings are displaced posteriorly, allowing the mediastinal edge to be more clearly defined.

BIBLIOGRAPHY

Swischuk LE: Two lesser known but useful signs of neonatal pneumothorax. AJR 127:623–627, 1976

FIG. 3-66. *(Upper left)* The left hemithorax in this infant is more hyperlucent than the right on this supine frontal chest radiograph. The left mediastinal edge is sharper and crisper than the right. *(Upper right)* Standard lateral view shows a larger volume of air layering over the anterior surface of the left lung (**arrows**). *(Lower left)* Supine view of another infant with hyperlucent hemithorax and sharpness of the left mediastinal edge. The findings could be misinterpreted as being due to rotation to the left. *(Lower right)* Standard lateral film confirms the presence of air anterior to the left lung (**arrows**). (Swischuk LE: Two lesser known but useful signs of neonatal pneumothorax. AJR 127:623–627, 1976. Copyright 1976. Reproduced by permission)

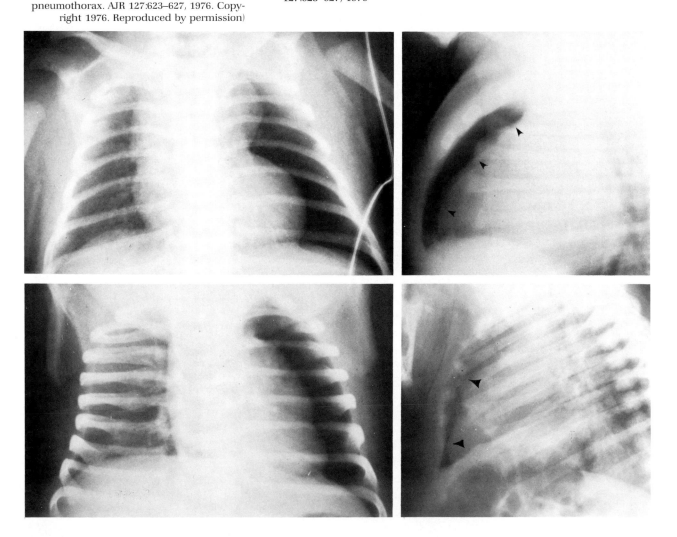

Iceberg (Thoracoabdominal) Sign

A sharply marginated mass visible through the diaphragm on either abdominal or chest radiographs must be in contact with air and thus lie at least partially in the thorax. Convergence of the lower lateral border of the mass toward the spine indicates that the bottom of the lesion is nearby and therefore that the mass is probably entirely thoracic. In contrast, lack of convergence or actual divergence of the lower border signifies an iceberg-like configuration, with a considerable segment hidden below in the abdomen (Fig. 3-67). Common examples of the iceberg sign include thoracoabdominal aneurysms, esophagogastric lesions, and azygos continuation of the inferior vena cava.

BIBLIOGRAPHY
Felson B: The mediastinum. Semin Roentgenol 4:41–58, 1969

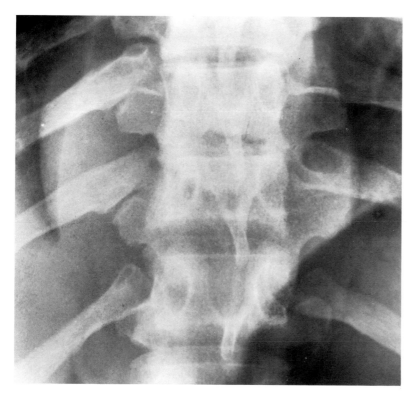

FIG. 3-67. In this patient with a paravertebral tuberculous abscess, there is lateral displacement of both right and left lower paravertebral lines, which diverge as they disappear into the abdomen.

Indrawn Pleura Sign

When a parenchymal mass of almost any cause is situated near the periphery of the lung, a line shadow may sometimes be seen extending from it to the visceral pleura. This is often associated with local indrawing of the pleura (Fig. 3-70). The indrawn pleura sign may be due to such causes as a fibrous scar subsequent to previous inflammatory disease or a zone of subsegmental atelectasis produced by bronchiolar obstruction secondary to the pulmonary mass. Because the sign has been reported in a large percentage of patients with alveolar cell carcinoma, this cell type should probably be suspected when the indrawn pleura sign is associated with a neoplastic process.

BIBLIOGRAPHY

Fraser RG, Pare JAP: Diagnosis of Diseases of the Chest. Philadelphia, WB Saunders, 1978

Simon G: Principles of Chest X-Ray Diagnosis. Philadelphia, FA Davis, 1956

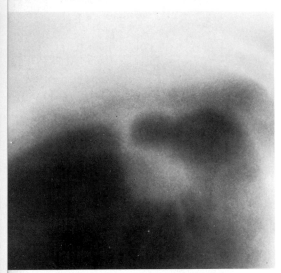

FIG. 3-70. Tomogram of the right upper lung demonstrates a line shadow extending from a peripheral parenchymal mass (squamous cell carcinoma) to the thickened and indrawn pleura.

FIG. 3-71. The anterior intercostal straight line of pleura and adjacent lung tissue closely follows the contour of the chest in this left oblique radiograph of a normal patient. (Schorr S, Aschner M: Intercostal lung bulging, a roentgen sign of emphysema in adults. Dis Chest 44:475–477, 1963)

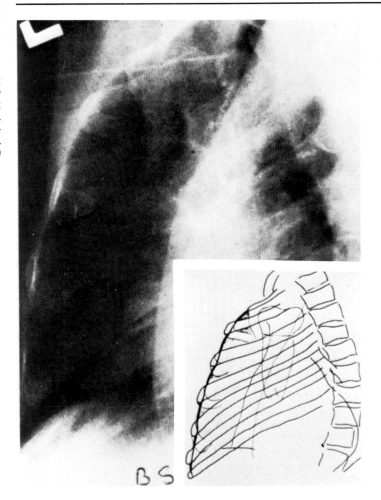

Intercostal Lung Bulging Sign

The pleural margin is normally relatively straight and regular and tends to follow the contour of the chest closely (Fig. 3-71). Ballooning of the lung in the intercostal spaces, especially on off-lateral or oblique views, has been reported as an early sign of pulmonary emphysema (Fig. 3-72). This intercostal lung bulging sign has been described in children as well as adults and has been reported to occur without any other radiographic signs of emphysema. However, the presence of intercostal bulging of the lung has also been described as a normal variant in nonemphysematous patients, some with severe wasting and some normal (Fig. 3-73 and 3-74). In these persons, the "sign" has been ascribed to a combination of x-rays striking the lung–intercostal interface tangentially and the normally increased intrusion of the lung into the interspace during maximum inspiration.

BIBLIOGRAPHY

Kattan KR, Spitz HB, Moskowitz M: Intercostal bulging of the lung without emphysema. AJR 112:542–545, 1971

Schorr S, Aschner M: Intercostal lung bulging, a roentgen sign of emphysema in adults. Dis Chest 44:475–477, 1963

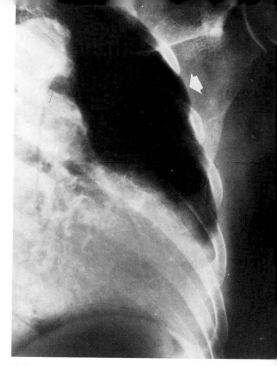

FIG. 3-73. Intercostal lung bulging (**arrow**) in a nonemphysematous, emaciated, elderly woman with carcinoma of the stomach. (Kattan KR, Spitz HB, Moskowitz M: Intercostal bulging of the lung without emphysema. AJR 112:542–545, 1971. Copyright 1971. Reproduced by permission)

FIG. 3-74. Lateral radiograph of a thin child with rheumatic fever shows prominent bulging of the intercostal spaces (**arrows**). (Kattan KR, Spitz HB, Moskowitz M: Intercostal bulging of the lung without emphysema. AJR 112:542–545, 1971. Copyright 1971. Reproduced by permission)

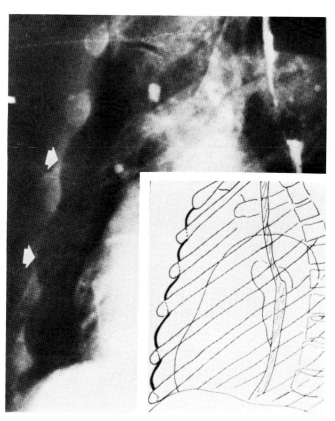

FIG. 3-72. Ballooning of the lung in the intercostal spaces (**arrows**) produces intercostal lung bulging in a patient with pulmonary emphysema. (Schorr S, Aschner M: Intercostal lung bulging, a roentgen sign of emphysema in adults. Dis Chest 44:475–477, 1963)

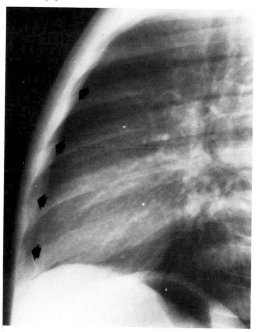

Juxtaphrenic Peak Sign

The juxtaphrenic peak, an indirect sign of upper lobe collapse, is usually seen on the posteroanterior radiograph as a small, sharply defined shadow projecting upward from the medial half of the hemidiaphragm at or near the highest point of the dome (Fig. 3-78). Its shape varies from that of a broad tent to a peak, steeple, or spire; occasionally, it is more rounded than angular. Rarely, there are twin peaks or even triple ones. The peak is often also visible in a lateral projection along the anterior half of the hemidiaphragm near its crest. The juxtaphrenic peak may be simulated by an interlobar fissure line adjacent to the right cardiophrenic angle, which is visible on frontal radiographs in about 5% of normal subjects (Fig. 3-79). Such a fissure line is rarely seen in the left lung. Although the mechanism of development of the juxtaphrenic sign is unclear, the appearance may occur when a segment of the basal pleura with its adipose tissue is retracted upward by the pull of increased negative pressure created by the collapse of an upper lobe. The smooth triangular shape and obliquity of the shadow strongly suggest that the apex of the tent is formed by an intrusion into a recess in the surface of the visceral pleura.

BIBLIOGRAPHY

Kattan KR, Eyler WR, Felson B: The juxtaphrenic peak in upper lobe collapse. Semin Roentgenol 15:187–193, 1980

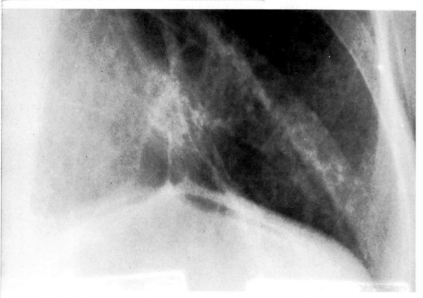

FIG. 3-78. Juxtaphrenic peak sign in left upper lobe collapse due to bronchogenic carcinoma. *(Top)* Posteroanterior film shows a heavy hilar density with silhouetting of the aortic knob and left heart border. Linear shadows extend upward from the crest of the elevated left hemidiaphragm. *(Bottom)* Closeup showing three fine, sharp spires, each extending from a small triangular wedge toward the lung root. The lines were thicker and less well defined in the lateral projection. (Kattan KR, Eyler WR, Felson B: The juxtaphrenic peak in upper lobe collapse. Semin Roentgenol 15:187–193, 1980. Reproduced by permission)

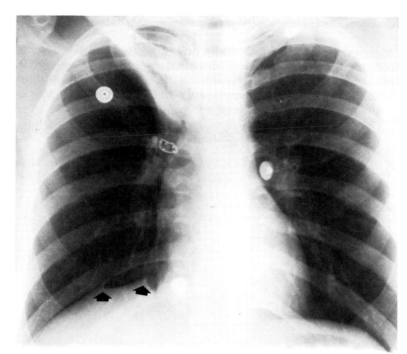

FIG. 3-79. (*Top*) Peaking at two sites (**arrows**) in an asthmatic woman with acute right upper lobe collapse. (*Bottom, left*) Closeup of (*top*). (*Bottom, right*) Normal radiograph obtained 1 day later. The medial peak has disappeared, but the lateral one, presumably representing the intersection of the inferior accessory fissure (**arrow**), persists. (Kattan KR, Eyler WR, Felson B: The juxtaphrenic peak in upper lobe collapse. Semin Roentgenol 15:187–193, 1980. Reproduced by permission)

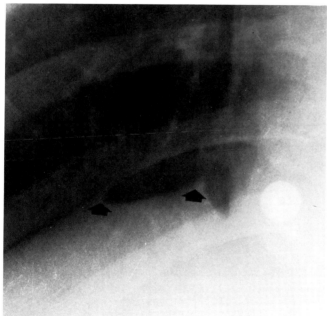

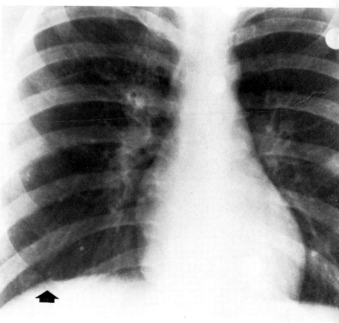

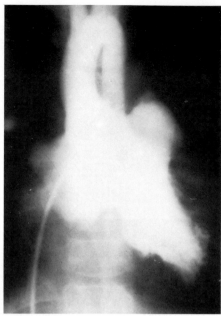

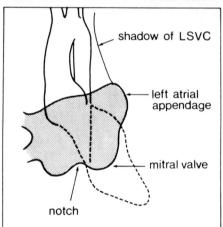

shadow of LSVC

left atrial
appendage

mitral valve

notch

Left Atrial Notch Sign

Persistence of the left superior vena cava is encountered in a number of children with congenital heart disease, and its preoperative diagnosis may be important to the cardiac surgeon. This persistent vessel can sometimes be identified on plain chest radiographs as a soft-tissue density in the upper left paramediastinum, though in young infants it often cannot be distinguished from a thymic shadow. Cardiac catheterization may demonstrate a notch in the inferior border of the left atrium (Fig. 3-82). This sign, which may be due to the dilated coronary sinus, has been reported to be diagnostic of a persistent left superior vena cava draining by way of the coronary sinus into the right atrium.

BIBLIOGRAPHY
Owen JP, Urquhart W: The left atrial notch: A sign of persistent left superior vena cava draining to the right atrium. Br J Radiol 52:855–861, 1979

FIG. 3-82. *(Top)* Film from a selective left ventricular angiogram and *(bottom)* corresponding line drawing demonstrate a notch on the inferior border of the left atrium in a patient with mitral regurgitation and widening of the left of the mediastinum due to a persistent left superior vena cava. (Owen JP, Urquhart W: The left atrial notch: A sign of persistent left superior vena cava draining to the right atrium. Br J Radiol 52:855–861, 1979)

Luftsichel Sign

The luftsichel is a crescentic paramediastinal translucency that is a sign of upper lobe collapse. It represents the interposition of the apex of the lower lobe between the mediastinum and the shrunken upper lobe, not mediastinal herniation as previously thought. The sign occurs more commonly on the left than the right. When the patient is erect, a left-sided luftsichel sign is associated with a sharp aortic knob border (Fig. 3-83); when the patient is supine, the border is obscured by silhouetting because the upper lobe falls backward in the recumbent position.

BIBLIOGRAPHY

Burgel E, Oleck HG: Über die rechtsseitige paramediastinale Luftsichel bei Oberlappenshrümpfung. Fortschr Geb Rontgenstr 93:160–163, 1960

Webber M, Davies P: The Luftsichel: An old sign in upper lobe collapse. Clin Radiol 32:271–275, 1981

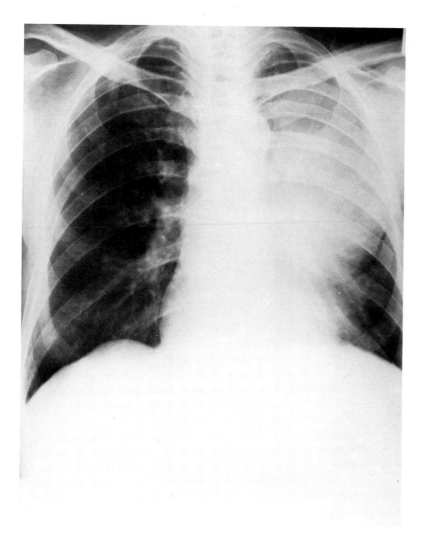

FIG. 3-83. In this patient with partial left upper lobe collapse, there is a paramediastinal translucency due to interposition of the apex of the lower lobe between the mediastinum and the shrunken upper lobe. The left heart border and hilum are obscured, and the left upper lobe bronchus is occluded. (Webber M, Davies P: The Luftsichel: An old sign in upper lobe collapse. Clin Radiol 32:271–275, 1981)

Medial Stripe Sign

In some cases of pneumothorax, free air accumulates around the lung (cloaking phenomenon). A medial collection of free air, especially when seen alone, may be misdiagnosed as a pneumomediastinum or pneumopericardium (Fig. 3-84). An indication that such air indeed represents a pneumothorax is that it is unilateral and extends almost parallel along the entire mediastinal edge (Fig. 3-85). This medial stripe sign frequently reaches the most inferior aspect of the cardiac silhouette, unlike pneumomediastinal air collections, which seldom reach this level and usually remain unilateral in distribution. Pneumopericardium can usually be readily distinguished because the collections are so large that the heart becomes completely surrounded by air. If the proper diagnosis is still in doubt, a lateral decubitus view with the involved side up should be obtained; air representing a medial pneumothorax shifts and rises to the top, whereas pneumomediastinal or pneumopericardial air remains unchanged.

BIBLIOGRAPHY
Swischuk LE: Two lesser known but useful signs of neonatal pneumothorax. AJR 127:623–627, 1976

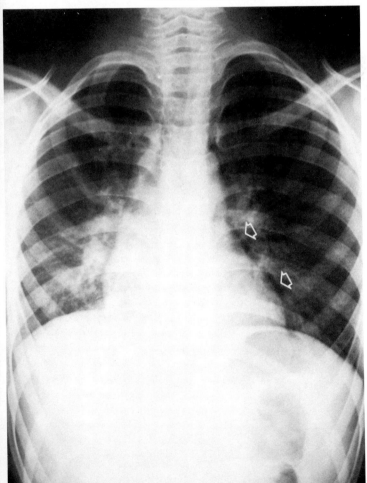

FIG. 3-84. A thin strip of free air along the left cardiac border (**arrows**) represents a medial pneumothorax, which could be confused with pneumomediastinum or pneumopericardium. (Swischuk LE: Emergency Radiology of the Acutely Ill or Injured Child. Baltimore, Williams & Wilkins, 1979)

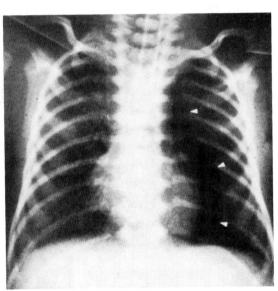

FIG. 3-85. Frontal chest radiograph demonstrates the medial stripe sign of medial pneumothorax. There is a wide stripe of free air along the medial aspect of the left lung extending along the entire mediastinum (**arrows**). The ipsilateral mediastinal edge is sharper than the right. (Swischuk LE: Two lesser known but useful signs of neonatal pneumothorax. AJR 127:623-627, 1976. Copyright 1976. Reproduced by permission)

Melting Sign

The melting sign is a characteristic resolution pattern of pulmonary infarcts on sequential chest radiographs that can be used to differentiate pulmonary infarcts from acute inflammatory and infectious disease processes involving the alveolar structures of the lung. The melting sign reflects a gradual reduction in size or shrinkage of the radiographic density, which retains the same general configuration seen on initial views (Fig. 3-86). There is resorption of the perimeters of the infarct with preservation of the pleural base. In contrast, the resolution of pneumonia tends to be patchy and is characterized by fading of the radiographic density throughout the entire involved area.

BIBLIOGRAPHY

Woesner ME, Sanders I, White GW: The melting sign in resolving transient pulmonary infarction. AJR 111:782–790, 1971

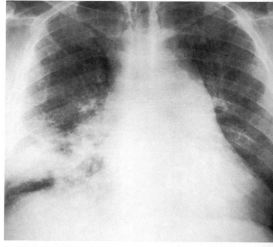

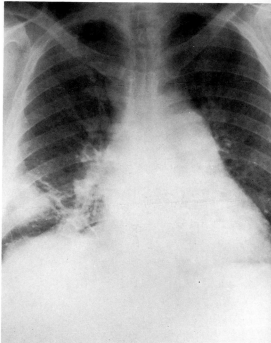

FIG. 3-86. *(Top)* On an anteroposterior radiograph made 3 days after the patient had undergone open heart surgery, a very irregular density is observed at the right base. The major differential diagnosis was between pneumonia and pulmonary embolization with infarction. *(Bottom)* On a film obtained 5 days later, the dense lesion is seen to have reduced in size yet to have retained the same general configuration seen on the initial view. The diagnosis of pulmonary embolism was confirmed on a radionuclide lung scan. (Woesner ME, Sanders I, White GW: The melting sign in resolving transient pulmonary infarction. AJR 111:782–790, 1971. Copyright 1971. Reproduced by permission)

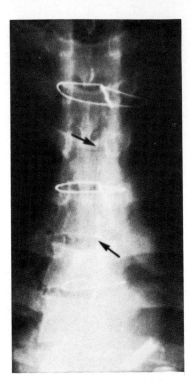

Midsternal Stripe Sign

Sternal dehiscence is a major complication of median sternotomy performed for surgical repair of the heart and great vessels. In one series, thin vertical lucent lines were seen in the immediate postoperative period in patients who later developed sternal dehiscence (Fig. 3-87). The absence of such a midsternal stripe sign in the postoperative film was reported to effectively rule out dehiscence. Therefore, the sign has been suggested as a tool in the identification of patients at high risk for this complication. Nevertheless, in this and other studies, the midsternal stripe sign has frequently been a transient phenomenon that has disappeared within a few days and has been unrelated to dehiscence (Fig. 3-88).

BIBLIOGRAPHY

Berkow AE, Demos TC: The midsternal stripe and its relationship to postoperative sternal dehiscence. Radiology 121:525, 1976

Escovitz ES, Okulski TA, Lapayowker MS: The midsternal stripe: A sign of dehiscence following median sternotomy. Radiology 121:521–524, 1976

FIG. 3-87. Anteroposterior chest radiograph obtained in the immediate postoperative period demonstrates a thin vertical lucent line **(arrows)** in a patient who later developed sternal dehiscence. (Escovitz ES, Okulski TA, Lapayowker MS: The midsternal stripe: A sign of dehiscence following median sternotomy. Radiology 121:521–524, 1976)

FIG. 3-88. Anteroposterior chest radiograph obtained on the third day after a coronary bypass procedure demonstrates a vertical lucent midsternal stripe **(arrow)** but no clinical evidence of dehiscence. (Berkow AE, Demos TC: The midsternal stripe and its relationship to postoperative sternal dehiscence. Radiology 121:525, 1976)

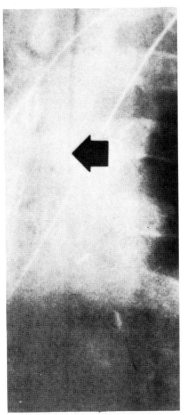

Migrating Staple Sign

Although pneumothorax is a common complication of thoracotomy, it may be difficult to demonstrate on postoperative portable chest films. If the thoracic surgeon uses a stapling device to suture the peripheral lung parenchyma, migration of the metal staples provides a radiographic sign of postoperative pneumothorax (Fig. 3-89). If the lung is fully expanded, the staples remain in the same location on serial chest films. When a pneumothorax develops, the lung parenchyma containing the staples collapses. As the amount of air in the pleural cavity increases, the lung tissue containing the metal staples retracts toward the hilum.

BIBLIOGRAPHY

Tegtmeyer CJ, Fu WR: A roentgenographic sign in the diagnosis of postoperative pneumothorax. J Can Assoc Radiol 24:76–77, 1973

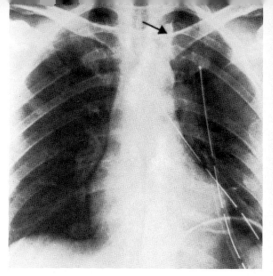

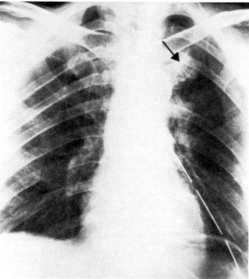

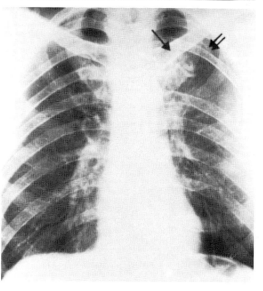

FIG. 3-89. *(Top)* Postoperative portable radiograph shows surgical staples (**arrow**) in the lung parenchyma. *(Center)* Radiograph 1 day later shows that the staples (**arrow**) have shifted toward the hilum, indicating a pneumothorax. The pleural edge is not seen. *(Bottom)* The pneumothorax is clearly visualized on a follow-up radiograph (**double arrow**). The staples (**single arrow**) are again seen in the new position. (Tegtmeyer CJ, Fu WR: A roentgenographic sign in the diagnosis of postoperative pneumothorax. J Can Assoc Radiol 24:76–77, 1973)

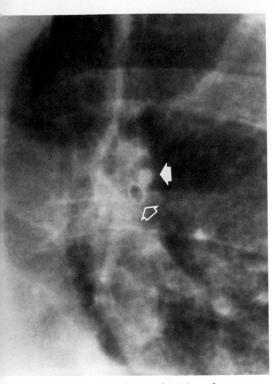

FIG. 3-90. The combination of an opaque central pulmonary artery seen on end (**closed arrow**) and the adjacent circular lucency of the accompanying bronchus (**open arrow**) produces the monocle sign.

Monocle Sign

A central pulmonary artery seen on end may appear sufficiently opaque to simulate a rounded calcified lymph node. However, the bronchus accompanying a central pulmonary artery shows an adjacent circular lucency, providing a means of differentiation (Fig. 3-90).

BIBLIOGRAPHY

Lillington GA, Jamplis RW: A Diagnostic Approach to Chest Diseases. Baltimore, Williams & Wilkins, 1977

Signs of Mucoid Impaction

Mucoid impaction refers to inspissation of tenacious mucoid sputum within one or more segmental or subsegmental bronchi. The condition predominantly involves the upper lobes and is often associated with asthma and bronchitis and occasionally with mucoviscidosis. On chest radiographs or conventional tomography, a mucoid impaction typically presents as an elongated opacity with undulating borders. A pair of impactions frequently forms a V, the apex of which is toward the hilus (V sign; Fig. 3-91). Involvement of numerous adjacent bronchi produces the cluster of grapes sign (Fig. 3-92).

BIBLIOGRAPHY

Tsai SH, Jenne JW: Mucoid impaction of the bronchi. AJR 96:953–961, 1966

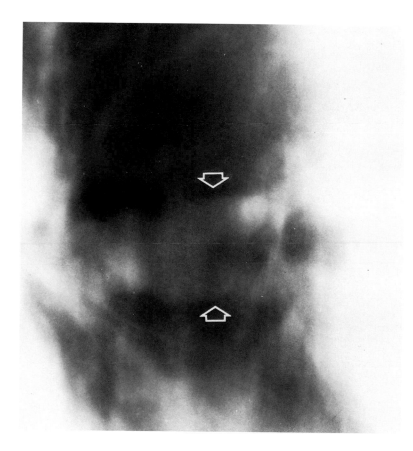

FIG. 3-91. Tomography of the lung demonstrates two mucoid impactions (**arrows**) in the lingula forming a V, the apex of which is toward the hilus. (Tsai SH, Jenne JW: Mucoid impaction of the bronchi. AJR 96:953–961, 1966. Copyright 1966. Reproduced by permission)

FIG. 3-92. Tomography of the lung demonstrates two mucoid impactions (**arrows**) in the superior segment of the right lower lobe. The scalloped borders suggest a cluster of grapes appearance. (Tsai SH, Jenne JW: Mucoid impaction of the bronchi. AJR 96:953–961, 1966. Copyright 1966. Reproduced by permission)

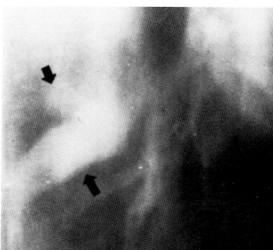

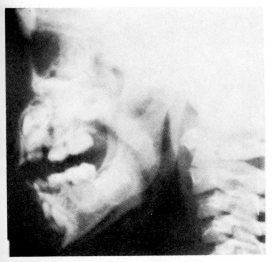

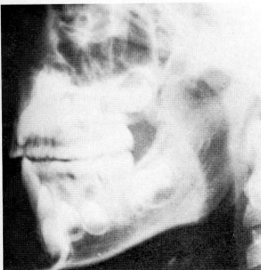

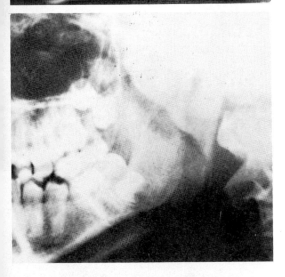

Neuhauser's Sign

Congenital agammaglobulinemia is an X-linked recessive trait (seen only in males) characterized by recurrent upper respiratory tract infection, extensive pulmonary parenchymal disease, and frequent sinusitis. The lymphoid tissue in persons with agammaglobulinemia, unlike that in normal patients, is devoid of plasma cells, and draining lymph nodes do not tend to enlarge in the normal way in response to local infection. Patients have a paradoxical absence of hilar node enlargement in the face of extensive pulmonary parenchymal disease and a striking deficiency of radiographically demonstrable adenoid tissue in the posterior nasopharynx (Neuhauser's sign; Fig. 3-93) despite recurrent upper respiratory tract infection and frequent sinusitis.

BIBLIOGRAPHY
Margulis AR, Feinberg SB, Lester RG et al: Roentgen manifestations of congenital agammaglobulinemia. Radiology 69:354–359, 1957
Rosen FS, Janeway CA: The gamma globulins. III. The antibody deficiency syndromes. N Engl J Med 275:709–715, 1966

FIG. 3-93. *(Top)* Lateral film of the nasopharynx of a 2-year-old boy with congenital agammaglobulinemia shows absence of normal lymphoid tissue. *(Center)* Lateral film of the nasopharynx of a 6-year-old boy with congenital agammaglobulinemia shows absence of normal lymphoid tissue. *(Bottom)* Lateral film of the nasopharynx of a normal child shows a normal amount of nasopharyngeal lymphoid tissue. (Margulis AR, Feinberg SB, Lester RG et al: Roentgen manifestations of congenital agammaglobulinemia. Radiology 69:354–359, 1957)

Obscured Outer Edge Sign

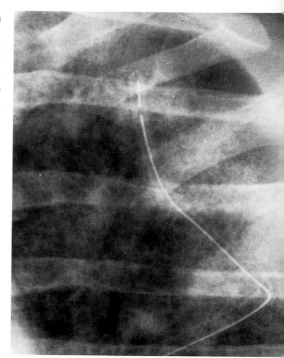

The ectopic location of an improperly placed pleural drainage tube used in the treatment of pneumothorax may not be appreciated on frontal radiographs of the chest. The extrapleural position of a chest tube may be identified by the obscured outer edge sign, a variant of the silhouette sign. The plastic material from which chest tubes are made, unless impregnated with a radiodense substance, has about the same density as soft tissue. Thus, a nonimpregnated tube lying within the pleural space and surrounded by free air or normally aerated lung should have a clearly defined edge because of the density difference between air and plastic (Fig. 3-94A). In contrast, if the tube lies within the chest wall, the similarity in density between the tube and the surrounding soft tissues often makes the outer edge of the tube invisible (Fig. 3-94B). When a nonopaque tube is projected over a pneumothorax or normally aerated lung on a frontal radiograph and its outer edge is invisible, an extrapleural location should be suspected and an appropriate oblique view obtained (Fig. 3-94C).

BIBLIOGRAPHY
Webb WR, Godwin JD: The obscured outer edge: A sign of improperly placed pleural drainage tubes. AJR 134:1062–1064, 1980

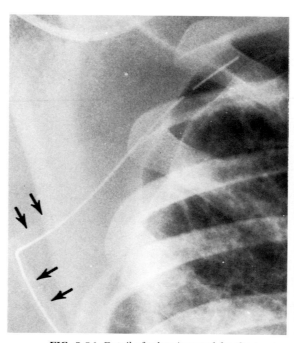

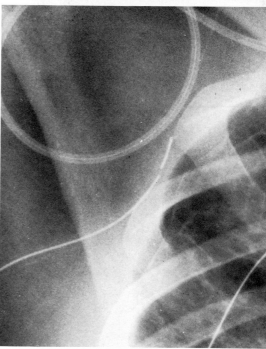

FIG. 3-94. Detail of tubes inserted for the treatment of pneumothoraces. *(Top)* The outer edge of the tube tip in the left apex is well defined by surrounding aerated lung. *(Left)* The outer edge of the tube in the right apex is well defined only in the extrathoracic portion of its course **(arrows).** The edge near the tip is obscured by chest wall soft tissues. *(Right)* An oblique view confirms the extrapleural location of the right apical tube. (Webb WR, Godwin JD: The obscured outer edge: A sign of improperly placed pleural drainage tubes. AJR 134:1062–1064, 1980. Copyright 1980. Reproduced by permission)

One—Two—Three Sign

The combination of right paratracheal and bilateral hilar lymph node enlargement has been described as a characteristic pattern of adenopathy in sarcoidosis (Fig. 3-95). Nevertheless, some authors report that paratracheal lymph node enlargement in sarcoidosis is far more often bilateral (Fig. 3-96) than right-sided only. This bilaterality can often be appreciated only on tomographic views; on routine frontal radiographs, the right paratracheal area is much more clearly visible than the left, which is obscured by the superimposed aorta and brachiocephalic vessels.

BIBLIOGRAPHY

Kirks DR, McCormick VD, Greenspan RH: Pulmonary sarcoidosis: Roentgenologic analysis of 150 patients. AJR 117:777–786, 1973

Theros EG: RPC of the month from the AFIP. Radiology 92:1557–1561, 1969

FIG. 3-95. *(Left)* Frontal and *(right)* lateral views of the chest demonstrate enlargement of the right and left hilar and right paratracheal lymph nodes, producing the classic pattern of adenopathy in sarcoidosis. (Taken from the Diagnostic Radiological Helath Sciences Learning Laboratory, as developed by the Radiological Health Sciences Education Project, University of California at San Francisco, under contract with the Bureau of Radiological Health, Food and Drug Administration, and in cooperation with the American College of Radiology)

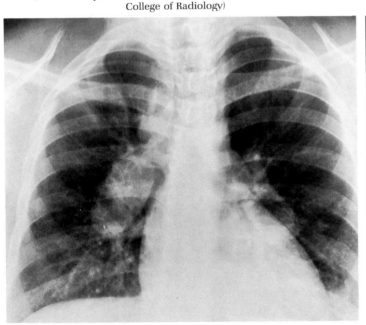
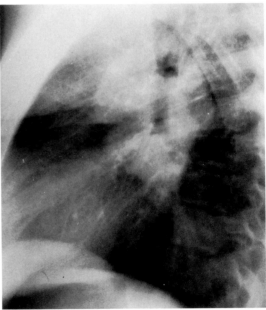
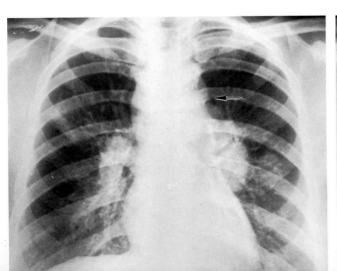
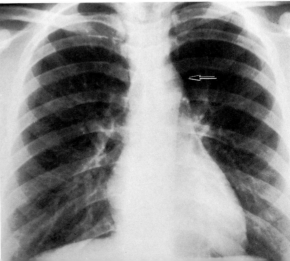

Paradoxical Movement of the Mediastinum Sign

In normal patients, chest fluoroscopy demonstrates narrowing of the mediastinal shadow during inspiration and enlargement of the shadow during expiration. In a patient with partial obstruction of air flow through the trachea or larynx, most often due to an impacted foreign body, the fluoroscopic pattern is the reverse of normal. The patient with partial upper airway obstruction has a decrease in intra-alveolar pressure and a more negative intrapleural pressure than normal. On inspiration (Fig. 3-97, *left*), the suction effect of the diaphragm increases, causing increased blood return to the heart and lungs and enlargement of the pulmonary vasculature and blood-containing structures of the mediastinum, especially on the venous side. During expiration, the intra-alveolar pressure increases, and the negative intrapleural pressure decreases. This squeezes the mediastinum and produces the radiographic pattern of a narrowed mediastinum, decreased pulmonary vasculature, and relative lucency of the lungs (Fig. 3-97, *right*), all the reverse of normal. Because conventional chest radiographs are often normal in patients with partial upper airway obstruction, fluoroscopic demonstration of paradoxical movement of the mediastinum may be the earliest diagnostic sign.

BIBLIOGRAPHY

Grünebaum M, Adler S, Varsano I: The paradoxical movement of the mediastinum: A diagnostic sign of foreign-body aspiration during childhood. Pediatr Radiol 8:213–218, 1979

Rigler LG: Functional roentgen diagnosis (Caldwell lecture 1958). AJR 82:1–24, 1959

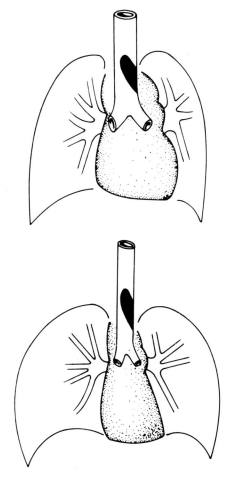

FIG. 3-97. Schematic drawing of the changes seen on radiographs in a patient in whom a foreign body is partially obstructing the tracheal lumen. *(Top)* On inspiration, there is widening of the mediastinal shadow and prominence of the pulmonary vasculature at the central part of the lungs. *(Bottom)* During the expiratory phase, the mediastinum narrows, and the pulmonary vasculature returns to normal. There is relative hyperinflation of the lungs. (Grünebaum M, Adler S, Varsano I: The paradoxical movement of the mediastinum: A diagnostic sign of foreign-body aspiration during childhood. Pediatr Radiol 8:213–218, 1979)

◀ **FIG. 3-96.** *(Left* Frontal chest radiograph demonstrates bilateral hilar and bilateral paratracheal lymphadenopathy in a patient with sarcoidosis. Enlargement of the left paratracheal lymph nodes **(arrow)** is evident as a soft-tissue density that silhouettes out the aortic arch. The pulmonary parenchyma is normal. *(Right)* Follow-up radiograph 2 years later is normal. There is no evidence of left paratracheal lymphadenopathy, and the aortic arch can be clearly identified **(arrow).** (Kirks DR, McCormick VD, Greenspan RH: Pulmonary sarcoidosis: Roentgenologic analysis of 150 patients. AJR 117:777–786, 1973. Copyright 1973. Reproduced by permission)

Pericardial Fat Tag Sign

A pneumothorax may be difficult to detect in critically ill patients examined in the supine or semierect position, because intrapleural air often assumes a subpulmonary position in recumbent patients even without underlying pulmonary disease. One reported specific sign of subpulmonary pneumothorax is the presence of lobulated, discrete densities of 1 cm to 1.5 cm seen adjacent to the cardiac apex (Fig. 3-98). These densities probably represent fat deposits lying on the pericardial surface. It is postulated that these fat tags become rounded and lobulated in the presence of a pneumothorax because they are no longer flattened by contact with the adjacent lung.

BIBLIOGRAPHY

Ziter FMH, Westcott JL: Supine subpulmonary pneumothorax. AJR 137:699–701, 1981

FIG. 3-98. Two patients with pericardial fat tags (**arrows**). Additional films demonstrated the presence of pneumothoraces.

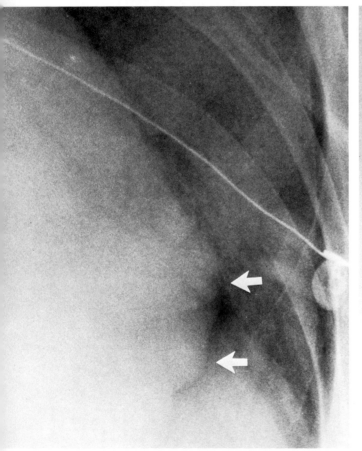

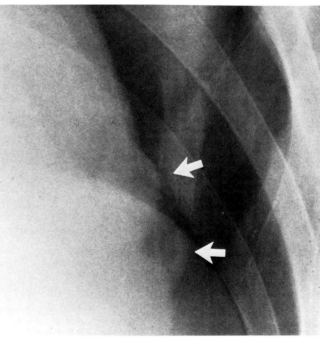

Pericardial Line Sign

In neonates with combined pneumopericardium and pneumomediastinum, a discrete line can often be seen extending inferolaterally from the pericardial reflection at the great vessels (Fig. 3-99). This pericardial line, composed of the parietal pericardium and a layer of fibrous tissue (the fibrous pericardium) lying between the air in the mediastinum and the pericardial air, is specific for pneumopericardium.

BIBLIOGRAPHY
Burt TB, Lester PD: Neonatal pneumopericardium. Radiology 142:81–84, 1982

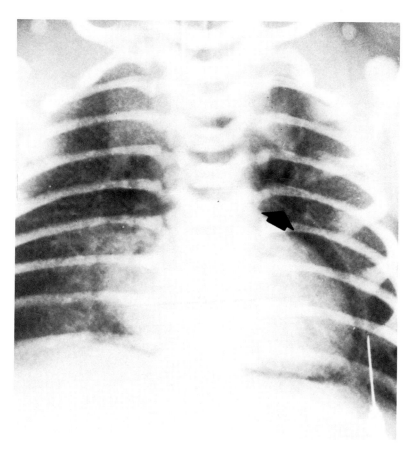

FIG. 3-99. The pericardium (**arrow**) is seen as a discrete line extending inferolaterally from the pericardial reflection and lying between the air in the mediastinum and the air in the pericardial sac. (Burt TB, Lester PD: Neonatal pneumopericardium. Radiology 142:81–84, 1982)

Phantom (Vanishing Tumor) Sign ▬▬▬▬▬

Interlobar effusion, especially in patients with heart failure, may cause a sharply defined elliptical or circular density that closely resembles a solid parenchymal tumor on frontal radiographs (Fig. 3-100). As the patient's cardiac status improves, the fluid density rapidly regresses (Fig. 3-101). Phantom tumors most often involve the minor fissure, though they may also be seen in the major fissure (Fig. 3-102). With subsequent attacks of heart failure, the fluid density tends to recur in the same area.

FIG. 3-100. *(Left)* Frontal and *(right)* lateral chest radiographs demonstrate a sharply defined elliptical density in the right midlung **(arrows)** resembling a solid parenchymal mass (Plantom tumor). Note the associated right pleural effusion and signs of pulmonary vascular congestion.

BIBLIOGRAPHY

Feder BH, Wilk SP: Localized interlobar effusion in heart failure: Phantom lung tumor. Dis Chest 30:289–297, 1956

Weiss W, Boucot KR, Gefter WI: Localized interlobar effusion in congestive heart failure. Ann Intern Med 38:1177–1186, 1953

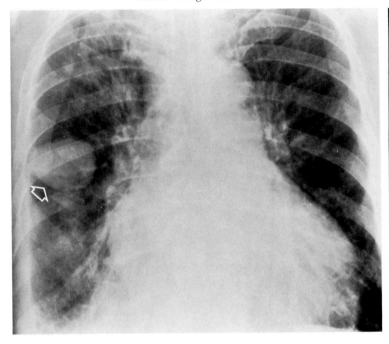

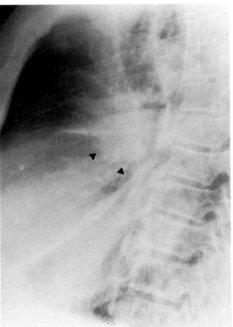

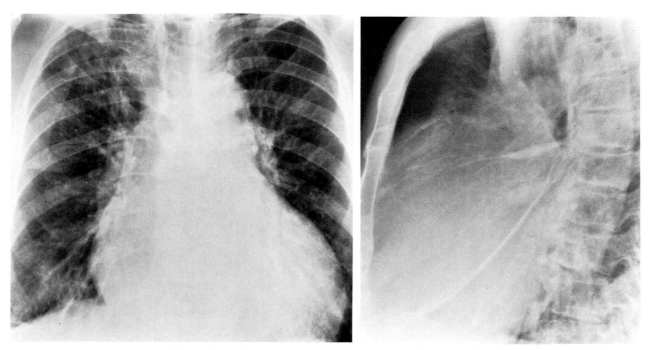

FIG. 3-101. *(Left)* Frontal and *(right)* lateral chest radiographs following improvement of the patient's cardiac status show rapid regression of the fluid density, clearly indicating the true nature of the phantom tumor.

FIG. 3-102. *(Left)* Frontal and *(right)* lateral chest radiographs demonstrate a phantom tumor (**arrow**) that developed in the lower portion of the major fissure following trauma. The lesion regressed completely within 1 week.

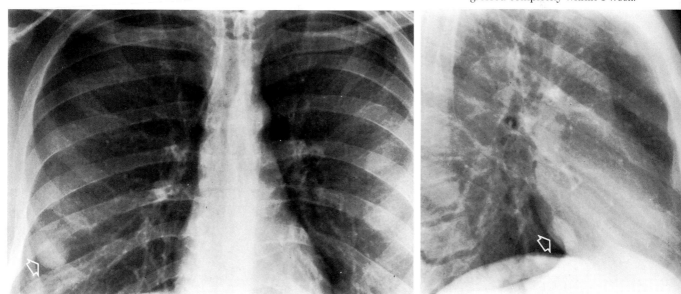

Pleuropulmonary Tail Sign

Several types of linear densities extending from a peripheral pulmonary lesion to the pleura (pleuropulmonary tails) have been described. A *pleural tail* is a thin, untapered linear density that arises from the lateral margin of a peripheral pulmonary nodule and terminates in a small triangular density at the pleural surface (Fig. 3-103). This appearance was originally regarded as pathognomonic of malignancy, primarily bronchioalveolar carcinoma (Fig. 3-104). A similar pattern, however, has been described in patients with various types of granulomatous disease. The *rabbit ears sign* has been defined as two or more thicker lines extending from a peripheral lesion to the pleura. A *participating tail* has been described as the total peripheral extension of one contour of a nodule in a configuration that is somewhat cone-shaped and gradually tapers toward the pleural surface (Fig. 3-105). Although this sign was originally reported as a radiographic sign of pulmonary granuloma, a similar pattern has been described with malignant processes.

The various pleuropulmonary tail signs appear to reflect thickened, fibrotic connective tissue septae with indrawing of the visceral pleura. In patients with malignant lesions, septal thickening results from fibrosis with or without tumor infiltration. A recent study has suggested that all three of these signs are nonspecific features of peripherally located pulmonary lesions and thus cannot be used to differentiate a malignant from a nonmalignant process. However, a tail sign may call attention to an otherwise obscure lesion, and transition from one type of sign to another has been reported as useful in evaluation of the activity of the process.

BIBLIOGRAPHY

Bryk D: The participating tail: A roentgenographic sign of pulmonary granuloma. Am Rev Respir Dis 100:406–408, 1969

Hill CA: "Tail" signs associated with pulmonary lesions: Critical reappraisal. AJR 139:311–316, 1982

Rigler LG: Bronchioloalveolar carcinoma of the lung: Report of new roentgenologic sign. International Congress of Radiology, Rome, September, 1965

Webb WR: The pleural tail sign. Radiology 127:309–313, 1978

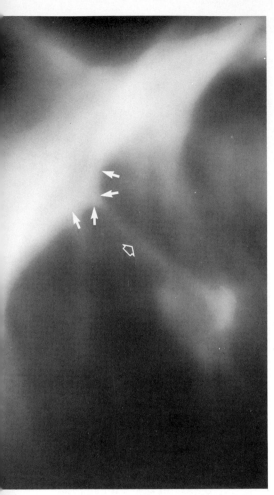

FIG. 3-103. Tomogram of the right upper lobe demonstrates a 1.5-cm granuloma associated with a 2.4-cm pleural tail (**open arrow**). The triangular densities (**closed arrows**) at the intersection of the tail and chest wall represent pleural dimpling. (Webb WR: The pleural tail sign. Radiology 127:309–313, 1978)

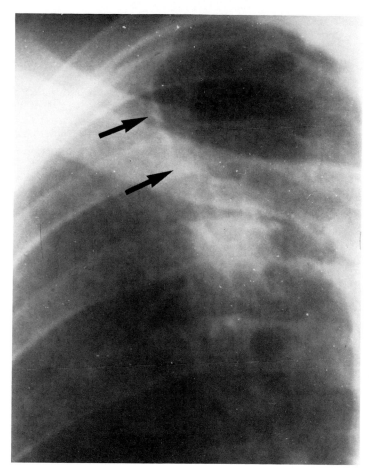

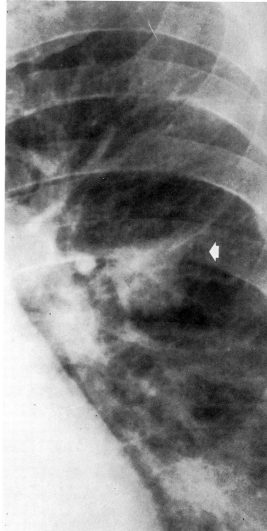

FIG. 3-104. Well-defined pleural tail (**arrows**) arising from a spiculated mass (bronchioalveolar carcinoma). (Webb WR: The pleural tail sign. Radiology 127:309–313, 1978)

FIG. 3-105. Granuloma in the superior segment of the left lower lobe with a participating tail. The lateral superior contour of the nodule extends in a gradually tapering fashion (**arrow**) and terminates in a line shadow that extends toward the pleural surface. (Bryk D: The participating tail: A roentgenographic sign of pulmonary granuloma. Am Rev Respir Dis 100:406–408, 1969)

Posterior Wedging Sign ▬▬▬▬

In patients with significant mitral insufficiency, cardiac fluoroscopy may demonstrate simultaneous splaying of the esophagus to the right and of the descending aorta to the left during ventricular systole. This posterior wedging sign is the result of sudden enlargement of the left atrium posteriorly and bilaterally caused by rapid filling, which in turn is primarily due to a large regurgitant flow from the left ventricle. The swiftly dilating left atrium thus becomes "wedged" between the two tubular structures, pushing them apart laterally and posteriorly (Fig. 3-106).

BIBLIOGRAPHY
Chen JTT, Lester RG, Peter RH: Posterior wedging sign of mitral insufficiency. Radiology 113:451–453, 1974

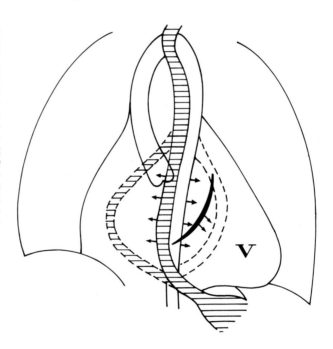

FIG. 3-106. Posterior wedging sign of severe mitral insufficiency. The descending aorta and esophagus *(shaded area)* may originally be close together in the midline. In systole, the esophagus is displaced to the right and the aorta to the left, as indicated by the **horizontal arrows.** The *heavy black stripe* between the two images of the aorta represents the atrioventricular groove. This groove contains a radiolucent fat line, which moves toward the apex of the left ventricle (**V**) during ventricular systole, (**oblique arrows**). The position of this line can be used for verification of the correct timing of the cardiac cycle when posterior wedging occurs. (Chen JTT, Lester RG, Posterior wedging sign of mitral insufficiency. Radiology 113:451–453, 1974)

Rat Tail Narrowing Sign

Bronchographic narrowing of a bronchus with lack of normal arborization as the bronchus extends peripherally (Fig. 3-107) has been described as a sign of carcinoma of the lung. Unfortunately, an identical rat tail narrowing appearance can also be seen in association with peripheral inflammatory processes. Asymmetric narrowing of a bronchus with irregular encroachment of the lumen (Fig. 3-108) is generally considered a good, though infrequent, sign of malignant disease. Invasion of the bronchus by tumor causes asymmetric narrowing before complete occlusion, unlike inflammatory narrowing as from tuberculosis, which almost always produces symmetric, smooth bronchial narrowing.

BIBLIOGRAPHY
Felson B: Chest Roentgenology. Philadelphia, WB Saunders, 1973
Rinker CT, Garrotto LJ, Lee KR et al: Bronchography: Diagnostic signs and accuracy in pulmonary carcinoma. AJR 104:802–807, 1968

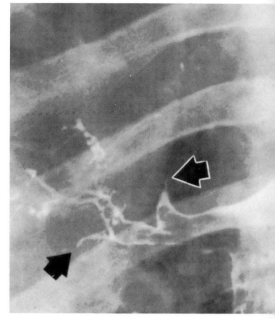

FIG. 3-107. Rattail involvement of bronchi of the right upper lobe (**arrows**) in a patient with bronchogenic carcinoma. (Felson B: Chest Roentgenology. Philadelphia, WB Saunders, 1973)

FIG. 3-108. Asymmetric narrowing of a bronchus (**arrow**) in a patient with bronchogenic carcinoma. (Rinker CT, Garrotto LJ, Lee KR et al: Bronchography: Diagnostic signs and accuracy in pulmonary carcinoma. AJR 104:802–807, 1968. Copyright 1968. Reproduced by permission)

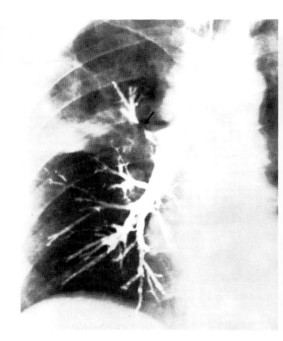

Reverse 5 Sign

Infants with the hypoplastic left heart syndrome have extremely small ascending aortas, no ascending aortic shadow, and usually an enlarged right atrium on frontal radiographs of the chest (Fig. 3-109). This combination produces a striking angulation where the vertical superior vena cava joins the bulbous right atrium, causing the right cardiac silhouette to have a reverse 5 appearance (Fig. 3-110). This sign is reported to be diagnostic of the hypoplastic left heart syndrome.

BIBLIOGRAPHY

Folger GM, Saied A: A new roentgenographic sign of hypoplastic left heart. Chest 64:298–302, 1973

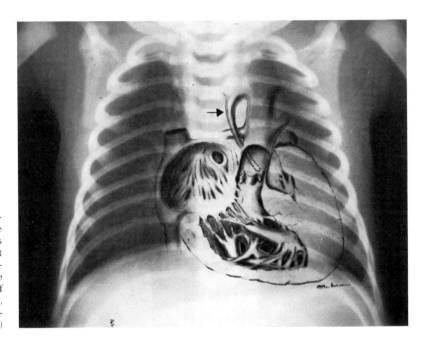

FIG. 3-109. Composite of a frontal chest radiograph and postmortem drawing of the same heart. Characteristic anatomic findings in a typical heart with the hypoplastic left heart syndrome are seen. The size and position of the ascending aorta (**arrow**) preclude its contributing to the right superior aspect of the cardiovascular silhouette. (Folger GM, Saied A: A new roentgenographic sign of hypoplastic left heart. Chest 64:298–302, 1973)

FIG. 3-110. Superimposition of the reverse 5 sign on a typical frontal chest radiograph of a patient with hypoplastic left heart syndrome. (Folger GM, Saied A: A new roentgenographic sign of hypoplastic left heart. Chest 64:298–302, 1973)

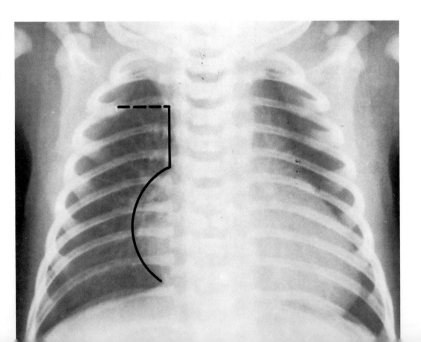

Right Paratracheal Stripe Sign

In normal patients, a thin stripe of water density (1–4 mm wide) is usually visible on posteroanterior chest radiographs between the tracheal air column and the adjacent right lung (Fig. 3-111). Widening of the right paratracheal stripe (to 5 mm or more) is reliable evidence of disease (Fig. 3-112). The differential diagnosis includes lymphadenopathy, mediastinal inflammation or hemorrhage, pleural thickening or effusion, and tracheal disease. In patients with blunt trauma to the chest, widening of the right paratracheal stripe is frequently associated with major arterial injury (Fig. 3-113); in contrast, patients with stripes of normal width have normal arteriograms (Fig. 3-114).

BIBLIOGRAPHY

Savoca CJ, Austin JMH, Goldberg HI: The right paratracheal stripe. Radiology 122:295–301, 1977

Woodring JH, Pulmano CM, Stevens RK: The right paratracheal stripe in blunt chest trauma. Radiology 143:605–608, 1982

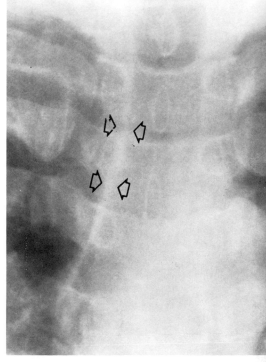

FIG. 3-111. Normal right paratracheal stripe (**arrows**) measuring less than 4 mm.

FIG. 3-112. Widened right paratracheal stripe (**arrows**) in a patient with tracheal carcinoma. (Savoca CJ, Austin JMH, Goldberg HI: The right paratracheal stripe. Radiology 122:295–301, 1977)

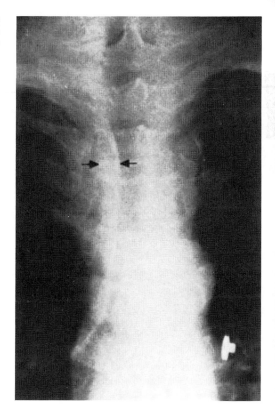

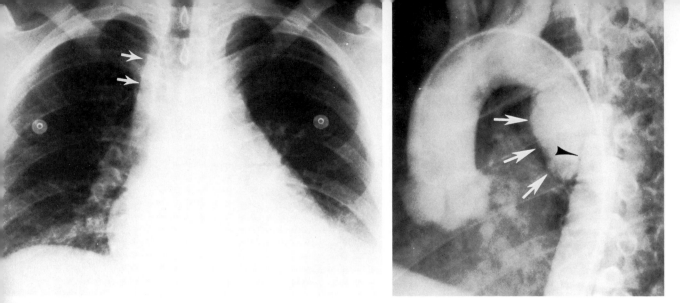

FIG. 3-113. *(Left)* Supine chest radiograph in a patient with blunt chest trauma. The right paratracheal stripe **(arrows)** measures 1 cm in width. *(Right)* Aortogram demonstrates a pseudoaneurysm at the level of the aortic isthmus **(arrows).** The **arrowhead** indicates an intimal flap. (Woodring JH, Pulmano CM, Stevens RK: The right paratracheal stripe in blunt chest trauma. Radiology 143:605–608, 1982)

FIG. 3-114. *(Left)* Supine chest radiograph in a patient with blunt chest trauma. Note the normal right paratracheal stripe **(arrows),** which is 2 mm wide. *(Right)* Aortogram shows that the aorta and its major branches are normal. (Woodring JH, Pulmano CM, Stevens RK: The right paratracheal stripe in blunt chest trauma. Radiology 143:605–608, 1982)

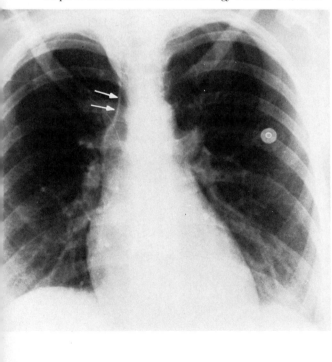

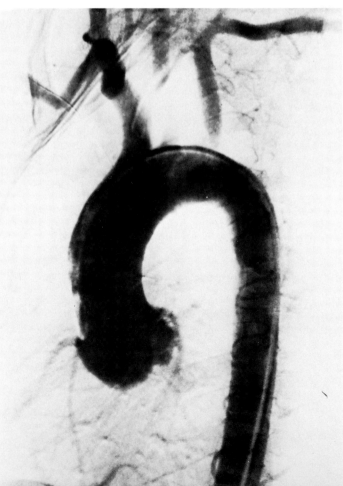

Rigler Notch Sign

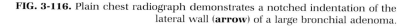

A notch or umbilication in the border of a solitary pulmonary nodule was originally described as a sign of primary or metastatic malignancy (Fig. 3-115). Often seen only on tomography, the notch was thought to be related to the site of entry of the major blood vessels supplying the malignant lesion. Unfortunately, an identical appearance is also commonly encountered in granulomatous and other lesions (Fig. 3-116) and is therefore no longer considered a valid sign.

BIBLIOGRAPHY
Felson B: Chest Roentgenology. Philadelphia, WB Saunders, 1973
Rigler LG: A new roentgen sign of malignancy in the solitary pulmonary nodule. JAMA 157:907, 1955
Rigler LG, Heitzman ER: Planigraphy in the differential diagnosis of the pulmonary nodule with particular reference to the notched sign of malignancy. Radiology 65:692–702, 1955

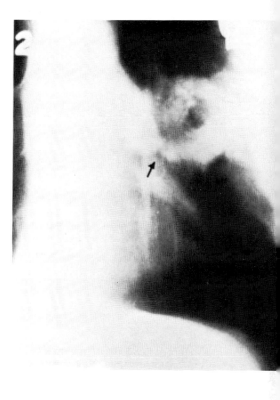

FIG. 3-115. Lung tomogram demonstrates an indentation of the inferior wall (**arrow**) of a large cavitating squamous cell carcinoma. (Rigler LG, Heitzman ER: Planigraphy in the differential diagnosis of the pulmonary nodule with particular reference to the notched sign of malignancy. Radiology 65:692–702, 1955)

FIG. 3-116. Plain chest radiograph demonstrates a notched indentation of the lateral wall (**arrow**) of a large bronchial adenoma.

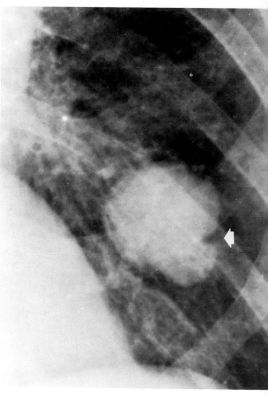

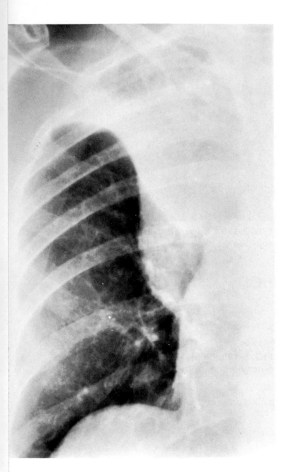

S Sign of Golden

A reverse S-shaped curve seen on frontal views in patients with collapse of the right upper lobe has been described as a sign of bronchogenic carcinoma (Fig. 3-122). The upper, laterally concave segment of the S is formed by the elevated minor fissure, whereas the lower medial convexity is produced by the tumor mass, which has caused bronchostenosis and is responsible for the collapse. Although the S sign of Golden is strongly suggestive of bronchogenic carcinoma, a similar appearance is occasionally caused by enlarged lymph nodes, mediastinal tumors, or bronchial metastases associated with lobar collapse.

BIBLIOGRAPHY
Felson B: Chest Roentgenology. Philadelphia, WB Saunders, 1973
Golden R: The effect of bronchostenosis upon the roentgen-ray shadows in carcinoma of the bronchus. AJR 13:21–30, 1925

FIG. 3-122. Typical reverse S-shaped curve (S sign of Golden) seen on a frontal chest radiograph in a patient with collapse of the right upper lobe associated with bronchogenic carcinoma.

Saber Sheath Trachea Sign

The saber sheath trachea is a rather fixed deformity of the intrathoracic trachea that is reported to be a sign of chronic obstructive pulmonary disease. In this condition, the coronal diameter of the intrathoracic trachea is half or less that of the sagittal diameter, and the shape of the trachea abruptly changes to a rounded configuration at the thoracic outlet (Fig. 3-123). The lateral walls of the trachea are usually thickened, and there is often evidence of ossification of the cartilaginous rings.

BIBLIOGRAPHY

Greene R, Lechner GL: "Saber-sheath" trachea: A clinical and functional study of marked coronal narrowing of intrathoracic trachea. Radiology 115:265–268, 1975

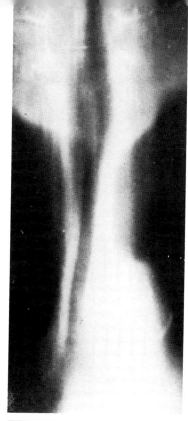

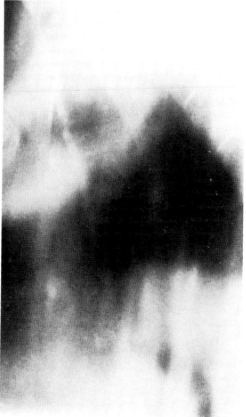

FIG. 3-123. *(Top)* Anteroposterior and *(bottom)* lateral tomographic sections through the intrathoracic trachea in a patient with chronic obstructive pulmonary disease. Note the severe coronal narrowing of the intrathoracic trachea with an abrupt change to a more rounded cross-sectional shape at the thoracic outlet. Calcific densities are present in the tracheal rings. (Greene R, Lechner GL: "Saber-sheath" trachea: A clinical and functional study of marked coronal narrowing of intrathoracic trachea. Radiology 115:265–268, 1975)

Scimitar Sign

The scimitar sign is a linear or curvilinear structure resembling a Turkish scimitar and representing partial anomalous pulmonary venous return below the diaphragm (Fig. 3-128). This anomalous vessel, which occurs most frequently on the right side, usually drains into the inferior vena cava but also has been reported to empty into the portal vein, into the hepatic vein, or directly into the lower part of the right atrium.

The scimitar sign may be seen in the hypoplastic lung syndrome, in which case it is associated with partial hypoplasia of the right lung and right pulmonary artery, dextrocardia, and anomalies of the right bronchial tree. Partial anomalous pulmonary return may also be associated with cardiovascular anomalies such as ventricular septal defect, tetralogy of Fallot, patent ductus arteriosus, coarctation of the aorta, persistence of the left superior vena cava, and pulmonary stenosis.

BIBLIOGRAPHY

Felson B: Chest Roentgenology. Philadelphia, WB Saunders, 1973

Neill CA, Ferencz C, Sabiston DC: The familial occurrence of hypoplastic right lung with systemic arterial supply and venous drainage "scimitar syndrome." Bull Johns Hopkins Hosp 107:1–15, 1960

FIG. 3-128. Two examples of curvilinear vascular pathways (**arrows**) resembling a Turkish scimitar.

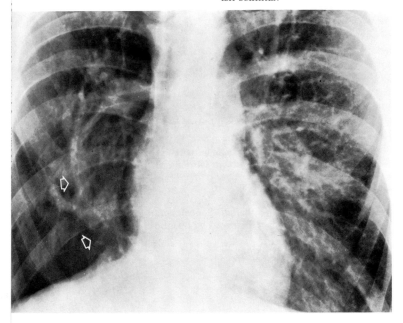
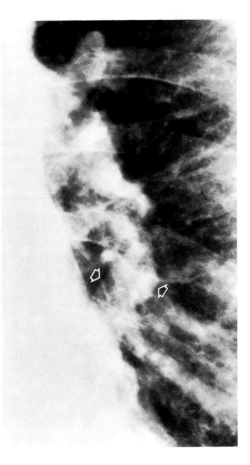

Semitic Nose Sign

Thymomas in the anterior part of the mediastinum have been reported to have a characteristic shape on plain chest radiographs. The tumor mass is said to typically have a straight upper border and a curved lower contour, resembling a beak-shaped "Semitic" nose (Fig. 3-129).

BIBLIOGRAPHY

Rosenthal T, Hertz M, Samra Y et al: Thymoma: Clinical and additional radiologic signs. Chest 65:428–430, 1974

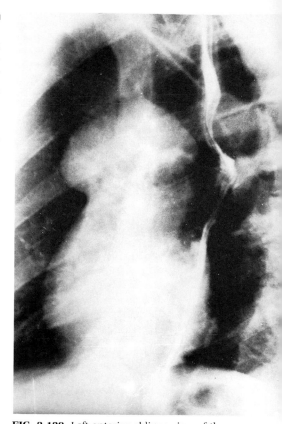

FIG. 3-129. Left anterior oblique view of the chest demonstrates an anterior mediastinal mass with a flat upper border and curved lower contour representing a thymoma. (Rosenthal T, Hertz M, Samra Y et al: Thymoma: Clinical and additional radiologic signs. Chest 65:428–430, 1974

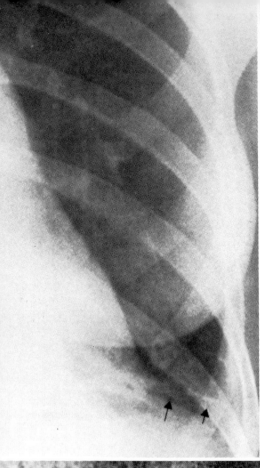

Sentinel Lines Sign

Sentinel lines, coarse linear densities at the base of the lung, may be a sign of adjacent lower lobe volume loss (Fig. 3-130). These basilar densities may be horizontal, oblique, or slightly curved. They may be concave upward and are most often seen at the left base, though they are occasionally right-sided or bilateral. The radiographic appearance is related to bending or kinking of the lower lung bronchi, which results in poor bronchial drainage and filling of the bronchi with mucus or in alveolar atelectasis distal to the kink (Fig. 3-131). It is important to differentiate sentinel lines from other well-known basal horizontal densities such as plate-like atelectasis and septal lines. Demonstration of sentinel lines should suggest the possibility of volume loss in the lower lobe; if the collapsed lower lobe reexpands, the sentinel lines disappear.

BIBLIOGRAPHY
Strickland B: "Sentinel lines"—An unusual sign of lower lobe contraction. Thorax 31:517–521, 1976

FIG. 3-130. *(Top)* Several horizontal linear densities are seen at the left base **(arrows).** The triangular density of a contracted lower lobe is just visible through the heart shadow. *(Bottom)* The linear densities correspond to the distal branches of the lingular bronchi outlined against a well-aerated background. The main lingular divisions are bent from the mechanical displacement of the contracted lower lobe. There is advanced bronchiectasis in the lower lobe. (Strickland B: "Sentinel lines" — An unusual sign of lower lobe contraction. Thorax 31:517–521, 1976)

FIG. 3-131. *(Left)* There is a group of horizontal curved lines at the left base **(arrow)** with concavity facing upward. *(Right)* The lower lobe is collapsed and fails to fill with contrast. The lingular bronchi are bronchiectatic, but the lobe is only partially contracted. The curved lines **(arrow)** represent the underfilled subdivisions of the lingular bronchi. (Strickland B: "Sentinel lines" — An unusual sign of lower lobe contraction. Thorax 31:517–521, 1976)

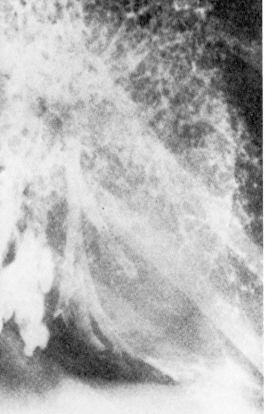

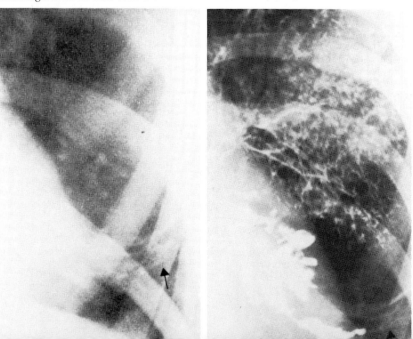

Shaggy Heart Sign

Coalescence of air–space consolidation contiguous to the heart may obscure the cardiac borders and produce the shaggy heart sign (Fig. 3-132). Although originally described as a common feature of the pulmonary disease in pertussis, especially in patients with severe and prolonged illness, the sign is not pathognomonic of pertussis and is more commonly seen with viral pulmonary infections (Fig. 3-133). A similar appearance can be seen in patients with asbestosis (Fig. 3-134), in whom combined parenchymal and pleural changes partially obscure the heart border and diaphragm.

BIBLIOGRAPHY
Barnhard HJ, Kniker WT: Roentgenologic findings in pertussis: With particular emphasis on the "shaggy heart" sign. AJR 84:445–450, 1960

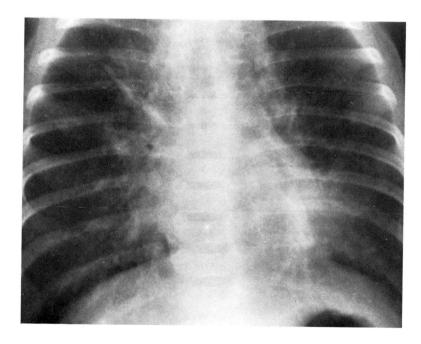

FIG. 3-132. Obscuration of the cardiac borders by contiguous air–space consolidation produces the shaggy heart sign in this patient with pertussis.

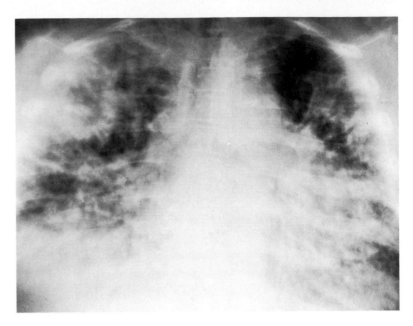

FIG. 3-133. Shaggy heart sign in a patient with severe viral pneumonia.

FIG. 3-134. *(Left)* Frontal radiograph of a 61-year-old asbestos miner demonstrates severe disorganization of lung architecture with generalized coarse reticulation, which has become confluent in the right base and obliterates the right hemidiaphragm. There is marked pleural thickening, particularly in the apical and axillary regions. A spontaneous pneumothorax is present on the left. *(Right)* Frontal radiograph obtained 4 months later demonstrates marked deterioration in the appearance of the chest and obliteration of the heart borders and diaphragm. Further loss of lung volume is also noted. (Fraser RG, Pare JAP: Diagnosis of Diseases of the Chest. Philadelphia, WB Saunders, 1979)

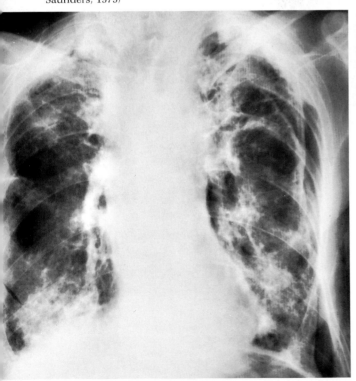

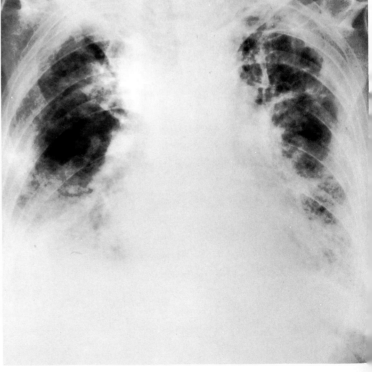

Sharp Edge Sign

In a supine infant with a pneumothorax, air rises to lie along the heart margins and produces a sharper than usual cardiac silhouette (Fig. 3-135). Similarly, the interface between a pneumothorax or loculated air and the diaphragm is sharper than an interface between the diaphragm and aerated lung (Fig. 3-136).

BIBLIOGRAPHY
Oestreich AE: Pediatric Radiology; Medical Outline Series. Garden City, NY, Medical Examination Publishing Co, 1977

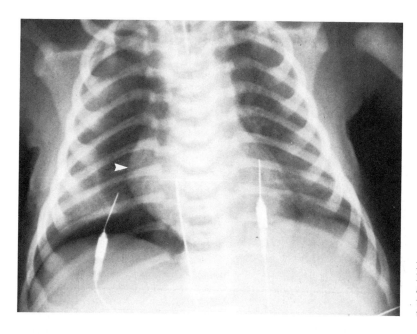

FIG. 3-135. Sharp margin of the cardiac silhouette (**arrowhead**) in a supine infant with a pneumothorax. A sharp edge sign involving the right hemidiaphragm is also seen. (Courtesy of Alan E. Oestrich, M.D.)

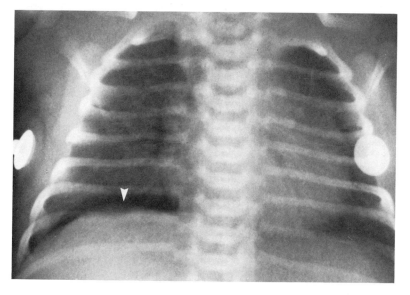

FIG. 3-136. Sharp edge sign (**arrowhead**) involving the right hemidiaphragm. (Courtesy of Alan E. Oestreich, M.D.)

Silhouette Sign

The usefulness of the silhouette sign, a major sign in pulmonary radiology, is based on the finding that an intrathoracic soft-tissue density touching a border of the heart, aorta, or diaphragm will obliterate that border on a chest radiograph and conversely, that an intrathoracic lesion that is not anatomically contiguous with a border of one of these structures will not obscure that border. The silhouette sign is invaluable in a determination of the anatomic location of a pulmonary parenchymal process. A lesion that obliterates part or all of a heart border is anterior in location and lies in the right middle lobe, lingula, anterior segment of an upper lobe, anterior mediastinum, lower end of the oblique fissure, or anterior portion of the pleural cavity (Figs. 3-137 and 3-138). In contrast, a density that overlaps but does not obliterate the heart border is posterior in location and lies in a lower lobe, posterior mediastinum, or posterior portion of the pleural cavity (Fig. 3-139). An uncommon exception in which loss of definition of the right heart border is not associated with right middle lobe disease is severe pectus excavatum (Fig. 3-140).

Silhouetting of the ascending aorta implies an anterior lesion, whereas a density that overlies but does not obliterate this border must lie posteriorly (Fig. 3-141). Silhouetting of the left border of the aortic knob (which lies posteriorly) implies a lesion in the apicoposterior segment of the left upper lobe or in the posterior mediastinum or pleura adjacent to this segment. A density overlapping but not obliterating the aortic knob must be anterior or far posterior (Fig. 3-142). Silhouetting of the lateral border of the descending thoracic aorta can be seen with lesions of the superior and posterior basal segments of the left lower lobe (Fig. 3-143) and as a result of pleural fluid along the mediastinum or an appropriately located mediastinal mass. Silhouetting of a hemidiaphragm not only suggests the presence of a lesion, but if seen only on the lateral view, may also indicate which hemithorax is the site of disease. It must be remembered, however, that the anterior portion of the left hemidiaphragm is normally silhouetted by the heart on the lateral view (see Fig. 3-139).

FIG. 3-137. *(Left)* Frontal chest radiograph demonstrates minimal obliteration of the lower part of the right heart border (**arrows**). *(Right)* Lateral view demonstrates collapse of the right middle lobe (**arrows**).

BIBLIOGRAPHY

Felson B: Chest Roentgenology. Philadelphia, WB Saunders, 1973
Felson B, Felson H: Localization of intrathoracic lesions by means of the PA roentgenogram: The silhouette sign. Radiology 55:363–374, 1950

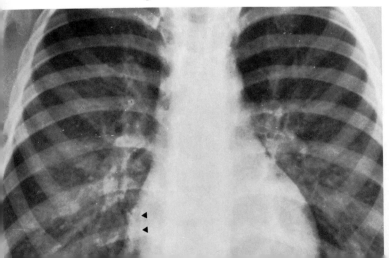
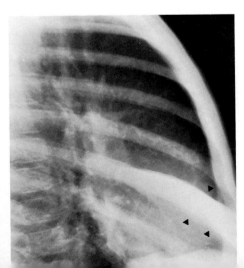

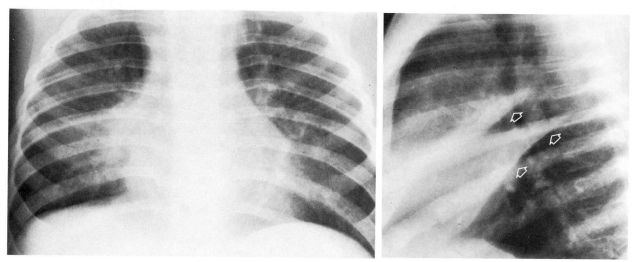

FIG. 3-138. *(Left)* Frontal chest radiograph demonstrates obliteration of both the right and left borders of the heart. *(Right)* Lateral view demonstrates collapse of both the right middle lobe and lingula **(arrows).**

FIG. 3-139. *(Left)* Frontal chest radiograph demonstrates a right lower lung density with preservation of the right heart border. The right hemidiaphragm is obscured. *(Right)* Lateral view confirms the presence of right lower lobe collapse (bronchogenic carcinoma) with posterior displacement of the major fissure **(1).** The elevated right hemidiaphragm **(2)** is obliterated posteriorly by the airless right lower lobe, and the anterior third of the left hemidiaphragm **(3)** is obscured by the bottom of the heart. The overlapping shadows of the back of the heart **(4)** which lies in the left thorax, and the right hemidiaphragm simulate interlobar effusion. (Felson B: Chest Roentgenology. Philadelphia, WB Saunders, 1973)

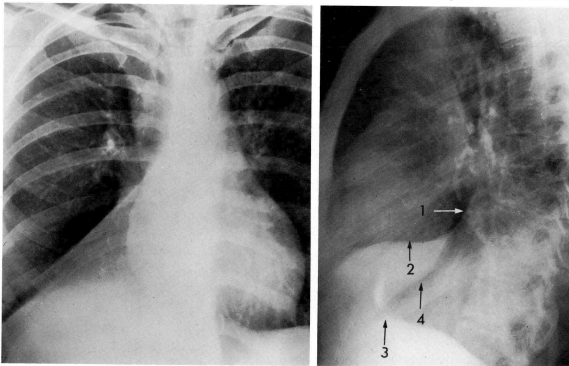

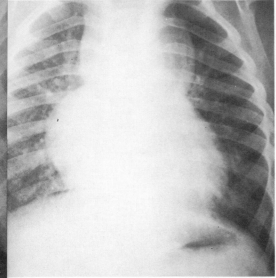

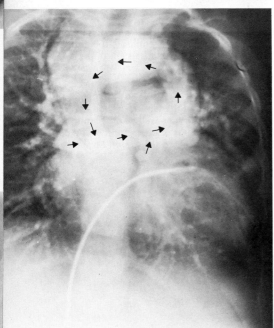

Snowman Sign

The snowman configuration is characteristic of type 1 total anomalous pulmonary venous return, in which the anomalous pulmonary veins unite to form a common trunk that enters the superior vena cava or azygos vein. Plain frontal chest radiographs show a characteristic snowman appearance (Fig. 3-144) produced by a combination of right atrial and right ventricular enlargement (bottom part of the snowman) and marked superior mediastinal widening caused by the anomalous pulmonary vein (upper part of the snowman). Occasionally, a similar appearance is produced in infants with a left-to-right shunt (such as ventricular septal defect) accompanied by abundant thymus tissue. The diagnosis of total anomalous pulmonary venous return is documented by arteriographic demonstration of the anomalous inverted-U-shaped vein responsible for the upper part of the snowman entering the superior vena cava.

BIBLIOGRAPHY

Swischuk LE: Plain Film Interpretation in Congenital Heart Disease. Baltimore, William & Wilkins, 1979

FIG. 3-144. *(Top)* Frontal chest radiograph of a patient with type 1 total anomalous pulmonary venous return demonstrates a snowman, or figure 8, heart with right atrial and right ventricular enlargement. Widening of the superior mediastinum is due to the large, anomalous inverted-U-shaped vein. Pulmonary vascularity is greatly increased. The large pulmonary artery is hidden in the superior mediastinal silhouette. *(Bottom)* Angiocardiogram in a patient with type 1 total anomalous pulmonary venous return demonstrates that all the pulmonary veins drain into the inverted-U-shaped vessel, which eventually empties into the superior vena cava **(arrows).** Widening of the mediastinum produced by this vessel causes the "snowman" heart. (Swischuk LE: Plain Film Interpretation in Congenital Heart Disease. Baltimore, Williams & Wilkins, 1979)

Spinnaker Sail (Angel Wings) Sign

Loculated air confined to one side of the anterior mediastinum causes elevation of the thymus and a crescentic configuration similar to that of a wind-blown spinnaker sail (Fig. 3-145). If the loculated anterior mediastinal air extends to both sides, elevation of both thymic lobes produces an angel wing configuration (Fig. 3-146).

BIBLIOGRAPHY

Moseley JE: Loculated pneumomediastinum in the newborn: Thymic "spinnaker sail" sign. Radiology 75:788–790, 1960

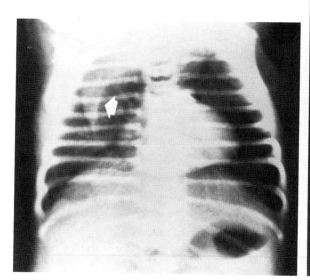
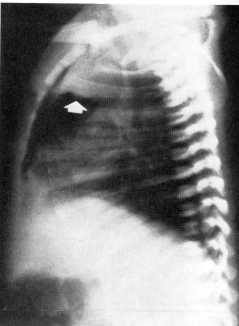

FIG. 3-145. *(Left)* The crescentic sail shadow extending out over the right lung (**arrow**) represents the displaced right lobe of the thymus in a newborn with pneumomediastinum. *(Right)* Lateral projection shows air in the anterior mediastinum lifting the thymus off the pericardium and great vessels (**arrow**). (Moseley JE: Loculated pneumomediastinum in the newborn: A thymic "spinnaker sail" sign. Radiology 75:788–790, 1960)

FIG. 3-146. *(Left)* Elevation of both thymic lobes by mediastinal air (**arrows**). *(Right)* Lateral projection shows the anterior mediastinal air lifting the thymus off the pericardium and great vessels (**arrows**).

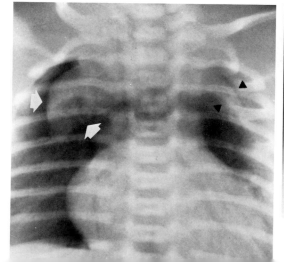
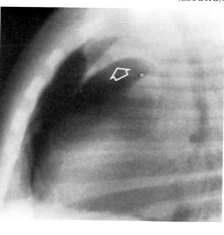

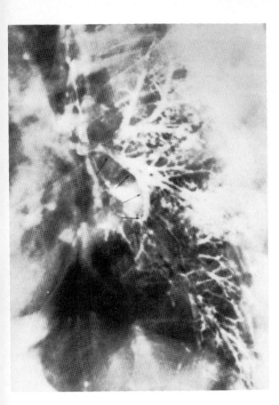

Stretched (Bent) Bronchus Sign

The stretched or bent bronchus sign is produced by a tumor mass that displaces a segment of the bronchus, leaving the proximal and terminal portions in their normal positions (Fig. 3-147). This sign may either indicate primary carcinoma or be evidence of secondary metastatic deposits. The appearance of bronchial stretching is an excellent indication of malignancy in hilar and midlung masses but is of less value when applied to peripheral lesions.

BIBLIOGRAPHY

Rinker CT, Garrotto LJ, Lee KR et al: Bronchography: Diagnostic signs and accuracy in pulmonary carcinoma. AJR 104:802–807, 1968

FIG. 3-147. Displacement of a segment of the bronchus by a tumor mass (**arrows**). The proximal and terminal portions of the bronchus remain in their normal positions. (Rinker CT, Garrotto LJ, Lee KR et al: Bronchography: Diagnostic signs and accuracy in pulmonary carcinoma. AJR 104:802–807, 1968. Copyright 1968. Reproduced by permission)

FIG. 3-148. *(Left)* Posteroanterior chest radiograph demonstrates multiple areas of cavitation. *(Center)* Left lateral decubitus film shows several thin-walled cystic areas with "suspended" central densities. Note the lack of gravitational shift. *(Far, right)* Close-up of the left lower lung. The target lesions represented septic pulmonary emboli *(Escherichia coli)* in this 3-year-old child with acute lymphatic leukemia. (Zelefsky MN, Lutzker LG: The target sign: A new radiologic sign of septic pulmonary emboli. AJR 129:453–455, 1977. Copyright 1977. Reproduced by permission)

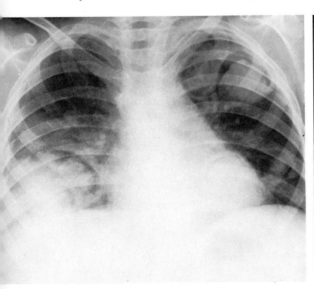

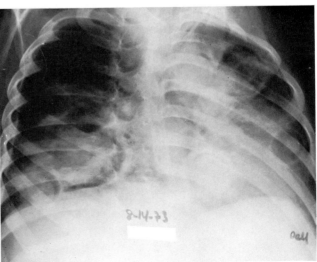

Target Sign

The target sign, a nodular density suspended in a thin-walled hyperlucent cavity, has been described as a radiographic sign of septic pulmonary emboli (Fig. 3-148). It is hypothesized that the central density represents a localized nidus of suppuration that is surrounded by overexpanded pulmonary lobules. The central suspension of density within the cystic space must be differentiated from the appearance of aspergillosis or tuberculosis, in which material within the cavity either changes position with gravity or adheres to one wall (Fig. 3-149).

BIBLIOGRAPHY

Zelefsky MN, Lutzker LG: The target sign: A new radiologic sign of septic pulmonary emboli, AJR 129:453–455, 1977

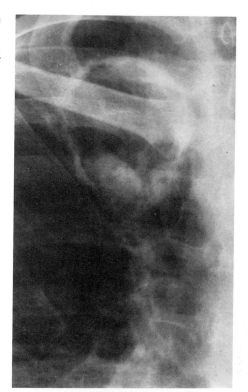

FIG. 3-149. Views of the upper half of the right lung from a frontal radiograph *(top)* and tomogram *(bottom)* demonstrate a rather thin-walled but irregular cavity in the paramediastinal zone. Situated within it is a smooth, oblong shadow of homogeneous density whose relationship to the wall of the cavity changes as the patient moves from *(top)* the erect to *(bottom)* the supine position. The cavity was tuberculous in origin, and the intracavitary mass was found to contain multiple mycelial threads characteristic of *Aspergillus*. (Fraser RG, Pare JAP: Diagnosis of Diseases of the Chest. Philadelphia, WB Saunders, 1978)

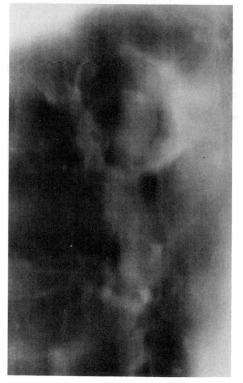

FIG. 3-148 *(Far, right).*

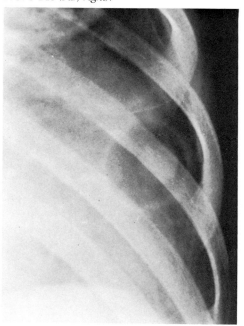

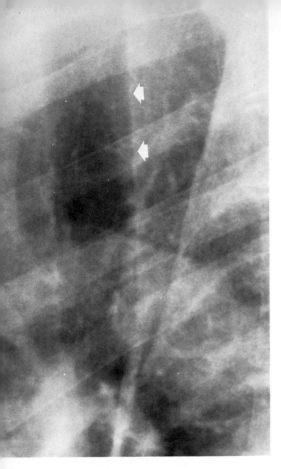

Thickened Posterior Tracheal Stripe Sign ▬▬▬

The posterior tracheal stripe is produced by the interface between the right posterior tracheal wall and the pleura covering that portion of the right upper lobe that lies in the right retrotracheal recess (Fig. 3-150). A thickened posterior tracheal stripe (wider than 4.5 mm) without an obstructed esophagus should suggest the possibility of carcinoma of the esophagus with tumor infiltration of the periesophageal lymphatic tissues (Fig. 3-151). In one study, the thickened posterior tracheal stripe sign appeared on routine lateral chest radiographs as early as 6 months before the development of symptoms in half of patients with esophageal carcinoma. A similar appearance has also been described in patients with esophageal obstruction (especially achalasia) and in patients with chronic obstructive or granulomatous pulmonary disease.

BIBLIOGRAPHY

Putman CE, Curtis AM, Westfried M et al: Thickening of the posterior tracheal stripe: A sign of squamous cell carcinomas of the esophagus. Radiology 121:533–536, 1976

FIG. 3-150. Thin posterior tracheal stripe (**arrows**) in a normal patient.

FIG. 3-151. Thickening of the posterior tracheal stripe (**arrows**) in two patients with carcinoma of the esophagus without obstruction. The figure on the *right* shows the posterior esophageal wall, which was extensively infiltrated by tumor. Decreased motility accounts for the air within the esophageal lumen. (Putman CE, Curtis AM, Westfried M et al: Thickening of the posterior tracheal stripe: A sign of squamous cell carcinoma of the esophagus. Radiology 121:533–536, 1976)

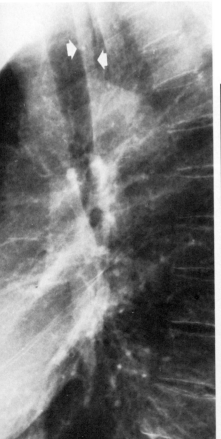

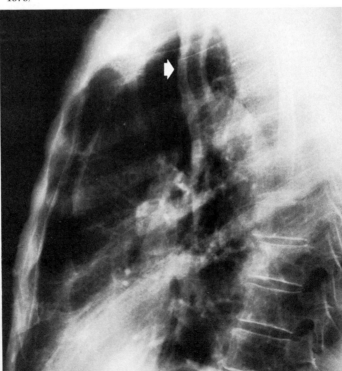

Third Mogul Sign

Mogul is a skiing term describing a mountainside mammilation of packed snow. Radiographically, the word has been used to depict a little hill that blends medially with the mediastinal silhouette and has a sharp lateral margin suggesting a serosal covering and therefore an extrapulmonary location (Fig. 3-152). On the left, the first mogul is paratracheal, above the carina, and usually represents the aorta. The second mogul is to the left of the carina, just above the left main stem bronchus, and should be the main pulmonary artery. The fourth mogul sits on the hemidiaphragm and usually represents the cardiac apex. The third mogul is an abnormal protuberance that sits on the left cardiac margin just below the left main stem bronchus and pulmonary artery (Fig. 3-153). This appearance suggests a large left atrial appendage, which is most commonly due to rheumatic heart disease but may also be seen with herniated left atrial appendage through a pericardial defect, disease of the chordae tendineae or papillary muscles, left atrial myxoma, or cardiomyopathy. Unusual causes include elevation of the left ventricle in tetralogy of Fallot, the uplifted outflow chamber of the right ventricle in Ebstein's malformation, the left-sided ascending aorta in corrected transposition, or the upper edge of an aneurysm of the heart or sinus of Valsalva.

BIBLIOGRAPHY
Daves ML: Skiagraphing the mediastinal moguls. New Physician, January, 19:49–54, 1970

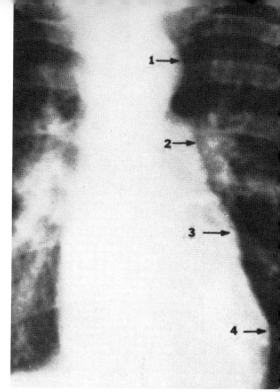

FIG. 3-152. Frontal chest radiograph demonstrates the four moguls on the left side of the mediastinum. The first mogul (**1**) is paratracheal; the second (**2**) is above the left main stem bronchus; the third (**3**) is below the bronchus; and the fourth (**4**) sits on the diaphragm. (Daves ML: Skiagraphing the mediastinal moguls. New Physician 19:49–54, 1970)

FIG. 3-153. *(Left)* Frontal chest film demonstrates a high third mogul in an adolescent with tetralogy and a large atrial septal defect. *(Right)* Right ventricular injection from an angiocardiogram demonstrates poststenotic dilatation of the infundibulum (**arrowheads**), which accounts for the high third mogul seen in the left-hand figure. Aortic filling occurs through the ventricular septal defect. (Daves ML: Skiagraphing the mediastinal moguls. New Physician 19:49–54, 1970)

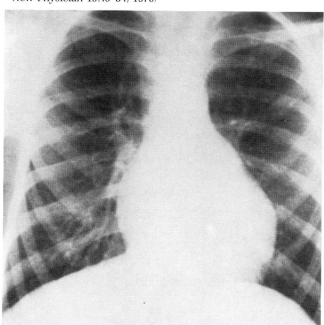

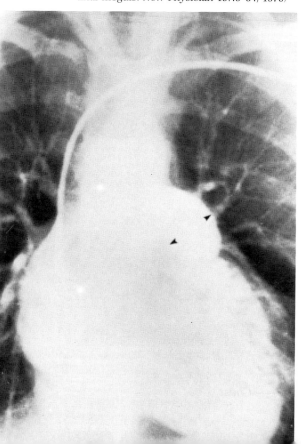

Thymic Wave Sign

The thymic wave sign is a subtle wavy appearance of the border of the normal soft thymus gland on frontal radiographs due to indentation by the costochondral junctions of the adjacent anterior ribs (Fig. 3-157). Presence of the thymic wave sign is an indication of a normal gland (Fig. 3-158); thymic tumors and other anterior mediastinal masses are firmer and cannot be easily indented by the anterior thoracic cage.

BIBLIOGRAPHY
Mulvey RB: The thymic "wave" sign. Radiology 81:834–838, 1963

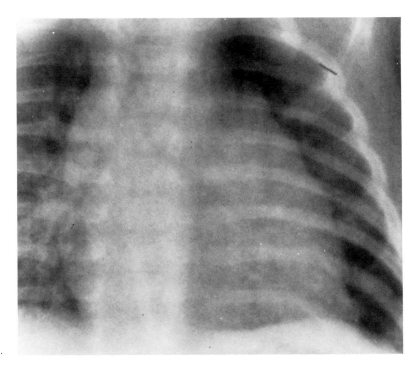

FIG. 3-157. Thymic wave sign.

FIG. 3-158. Dramatic example of the thymic wave sign. The apparent mass represents the normal compressible gland rather than a neoplastic process.

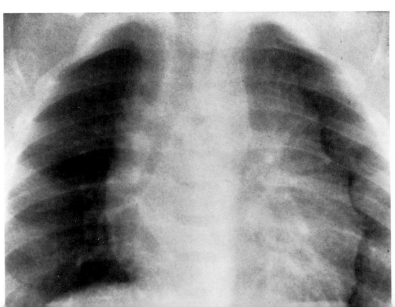

Top of the Knob Sign

Obliteration of the top of the aortic knob may be a secondary sign of left lower lobe collapse. This sign is associated with a relatively vertical shadow (interface) in the left upper mediastinum that is continuous below with the left border of the pericardium and may be visible through and even above the left clavicle (Fig. 3-159). Following re-expansion of the lung, the knob appears normal.

BIBLIOGRAPHY

Kattan KR: Upper mediastinal changes in lower lobe collapse. Semin Roentgenol 15:183–186, 1980

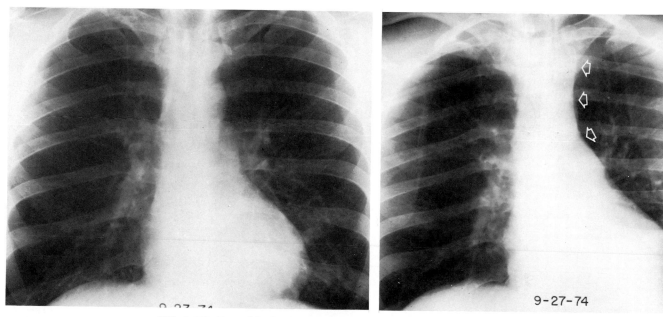

FIG. 3-159. Top-of-the-knob sign (and flat waist sign) in a drug addict with endocarditis and left lower lobe collapse from pneumonia. *(Left)* Normal chest. The pulmonary segment of the heart is concave, and most of the top of the aortic knob is visible. *(Right)* Four days later, there is collapse of the lower lobe behind the heart, as indicated by increased opacity of the left side of the heart, loss of the silhouette of the medial half of the left hemidiaphragm, obscuration of left lower lobe vascularity, and a lowered left hilum. The pulmonary outflow tract is now straight. There is also an almost vertical interface in the left upper mediastinum that obliterates the top of the aortic knob and is continuous below with the left pericardial border **(arrows).** (Kattan KR: Upper mediastinal changes in lower lobe collapse. Semin Roentgenol 15:183–186, 1980)

Tram Line Sign

Parallel or slightly tapering line shadows outside the boundary of the pulmonary hila are often called *tram lines* (Fig. 3-160). In patients with chronic bronchitis or asthmatics with repeated infections, tram lines have been attributed to thickening of the bronchial wall. The most common cause of these tubular shadows is bronchiectasis, in which the lines probably represent a combination of thickened bronchial walls, peribronchial fibrosis, and alveolar collapse. The width of the air column separating the parallel lines depends on the severity of the bronchial dilatation. Tram lines can also be seen in a small percentage of normal persons with no respiratory symptoms.

BIBLIOGRAPHY

Fraser RG, Pare JAP: Diagnosis of Diseases of the Chest. Philadelphia, WB Saunders, 1979

FIG. 3-160. *(Left)* Full and *(right)* coned views of the right lower lung in a patient with chronic bronchitis demonstrate parallel line shadows outside the boundary of the pulmonary hilum.

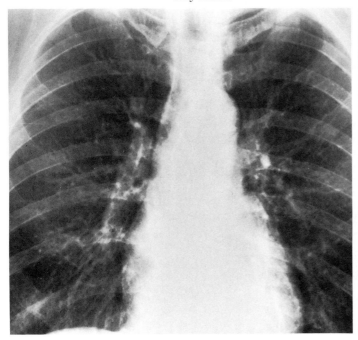
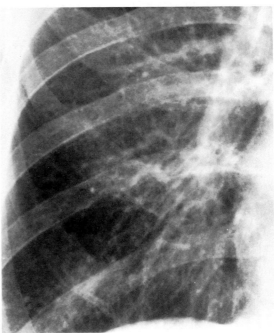

Tumor Track Sign

A track of density extending from a peripheal pulmonary mass to the hilum has been reported by some authors as a common sign of malignancy (Fig. 3-161). These tracks are said to consist of a mixture of peribronchial and perivascular fibrosis and infiltration by tumor elements. Other authors have concluded that such communicating tracks are quite uncommon in cases of peripheral carcinoma. A similar appearance has been described in both infectious and neoplastic lesions. The tumor track sign is thus of limited value in differential diagnosis.

BIBLIOGRAPHY

Fraser RG, Pare JAP: Diagnosis of Diseases of the Chest. Philadelphia, WB Saunders, 1978

Marmorshtain SI: Roentgenologic diagnosis of peripheral lung cancer. Vopr Onkol (Leningrad) 2:562–573, 1956

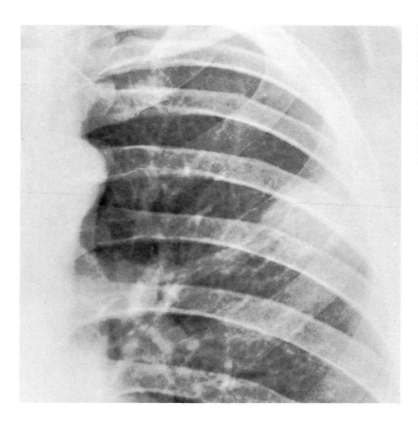

FIG. 3-161. Frontal radiograph of the upper half of the left lung demonstrates a poorly defined homogeneous mass situated in the axillary portion of the lung. The mass represents a bronchogenic carcinoma. Extending from the medial aspect of the mass to the hilum are a group of line shadows that were proved on resection to be caused by neoplasm extending along the bronchovascular bundles, predominantly in the lymphatics. (Fraser RG, Pare JAP: Diagnosis of Diseases of the Chest. Philadelphia, WB Saunders, 1978)

Upper Triangle Sign

A triangular shadow in the right upper lung, continuous with the mediastinum and with its apex pointing toward the right hilus, has been described as an indirect sign of right lower lobe collapse (Fig. 3-162). This sign appears to represent a partial shift of the upper anterior mediastinum to the right (Fig. 3-163) and may be mistaken for right upper lobe collapse or infiltrate.

BIBLIOGRAPHY
Kattan KR, Felson B, Holder LE et al: Superior mediastinal shift in right-lower-lobe collapse: The "upper triangle sign." Radiology 116:305–309, 1975

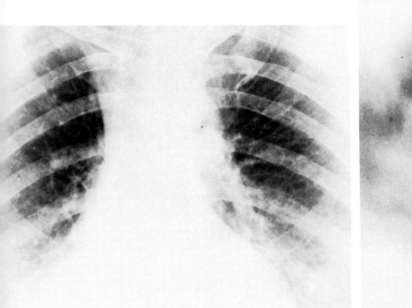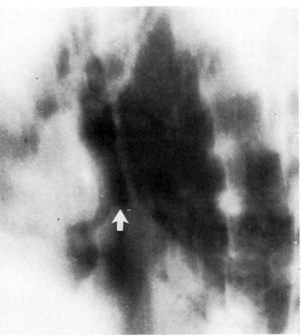

FIG. 3-162. *(Left)* Posteroanterior chest film demonstrates the usual signs of right lower lobe collapse, with the additional finding of a triangular shadow along the right side of the upper mediastinum. The apex of the shadow is at the hilus, and the base is at the level of the clavicle. The trachea is displaced to the right. *(Right)* Right posterior oblique tomogram of the right lung root and mediastinum demonstrates a bronchial adenoma obstructing the right lower lobe bronchus **(arrow).** No abnormality was found in the right upper lung at thoracotomy. (Kattan KR, Felson B. Holder LE et al: Superior mediastinal shift in right-lower-lobe collapse: The "upper triangle sign." Radiology 116:306–309, 1975)

FIG. 3-163. *(Left)* Posteroanterior chest film in a young woman who experienced severe postpartum dyspnea shows collapse of the right middle and lower lobes. The heart and mediastinum are shifted to the right. A large upper triangle sign is clearly seen. *(Right)* On a prior chest radiograph taken 4 months before delivery, the position and configuration of the mediastinum are normal. A subsequent follow-up film also showed a normal appearance. (Kattan KR, Felson B, Holder LE et al: Superior mediastinal shift in right-lower-lobe collapse: The "upper triangle sign." Radiology 116:305–309, 1975)

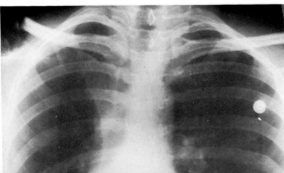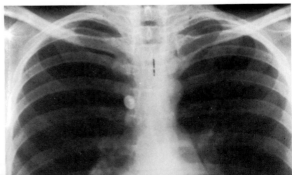

V Sign

In a patient with a small pneumothorax, two intersecting lines forming a V, the apex of which points laterally, can often be seen deep in the lateral costophrenic angle (Fig. 3-164). This V-shaped configuration is due to the x-ray beam striking the peripheral portion of the thorax obliquely rather than tangentially, thus projecting the anterior and posterior surfaces of the air–fluid level into different planes. Since neither line is perfectly parallel to the floor, they appear radiographically as two limbs of a V.

BIBLIOGRAPHY

Felson B: Chest Roentgenology. Philadelphia, WB Saunders, 1973

FIG. 3-164. Two intersecting lines (**lower arrows**) form a V, the apex of which is directed laterally on this frontal chest radiograph of a patient with pneumothorax. This appearance represents an air–fluid level in which the x-ray beam strikes the surface of the fluid obliquely. The triangular inferior pulmonary ligament (**upper arrow**) preserves the shape of the base of the collapsed lung. (Felson B: Chest Roentgenology. Philadelphia, WB Saunders, 1973)

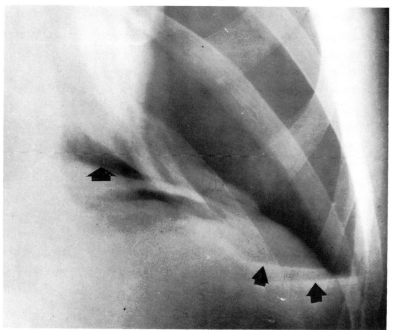

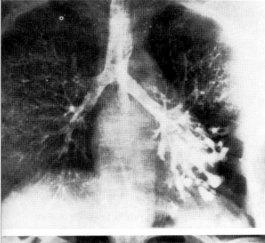

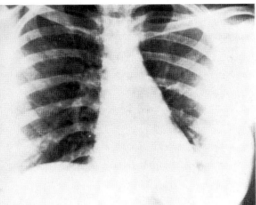

Vascular Plethora Sign

Severe basal bronchiectasis results in regional high vascular pressure and diversion of blood flow to the uninvolved portion of the lung through bronchopulmonary anastomoses (Fig. 3-167). This upper lobe vascular plethora may be unilateral or bilateral and is one of the signs of bronchiectasis involving the lung bases (Fig. 3-168).

BIBLIOGRAPHY
Solomon A, Hertz M: Unilateral vascular plethora: A sign in advanced unilateral basal bronchiectasis. Heart Lung 7:810–812, 1978

FIG. 3-167. *(Top)* Bronchogram showing saccular bronchiectasis in the left lower lobe. *(Bottom)* The left upper lobe vessels show substantial fullness in comparison to the normal, underfilled right upper lobe. (Solomon A, Hertz M: Unilateral vascular plethora: A sign in advanced unilateral basal bronchiectasis. Heart Lung 7:810–812, 1978)

FIG. 3-168. *(Left)* Bronchogram showing left basal bronchiectasis. *(Right)* Plain chest radiograph shows vascular plethora in the left upper lung. (Solomon A, Hertz M: Unilateral vascular plethora: A sign in advanced unilateral basal bronchiectasis. Heart Lung 7:810–812, 1978)

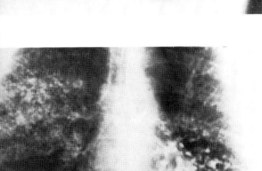

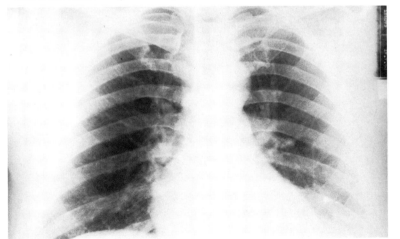

Vertebral Fade-Off Sign

On lateral chest radiographs, the overall density posteriorly tends to decrease from the level of the upper thoracic spine to that of the diaphragm (Fig. 3-169). The vertebral fade-off sign is any alteration in this typical pattern, specifically an area of increased density near the base of the lung representing an underlying area of pulmonary consolidation (Fig. 3-170).

FIG. 3-169. Normal *(left)* frontal and *(right)* lateral chest radiographs. Note that the overall density posteriorly tends to decrease from the level of the upper thoracic spine to that of the diaphragm.

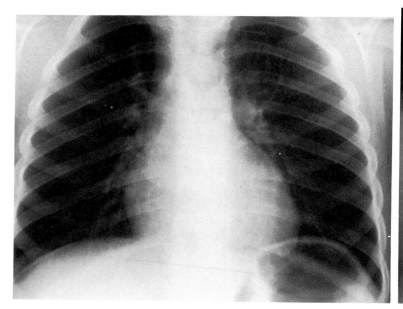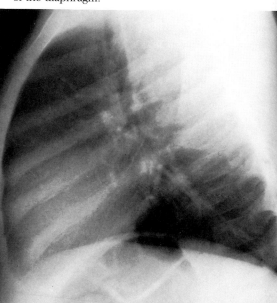

FIG. 3-170. *(Left)* Frontal and *(right)* lateral chest radiographs of the same patient following development of a left lower lobe pneumonia (**arrow**). The posterior density is now increased at the lower thoracic levels, indicating the underlying area of pulmonary consolidation.

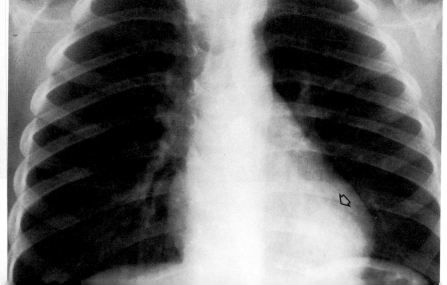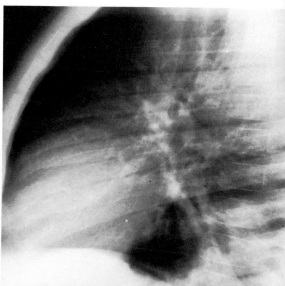

Westermark's Sign

Westermark's sign is a manifestation of local pulmonary oligemia distal to a large-vessel pulmonary embolism. The reduction in blood volume, without substantial change in air or tissue volume, causes relative lucency of the involved portion of lung (Fig. 3-175). This finding is best seen when oligemia due to deprivation of pulmonary arterial supply to a major part or all of a lung is contrasted with increased pulmonary arterial blood flow to the unoccluded lung. Westermark's sign is often seen in conjunction with enlargement of the ipsilateral main pulmonary artery (Fleischner's sign; see Fig. 3-52).

BIBLIOGRAPHY
Westermark N: On the roentgen diagnosis of lung embolism. Acta Radiol 19:357–372, 1938

FIG. 3-175. (A) Baseline chest radiograph. (B) Hyperlucency of the left upper lobe coincides with the onset of the patient's symptoms. (C) Arteriogram performed the same day as that in (B) demonstrates an occluding clot in the left upper lobe and multiple emboli in the right lung. (Julien P: Pulmonary embolism. In Eisenberg RL, Amberg JR (eds): Critical Diagnostic Pathways in Radiology: An Algorithmic Approach. Philadelphia, JB Lippincott, 1981)

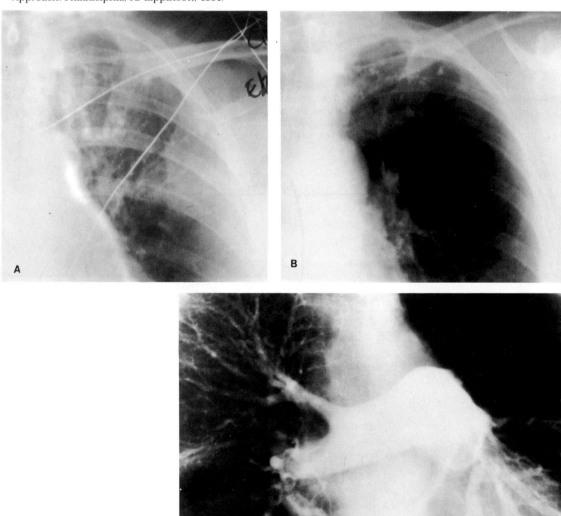

4

Bone

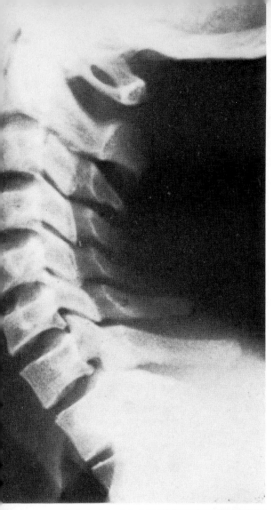

Acute Kyphosis Sign

Disruption of the posterior ligamentous structures following flexion injury to the cervical spine can damage the spinal cord and cause paralysis without any radiographic evidence of fracture or dislocation. The normal cervical spine is lordotic in the neutral position, showing a smooth anterior convex curve on lateral radiographs (Fig. 4-1). Kyphotic angulation localized to one level of the cervical spine (acute kyphosis sign; Fig. 4-2) indicates damage to the posterior spinal ligaments and potential vertebral instability caused by traumatic hyperflexion of the neck.

BIBLIOGRAPHY
Scher AT: Ligamentous injury to the cervical spine—Two radiological signs. S Afr Med J 53:802–804, 1978

FIG. 4-1. Lateral radiograph of the cervical spine of a normal patient demonstrates a smooth anterior convex curve. (Scher AT: Ligamentous injury to the cervical spine—Two radiological signs. S Afr Med J 53:802–804,1978)

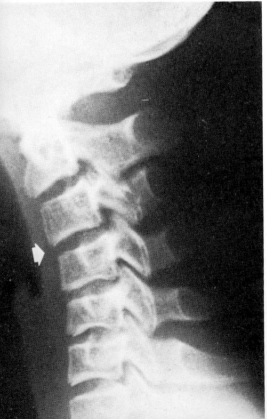

FIG. 4-2. Acute kyphotic angulation at the C3-C4 level (**arrow**) after whiplash injury to the neck. This appearance indicates damage to the posterior spinal ligaments and potential vertebral instability. (Scher AT: Ligamentous injury to the cervical spine—Two radiological sign. S Afr Med J 53:802–804,1978)

Antral Bowing Sign

Anterior bowing of the posterior wall of the maxillary sinus has been described as a characteristic plain radiographic finding in patients with juvenile angiofibroma, the most common benign tumor of the nasopharynx (Fig. 4-3). A similar appearance of widening of the pterygopalatine fossa with anterior bowing of the posterior wall of the maxillary antrum (Fig. 4-4) has also been reported on computed tomographic scans of patients with this lesion. However, the antral bowing sign is not pathognomonic of juvenile angiofibroma; it can also occur with other slow-growing, noninvasive lesions involving the retromaxillary region, such as lymphoepithelioma (Fig. 4-5, *top*), schwannoma (Fig. 4-5, *bottom*), and fibrous histiocytoma.

BIBLIOGRAPHY

Holman CB, Miller WE: Juvenile nasopharyngeal fibroma: Roentgenologic characteristics. AJR 94:292–298, 1965

Som PM, Shugar JMA, Cohen BA et al: The nonspecificity of the antral bowing sign in maxillary sinus pathology. J Comput Assist Tomogr 5:350–352, 1981

Weinstein MA, Levine H, Duchesneau PM et al: Diagnosis of juvenile angiofibroma by computed tomography. Radiology 126:703–705, 1978

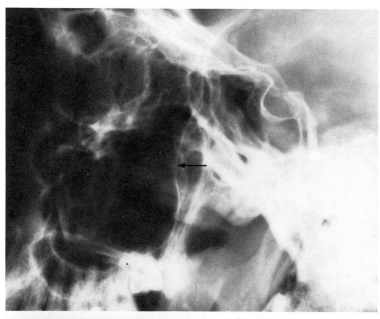

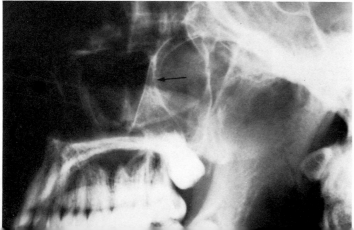

FIG. 4-3. Anterior bowing of the posterior maxillary antral wall (**arrows**) on plain radiographs of two patients with juvenile nasopharyngeal angiofibroma. (Holman CB, Miller WE: Juvenile nasopharyngeal fibroma: Roentgenologic characteristics. AJR 94:292–298,1965. Copyright 1965. Reproduced by permission)

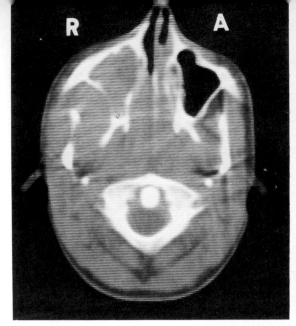 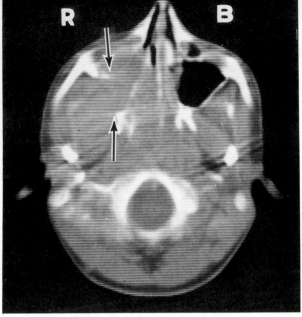

FIG. 4-4. *(Left)* Computed tomography demonstrates anterior displacement of the posterior wall of the right maxillary sinus in a 15-year-old boy with juvenile angiofibroma. The entire nasopharynx, right maxillary sinus, and all but the most anterior portion of the nasal fossa are filled with tumor. *(Right)* On a section 13 mm superior to that seen in the *(left)* figure the tumor has expanded the right pterygopalatine fossa and canal **(arrows).** (Weinstein MA, Levine H, Duchesneau PM et al: Diagnosis of juvenile angiofibroma by computed tomography. Radiology 126:703–705,1978)

FIG. 4-5. Antral bowing sign occurring with slow-growing, noninvasive lesions other than juvenile angiofibroma involving the retromaxillary region. *(Left)* Lateral plain film of skull demonstrates a large, homogeneous soft-tissue nasopharyngeal mass with anterior displacement of the posterior wall of the maxillary sinus **(arrow)** in a patient with a lymphoepithelioma. *(Right)* Computed tomography demonstrates a right retromaxillary mass (schwannoma) with smooth anterior bowing of the intact posterior antral wall **(arrow).** (Som PM, Shugar JMA, Cohen BA et al: The nonspecificity of the antral bowing sign in maxillary sinus pathology. J Comput Assist Tomogr 5:350–352,1981)

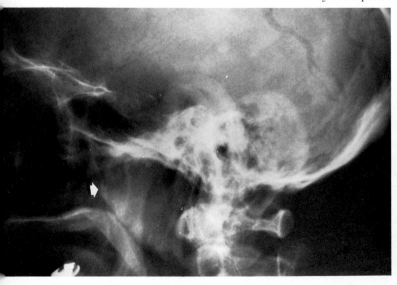 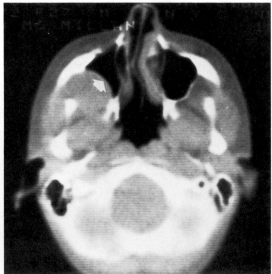

Beaten Brass Sign

The beaten brass appearance of the skull represents a marked increase in the convolutional pattern of the cranial bones (Fig. 4-6) caused by premature closure of several major sutures and resultant elevation of intracranial pressure.

BIBLIOGRAPHY
Rabinowitz JG: Pediatric Radiology. Philadelphia, JB Lippincott, 1978

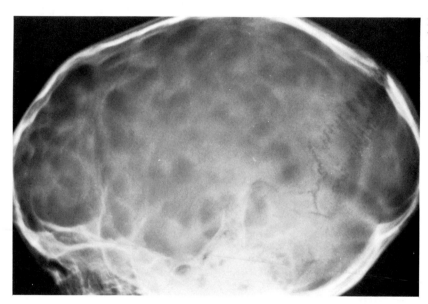

FIG. 4-6. Lateral view of the skull in a patient with premature closure of several sutures demonstrates prominence of convolutional markings.

Bite Sign

A large defect in the end of the proximal femur, looking as though a bite had been taken out of it (Fig. 4-7), is a radiographic finding of aseptic necrosis. The appearance is due to fragmentation, compression, and resorption of necrotic bone complicating the vascular insufficiency.

BIBLIOGRAPHY

Martel W, Sitterley BH: Roentgenologic manifestations of osteonecrosis. AJR 106:509–522, 1969

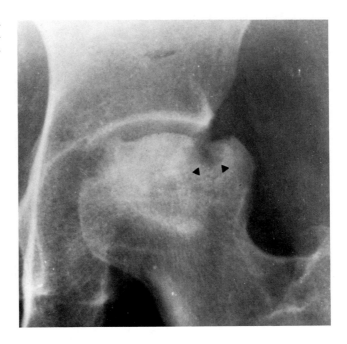

FIG. 4-7. Aseptic necrosis of the hip produces a large defect in the end of the proximal femur (**arrows**).

Blade of Grass Sign

The destructive phase of Paget's disease typically begins at the end of a bone or at an apophysis (*e.g.*, greater trochanter, tibial tubercle) and extends along the shaft. This results in an area of radiolucency that ends in a characteristic sharply marginated angular configuration (blade of grass sign; Fig. 4-8).

BIBLIOGRAPHY
Greenfield GB: Radiology of Bone Diseases. Philadelphia, JB Lippincott, 1980

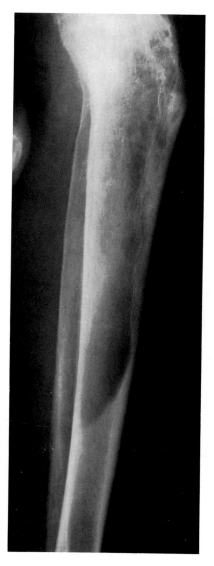

FIG. 4-8. Sharply demarcated radiolucency with angular configuration extending from the proximal tibia and involving two thirds of the shaft. This blade of grass sign represents the destructive phase of Paget's disease. Accentuation of the trabecular pattern at the proximal aspect of the tibia may also be seen. (Greenfield GB: Radiology of Bone Diseases. Philadelphia, JB Lippincott, 1980)

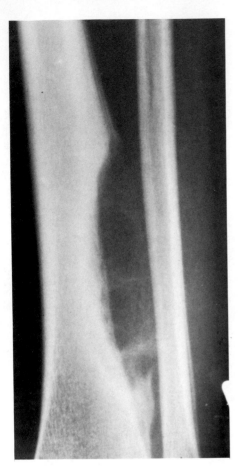

FIG. 4-9. Blister of bone sign.

Blister of Bone Sign

The blister of bone sign, a saccular protrusion of the cortex with multiple fine septae internally, is a characteristic appearance of aneurysmal bone cyst (Fig. 4-9). The thin shell of the lesion may fracture, causing extravasation of blood into the adjoining tissues.

BIBLIOGRAPHY
Meschan I: Analysis of Roentgen Signs in General Radiology. Philadelphia, WB Saunders, 1973

Boutonnière Deformity

The combination of flexion deformities of the proximal interphalangeal joints and hyperextension deformities of the distal interphalangeal joints results in a boutonnière deformity (Fig. 4-10), so named because the digit is held as if securing a carnation in a lapel (*boutonnière* is the French term for buttonhole). This pattern is most commonly seen in rheumatoid arthritis but can also appear in systemic lupus erythematosus or Jaccoud's (post-rheumatic fever) arthritis. On anteroposterior views, foreshortening of the phalanges and obscuration of the proximal interphalangeal joints are seen (Fig. 4-11).

BIBLIOGRAPHY

Forrester DM, Brown JC, Nesson JW: The Radiology of Joint Disease. Philadelphia, WB Saunders, 1978

FIG. 4-10. Flexion of the proximal interphalangeal joint and hyperextension of the distal interphalangeal joint result in a boutonnière deformity in this patient with systemic lupus erythematosus. (Forrester DM, Brown JC, Nesson JW: The Radiology of Joint Disease. Philadelphia, WB Saunders, 1978)

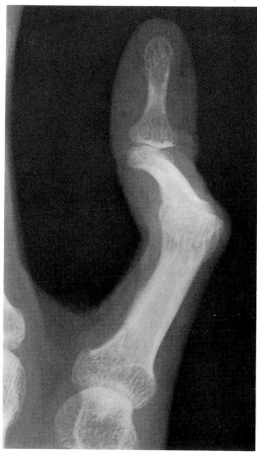

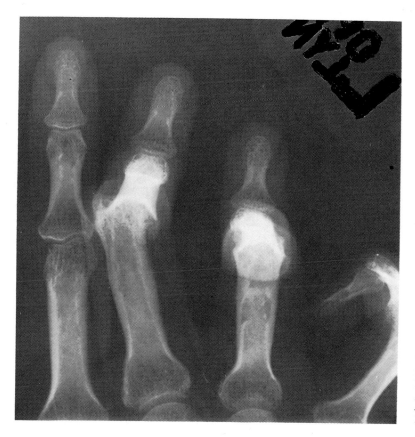

FIG. 4-11. On anteroposterior projection, boutonnière deformities of the third and fourth digits cause foreshortening of the phalanges and obscure the proximal interphalangeal joints. (Forrester DM, Brown JC, Nesson JW: The Radiology of Joint Disease. Philadelphia, WB Saunders, 1978)

Brim Sign

The brim sign consists of thickening of the pelvic brim or arcuate line (iliopectineal line) in Paget's disease of the pelvis (Fig. 4-12). This appearance is probably due to an osteoblastic reaction to altered bone stresses caused by destruction of the lamellae in the pelvis, with the resulting ridge of new bone around the pelvic brim adding to the normal sclerotic density of the area. The brim sign is found in a large majority of patients with Paget's disease of the pelvis and may aid in the differentiation of this condition from metastatic osteoblastic metastases, in which thickening of the ileopectineal line rarely occurs.

BIBLIOGRAPHY
Marshall TR, Ling JT: The brim sign: A new sign found in Paget's disease (osteitis deformans) of the pelvis. AJR 90:1267–1270, 1963

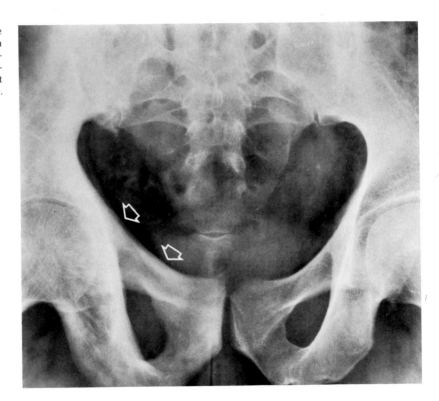

FIG. 4-12. Thickening of the ileopectineal line on the right (**arrows**) in a patient with Paget's disease of the pelvis. Note the difference in the thickness of the pelvic brim between the involved right side and normal left side.

Bulging Tumor Sign

A smooth tumor bulge into the sphenoid sinus, associated with hyperostosis, has been reported as a plain film radiographic sign of parasellar meningioma (Fig. 4-13). A tumor bulge without hyperostosis has been described in pituitary adenoma (Fig. 4-14).

BIBLIOGRAPHY

Gifford ID, Goree JA, Jimenez JP: Tumor bulge into the sphenoid sinus: A roentgen sign of parasellar meningioma. AJR 112:324–328, 1971

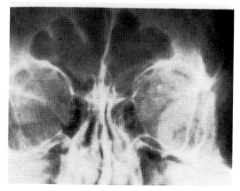

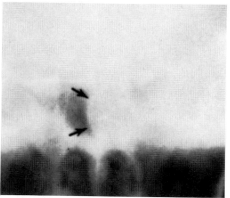

FIG. 4-13. *(Top)* Frontal skull radiograph demonstrates only a radiodensity of the left sphenoid wings. This finding is of questionable significance. *(Bottom)* Frontal sphenoid tomogram shows a tumor bulge into the sphenoid sinus **(arrows).** This bulge represents a sphenoid ridge meningioma extending to the cavernous sinus. (Gifford ID, Goree JA, Jimenez JP: Tumor bulge into the sphenoid sinus: A roentgen sign of parasellar meningioma. AJR 112:324–328,1971. Copyright 1971. Reproduced by permission)

FIG. 4-14. Lateral tomogram of the sella turcica demonstrates a tumor bulge into the sphenoid sinus **(arrows)** without hyperostosis in a patient with a chromophobe adenoma. (Gifford ID, Goree JA, Jimenez JP: Tumor bulge into the sphenoid sinus: A roentgen sign of parasellar meningioma. AJR 112:324–328,1971. Copyright 1971. Reproduced by permission)

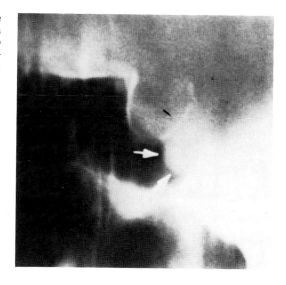

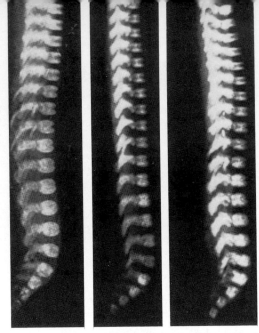

FIG. 4-15. (*Above*) Lateral radiographs of three normal infant spines. The anterior notches are clearly seen on the margins of the vertebral bodies in the thoracic and upper lumbar regions. (Naik DR: A sign of spina bifida cystica on lateral radiographs of the spine. Clin Radiol 23:193–195,1972)

Bullet-Nosed Vertebra Sign

The normal infant vertebral body appears ovoid on lateral radiographs and has a notch midway down its anterior margin (Fig. 4-15). In patients with meningomyelocele (spina bifida cystica), the anterior margin of the vertebral body becomes rounded or bullet-nosed (Fig. 4-16). This appearance in cases of meningomyelocele is probably due to the lack of a normal neural tube, which is essential for initiation of vertebral cartilage formation and may also influence molding of the normal vertebrae. The site at which the normal anterior notching disappears coincides with the upper level of the anatomic lesion. This is a useful confirmatory sign of the level of the bony abnormality, especially in patients with pronounced kyphosis, in whom interpretation is difficult on frontal radiographs because of considerable overlap of bony landmarks (Fig. 4-17). The anterior margin of the vertebral body may show a rounded outline at the L4 and L5 levels in normal infants, and the sign is thus of no value at these levels.

BIBLIOGRAPHY
Naik DR: A sign of spina bifida cystica on lateral radiographs of the spine. Clin Radiol 23:193–195, 1972

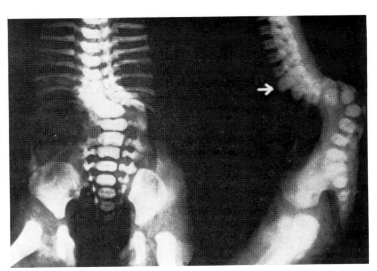

FIG. 4-17. (*Above, left*) Anteroposterior and (*right*) lateral radiographs of a case of spina bifida cystica. Kyphoscoliosis causes overlap of the bony landmarks on the frontal view. The upper level of the lesion can be identified on the lateral radiograph by demonstration of the disappearance of the anterior notch (**arrow**). (Naik DR: A sign of spina bifida cystica on lateral radiographs of the spine. Clin Radiol 23:193–195,1972)

FIG. 4-16. (*Above*) Lateral radiographs of spina bifida cystica spines. The (**arrows**) show the levels at which the anterior margins become rounded with disappearance of the anterior notches. These are also the upper levels of spina bifida cystica as diagnosed clinically and on anteroposterior radiographs. (Naik DR: A sign of spina bifida cystica on lateral radiographs of the spine. Clin Radiol 23:193–195,1972)

Button Sequestrum Sign

A button sequestrum of the skull is a round, lucent calvarial defect with a bony density (sequestrum) in its center. The term *button sequestrum* was first used to describe an unusual radiographic manifestation of eosinophilic granuloma (Fig. 4-18). Although most commonly seen in that disorder, this radiographic appearance has also been described in infectious osteitis (tuberculosis, *Staphylococcus* [Fig. 4-19]), metastatic carcinoma, radiation necrosis, meningioma (Fig. 4-20), dermoid cyst, and benign bone tumors, as well as following a ventriculoatrial shunt.

BIBLIOGRAPHY

Sholkof SD, Mainzer F: Button sequestrum revisited. Radiology 100:649–652, 1971

Wells PO: The button sequestrum of eosinophilic granuloma of the skull. Radiology 67:746–747, 1956

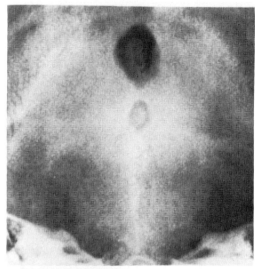

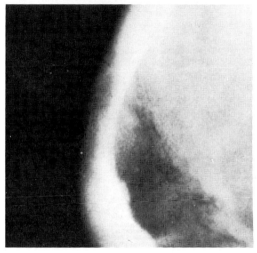

FIG. 4-18. Eosinophilic granuloma. *(Top)* Central retained bone is seen in each of two midline parietal lesions. *(Bottom)* A lateral view shows the intradiploic nature of the lesion. (Sholkoff SD, Mainzer F: Button sequestrum revisited. Radiology 100:649–652,1971)

FIG. 4-19. Staphylococcal osteomyelitis. A central nidus is seen within each of the multiple round lytic lesions. (Sholkoff SD, Mainzer F: Button sequestrum revisited. Radiology 100:649–652,1971)

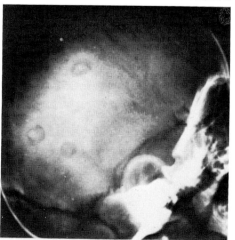

FIG. 4-20. Meningioma. The lucent lesion is irregularly marginated. Residual bone remains in the center. (Sholkoff SD, Mainzer F: Button sequestrum revisited. Radiology 100:649–652,1971)

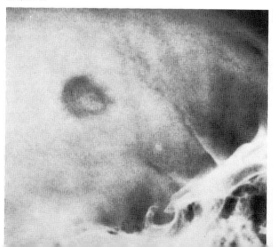

Carpal Sign

The carpal angle is that measured at the intersection of two tangents, the first touching the proximal contour of the navicular and lunate bones and the second touching the triquetral and lunate bones. In normal subjects, the angle measures approximately 130° (Fig. 4-21; *top*); in most patients with gonadal dysgenesis, the carpal angle measures 117° or less (Fig. 4-21, *bottom*).

BIBLIOGRAPHY
Kosowicz J: The roentgen appearance of the hand and wrist in gonadal dysgenesis. AJR 93:354–361, 1965

FIG. 4-21. *(Top)* In a normal subject, the bones of the proximal carpal row form a slight arch. Two lines drawn tangential to the contours of these bones form a normal carpal angle of 134°. *(Bottom)* In a patient with gonadal dysgenesis, the bones of the proximal carpal row are angularly arranged, and the carpal angle is only 108°. (Kosowicz J: The roentgen appearance of the hand and wrist in gonadal dysgenesis. AJR 93:354–361,1965. Copyright 1965. Reproduced by permission)

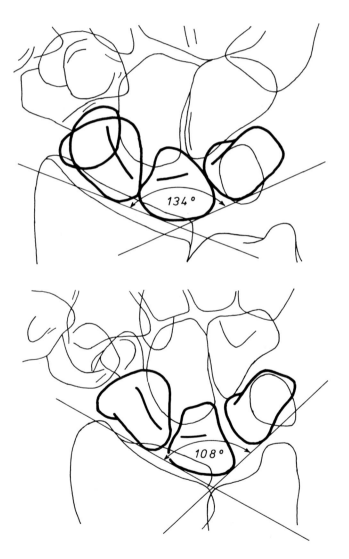

Catlin Mark

Posteriorly on each side of the sagittal suture, the parietal bones may normally contain a small opening through which an emissary vein passes (Fig. 4-22). These symmetric foramina are usually small but occasionally as large as several centimeters in diameter. Enlarged parietal foramina tend to be hereditary and are thus sometimes referred to as the *Catlin mark*, in honor of the 56 members of the Catlin family who first demonstrated this phenomenon.

BIBLIOGRAPHY
Goldsmith WM: The Catlin mark: The inheritance of an unusual opening in the parietal bones. J Hered 13:69–71, 1922
Murphy J, Gooding CA: Evolution of persistently enlarged parietal foramina. Radiology 97:391–392, 1970

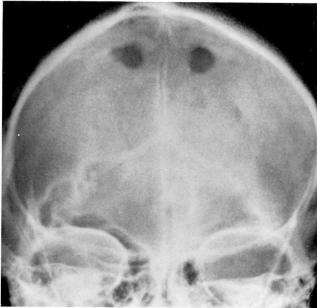

FIG. 4-22. Two examples of enlarged parietal foramina.

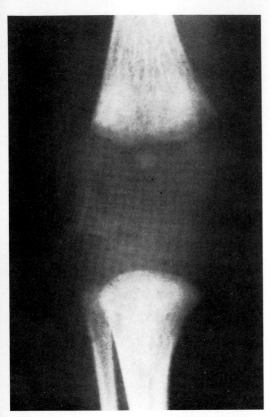

FIG. 4-23. Enlargement of a knee radiograph in a 1-day-old female with a maternal history of rubella demonstrates the celery stick sign. (Singleton EB, Rudolph AJ, Rosenberg HS et al: The roentgenographic manifestations of the rubella syndrome in newborn infants. AJR 97:82–91, 1966. Copyright 1966. Reproduced by permission)

Celery Stick Sign

In infants whose mothers had rubella during the first trimester of pregnancy, the architecture of the metaphysis and adjacent diaphysis of long bones is disorganized. This produces a characteristic pattern of alternating dense and lucent longitudinal striations (celery stick sign; Fig. 4-23). Although usually a reflection of maternal rubella infection, similar changes have been described in cytomegalic inclusion disease.

BIBLIOGRAPHY

Rabinowitz JG, Wolf BS, Greenberg EI et al: Osseous changes in rubella embryopathy (congenital rubella syndrome). Radiology 85:494–500, 1965

Singleton EB, Rudolph AJ, Rosenberg HS: The roentgenographic manifestations of the rubella syndrome in newborn infants. AJR 97:82–91, 1966

Williams HJ, Carey LS: Rubella embryopathy: Roentgenologic features. AJR 97:92–99, 1966

Cocktail Sausage Sign

The cocktail sausage sign is a manifestation of diffuse soft-tissue swelling of a toe (Fig. 4-24, *top*). It is often associated with periosteal reaction (Fig. 4-24, *bottom*) and is a classic clinical and radiographic sign of the rheumatoid variants.

BIBLIOGRAPHY
Forrester DM, Brown JC, Nesson JW: The Radiology of Joint Disease. Philadelphia, WB Saunders, 1978

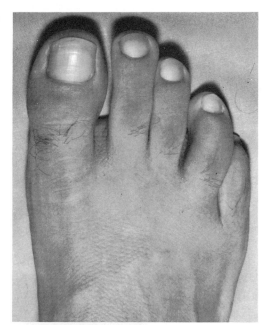

FIG. 4-24. *(Top)* Photograph of the foot of a patient with Reiter's syndrome shows diffuse swelling of a digit. *(Bottom)* Radiograph shows periosteal reaction accompanying the diffuse swelling. (Forrester DM, Brown JC, Nesson JW: The Radiology of Joint Disease. Philadelphia, WB Saunders, 1978)

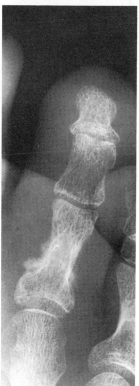

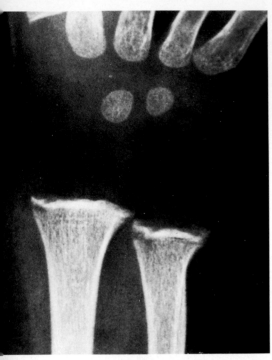

Corner Sign

In infantile scurvy a zone of radiolucency (Truemmerfeld zone) forms, giving the appearance of a double epiphysis. Initially, there may be a small area of rarefaction involving the cortex and spongiosa only at the margins just proximal to the metaphysis, producing the corner sign of scurvy (Fig. 4-25).

BIBLIOGRAPHY
Greenfield GB: Radiology of Bone Disease. Philadelphia, JB Lippincott, 1980
Park EA: Recognition of scurvy with especial reference to early x-ray changes. Arch Dis Child 10:265, 1935

FIG. 4-25. A small area of rarefaction at the margins of the distal radius and ulna is seen in this patient with scurvy. Note the characteristic "white line" of scurvy at the distal margin of the bone. (Edeiken J: Roentgen Diagnosis of Diseases of Bone. Baltimore, Williams & Wilkins, 1981. Copyright 1981. Reproduced by permission)

Cortical Ring Sign (Mandibular)

Fractures of the mandibular condylar process can be difficult to diagnose on standard radiographs because of the superimposition of bony structures and frequent difficulty in patient positioning. A dense cortical ring in the region of the mandibular neck on standard lateral mandibular or skull films indicates the presence of an anteromedially dislocated condylar neck fracture (Fig. 4-26). This cortical ring sign is seen in condylar neck fractures as a result of medial displacement of the condyle. If there is angulation of 60° or greater, the cortex of the dislocated part of the condylar neck can be oriented horizontally and seen axially as a dense ring on a true lateral view.

BIBLIOGRAPHY

Cacciarelli AA, Tabor HD: The cortical ring: A sign of anteromedial fracture dislocation of the mandibular condylar neck. AJR 138:355–356, 1982

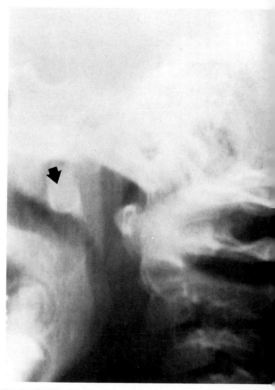

FIG. 4-26. *(Top)* Detail from a lateral skull film demonstrates a dense cortical ring (**arrow**) produced by a dislocated mandibular condyle and neck. *(Bottom)* A steep Towne's view demonstrates medial dislocation of the left condylar head and neck (**arrow**). This fracture was not seen well on the standard Towne's view of the skull series. (Cacciarelli AA, Tabor HD: The cortical ring: A sign of anteromedial fracture dislocation of the mandibular condylar neck. AJR 138:355–356, 1982. Copyright 1982. Reproduced by permission)

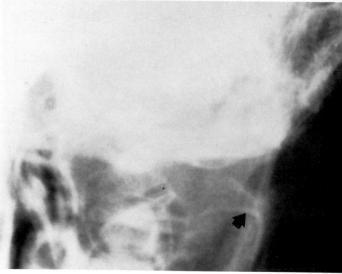

Cortical Ring Sign (Navicular)

Rotatory subluxation of the carpal navicular may occur as an isolated traumatic lesion, in association with lunate or perilunate dislocation, or as a complication of rheumatoid arthritis. In addition to widening of the space between the navicular and lunate bones, there may be a virtually pathognomonic cortical ring shadow seen within the navicular outline on the posteroanterior view (Fig. 4-27). This ring is caused by foreshortening of the volarly rotated navicular, which allows the cortex of the waist of the abnormally oriented navicular to be seen on end. The sign is easily recognized, because the hook of the hamate presents the only normal cortical ring shadow in the posteroanterior view of the wrist.

BIBLIOGRAPHY

Crittenden JJ, Jones DM, Santarelli AG: Bilateral rotational dislocation of the carpal navicular. Radiology 94:629–630, 1970

FIG. 4-27. *(Left)* Frontal and *(right)* lateral views of the wrist demonstrate rotational dislocation of the navicular producing the cortical ring sign. (Crittenden JJ, Jones DM, Santarelli AG: Bilateral rotational dislocation of the carpal navicular. Radiology 94:629–630,1970)

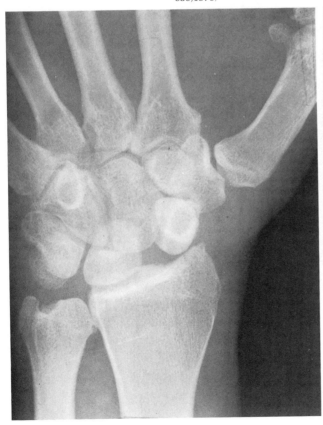
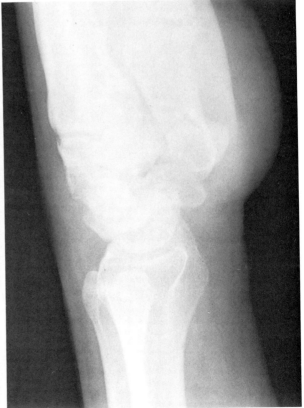

Cotton Wool Sign

In advanced Paget's disease of the skull, irregular areas of sclerosis may be seen in the thickened diploe, giving a characteristic cotton wool appearance (Fig. 4-28).

BIBLIOGRAPHY
Greenfield GB: Radiology of Bone Disease. Philadelphia, JB Lippincott, 1980

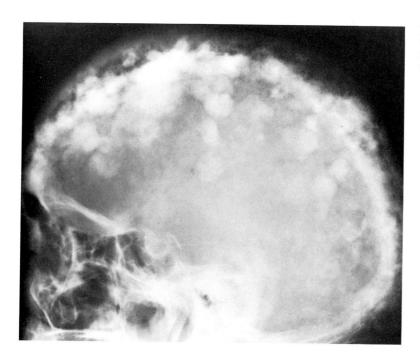

FIG. 4-28. Irregular areas of sclerosis produce the characteristic cotton wool appearance in this patient with advanced Paget's disease of the skull.

Crescent Sign

The first sign of structural failure in the femoral capital epiphysis due to ischemic necrosis is the development of a radiolucent subcortical band representing a fracture line (Fig. 4-29). The crescent sign is often shown more readily if traction is applied to the hip as the radiograph is obtained, because gas tends to collect in the subchondral area as a result of a vacuum phenomenon (Fig. 4-30). The subchondral lucent line is frequently seen before the characteristic subchondral sclerosis becomes evident. A similar crescent-shaped lucency has also been described with ischemic necrosis of the head of the humerus.

BIBLIOGRAPHY

Martel W, Poznanski AK: The effect of traction on the hip in osteonecrosis: A comment on the "radiolucent crescent line." Radiology 94:505–508, 1970

Norman A, Bullough P: The radiolucent crescent line: An early diagnostic sign of avascular necrosis of the femoral head. Bull Hosp Joint Dis 24:99–104, 1963

FIG. 4-29. Arc-like radiolucent subcortical band in a patient with ischemic necrosis of the femoral head. (Edeiken J: Roentgen Diagnosis of Diseases of Bone. Baltimore, Williams & Wilkins, 1981. Copyright 1981. Reproduced by permission)

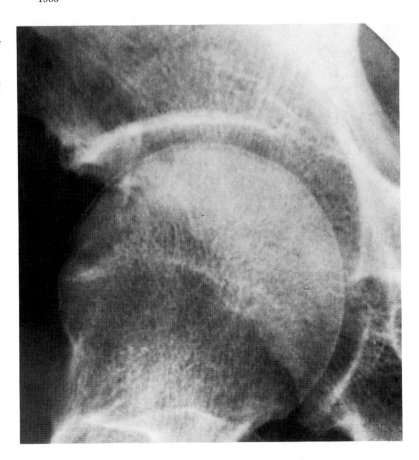

FIG. 4-30. Crescent-shaped subchondral lucency in a patient with ischemic necrosis of the femur. (Edeiken J: Roentgen Diagnosis of Diseases of Bone. Baltimore, Williams & Wilkins, 1981. Copyright 1981. Reproduced by permission)

Cupid's Bow Contour

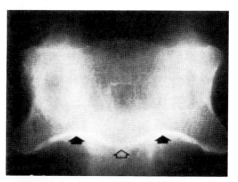

Cupid's bow contour is the name applied to a normal concavity on the inferior aspect of the third, fourth, and fifth lumbar vertebral bodies. On the frontal view, smooth parasagittal concavities on the undersurface of the vertebrae resemble a bow pointing cephalad (Fig. 4-31, *left*). On lateral views, the vertebral depressions are located posteriorly (Fig. 4-31, *right*). This normal contour of the end-plate (Fig. 4-32) should not be confused with other vertebral body anomalies of clinical importance, most of which are widespread and involve both the superior and inferior surfaces.

BIBLIOGRAPHY

Dietz GW, Christensen EE: Normal "Cupid's bow" contour of the lower lumbar vertebrae. Radiology 121:577–579, 1976

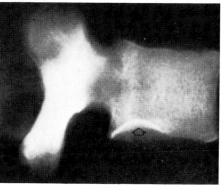

FIG. 4-31. (*Top*) Anteroposterior and (*bottom*) lateral tomograms of a lower lumbar vertebra reveal parasagittal cavities in the inferior end-plate of the centrum. The contour of the cortex in frontal projection simulates a Cupid's bow, the handgrip of the bow (**open arrow**) being in the midline and the extremities of the bow (**solid arrows**) forming a smooth arc in a cephalad direction. The lateral tomogram, cut to the left of the midline, demonstrates the posterior position of the concavities (**arrow**). (Dietz GW, Christensen EE: Normal "Cupid's bow" contour of the lower lumbar vertebrae. Radiology 121:577–579, 1976)

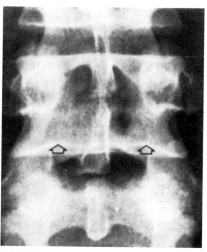

FIG. 4-32. Radiographs of the lumbar spine in two patients demonstrate variation in the severity of the Cupid's bow contour (**arrows**). (Dietz GW, Christensen EE: Normal "Cupid's bow" contour of the lower lumbar vertebrae. Radiology 121:577–579, 1976)

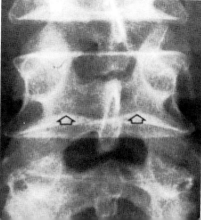

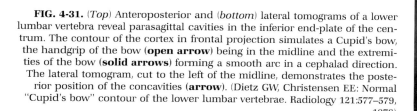

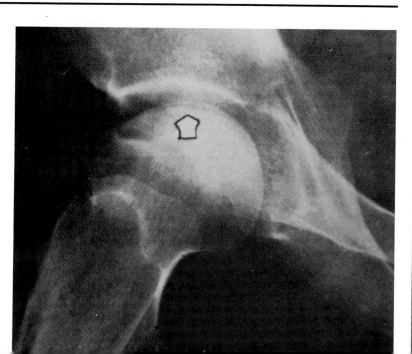

Disappearing Ellipse Sign

A linear nondepressed skull fracture may be seen as two connecting lines, because slight angulation of the x-ray beam results in separate visualization of the fracture as it crosses the outer table and then the inner table. These two lucent lines rejoin at points at which the table fractures superimpose, forming an elliptical shape (Fig. 4-33, *top*). A second projection may result in superimposition of the inner and outer table fractures with disappearance of the elliptical configuration (Fig. 4-33, *bottom*). Demonstration of this disappearing ellipse sign may be of value in the differentiation of a linear skull fracture from a vascular groove.

BIBLIOGRAPHY

Rhea JT: The disappearing ellipse: A new sign of a linear skull fracture. J Trauma 20:327–328, 1980

FIG. 4-33. *(Top)* Lateral view showing a linear fracture that appears to branch and rejoin, forming an elongated elliptical shape **(arrows).** *(Bottom)* Oblique view results in superimposition of the fracture lines **(arrow)** and disappearance of the ellipse. (Rhea JT: The disappearing ellipse: A new sign of a linear skull fracture. J Trauma 20:327–328,1980)

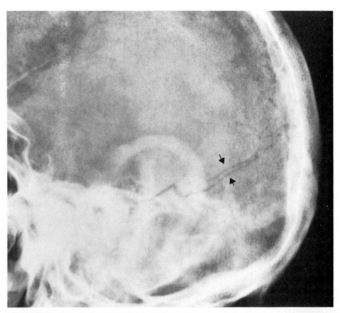

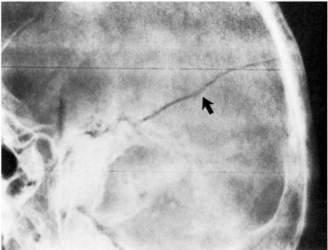

Displaced Spinolaminar Line Sign

The spinolaminar line is a smooth, gentle curve connecting the cortices of the posterior spinal canal of the cervical vertebrae. It is formed by the junction of the two laminar arches, seen in profile. Displacement of the spinolaminar line at any level is abnormal and is often an indication of subtle traumatic vertebral damage (Fig. 4-34). This is of particular importance in fractures of the upper cervical spine, which frequently are not associated with a neurologic deficit and are thus difficult to diagnose. The only nonpathologic cause of displacement of the spinolaminar line is a congenital anomaly of no clinical significance, found in about 10% of the population, in which the neural arch of C2 is elongated, causing some slight posterior displacement of the spinolaminar line at C2.

BIBLIOGRAPHY
Scher AT: Displacement of the spinolaminar line—A sign of value in fractures of the upper cervical spine. S Afr Med J 56:58–61, 1979

FIG. 4-34. *(Left)* Full and *(right)* coned lateral radiographs of the cervical spine. The full view demonstrates anterior displacement of the spinolaminar line of C1 (**upper arrow**) relative to that of C2 (**lower arrow**) and of the other cervical vertebrae in a patient with traumatic anterior displacement of C1. (Scher AT: Displacement of the spinolaminar line—A sign of value in fractures of the upper cervical spine. S Afr Med J 56:58–61,1979)

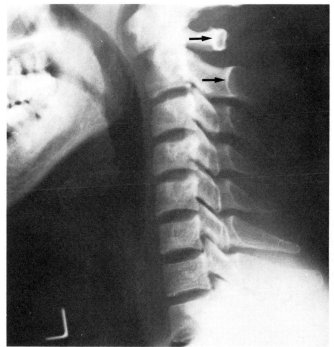
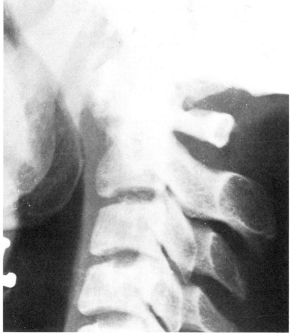

Divergent Spinous Processes Sign

Injury to the cervical spine may cause ligamentous damage severe enough to injure the spinal cord and produce paralysis but not severe enough to produce radiographic evidence of fracture or dislocation. In the normal cervical spine, the long axes of the spinous processes are related in such a way that lines drawn through them tend to converge at a central point posterior to the neck (Fig. 4-35). Following severe flexion injury to the cervical spine, marked divergence of lines drawn through the long axes of the spinous processes suggests severe underlying soft-tissue and posterior ligamentous damage (Fig. 4-36).

BIBLIOGRAPHY
Scher AT: Ligamentous injury to the cervical spine—Two radiological signs. S Afr Med J 53:802–804, 1978

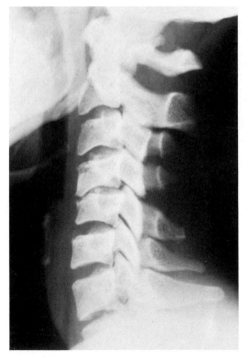

FIG. 4-35. Line drawing of a normal cervical spine shows that lines projected through the long axes of the spinous processes tend to converge. (Scher AT: Ligamentous injury of the cervical spine—Two radiological signs. S Afr Med J 53:802–804,1978)

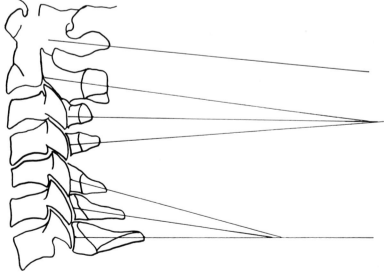

FIG. 4-36. *(Left)* lateral radiograph and *(right)* corresponding line drawing of the cervical spine of a patient who had sustained spinal cord injury. There is divergence of the spinous processes of C4 and C5, indicating posterior ligamentous damage. (Scher AT: Ligamentous injury of the cervical spine—Two radiological signs. S Afr Med J 53:802–804,1978)

Double Outline Sign

Extension–flexion injuries of the cervical spine may produce compression fractures of the articular mass leading to partial collapse. On lateral radiographs, the normal articular mass may be superimposed over the smaller image of the collapsed articular mass, producing a double outline sign (Fig. 4-37). Demonstration of this sign requires a true lateral view; small degrees of obliquity do not produce superimposition of the normal articular masses.

BIBLIOGRAPHY
Smith GR, Beckly DE, Abel MS: Articular mass fracture: A neglected cause of post-traumatic neck pain? Clin Radiol 27:335–340, 1976

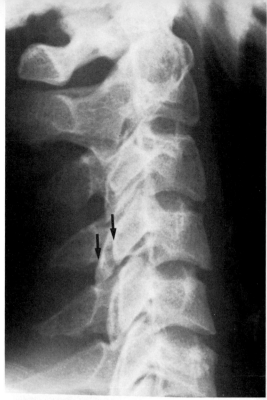

FIG. 4-37. *(Top)* Lateral view of the cervical spine demonstrates the double outline sign (**arrows**) and a defect in the inferior facet of the involved articular process. *(Bottom)* Tomography confirms the presence of a fracture of the articular process (**arrowheads**). (Harris JH, Harris WH: The Radiology of Emergency Medicine. Baltimore, Williams & Wilkins, 1981. Copyright 1981. Reproduced by permission)

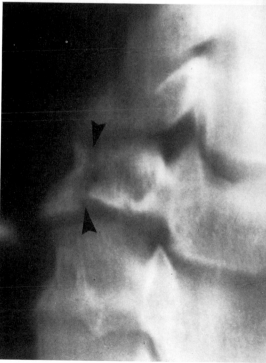

Double Spinous Process Sign

Clay shoveler's fracture represents an avulsion type of fracture of a spinous process in the lower cervical or upper thoracic region. The fracture was so named because it is frequently sustained by men working on heavy soil or clay, who at the time of thrusting a loaded shovel upward experience a sharp pain high between the shoulder blades. This type of fracture is difficult to demonstrate on emergency cross-table lateral radiographs because the shoulders frequently obscure the lower cervical spine. The diagnosis can be established with conventional anteroposterior views of the cervical spine by identification of a double shadow of the spinous process due to caudad displacement of the avulsed fragment (Fig. 4-38). This double spinous process sign must be differentiated from a bifid spinous process (Fig. 4-39), which usually lies at higher levels on a horizontal or almost horizontal plane.

BIBLIOGRAPHY

Cancelmo JJ: Clay shoveler's fracture: A helpful diagnostic sign. AJR 115:540–543, 1972

Zanca P, Lodmell EA: Fracture of spinous processes: New sign for recognition of fractures of cervical and upper dorsal spinous processes. Radiology 56:427–492, 1951

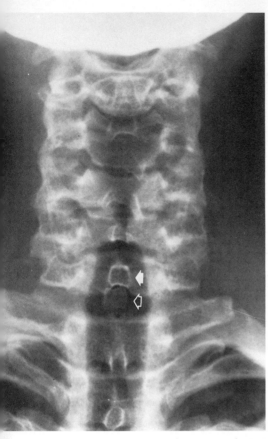

FIG. 4-38. Clay shoveler's fracture producing the double spinous process sign as a result of caudad displacement of the avulsed fragment (**open arrow**) with respect to the normal position of the major portion of the spinous process (**closed arrow**).

FIG. 4-39. Bifid spinous process (**arrow**) with both segments lying on a horizontal plane. (Cancelmo JJ: Clay shoveler's fracture: A helpful diagnostic sign. AJR 115:540– 543, 1972.) Copyright 1972. Reproduced by permission)

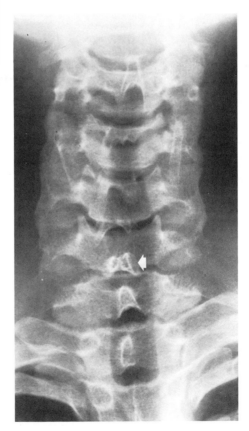

Doughnut Lesion

The calvarial doughnut lesion is a benign, asymptomatic entity, usually a coincidental finding on routine skull films, that appears as a relatively well defined area of radiolucency surrounded by a very dense region of sclerotic bone (Fig. 4-40). The doughnut lesion often contains densities of various sizes within the central area of radiolucency (Fig. 4-41). The calvarial doughnut lesion must be differentiated from button sequestrum or intradiploic epidermoid. The former has no sclerotic margin and is often associated with pain or soft-tissue abnormalities in the region of the bony lesion; the latter does not contain any central area of density.

BIBLIOGRAPHY

Keats TE, Holt JF: The calvarial "doughnut lesion": A previously undescribed entity. AJR 105:314–318, 1969

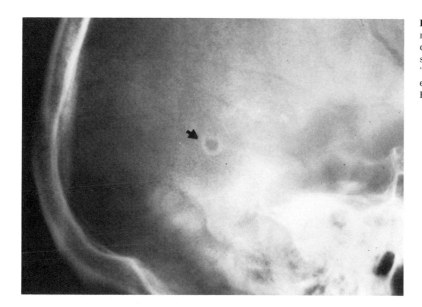

FIG. 4-40. Typical appearance of the doughnut lesion (**arrow**), a well-defined area of radiolucency surrounded by a dense region of sclerotic bone. (Keats T, Holt JF: The calvarial "doughnut lesion": A previously undescribed entity. AJR 105:314–318, 1969. Copyright 1969. Reproduced by permission)

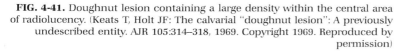

FIG. 4-41. Doughnut lesion containing a large density within the central area of radiolucency. (Keats T, Holt JF: The calvarial "doughnut lesion": A previously undescribed entity. AJR 105:314–318, 1969. Copyright 1969. Reproduced by permission)

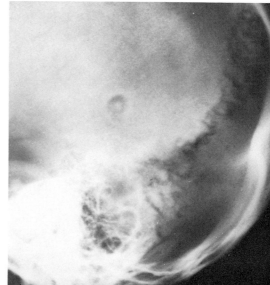

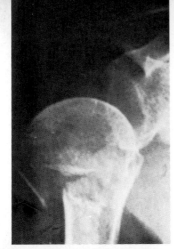

Drooping Shoulder Sign ▬▬▬▬▬

Inferior subluxation of the humeral head, often associated with a fracture, is a relatively benign condition that must be differentiated from the more serious true fracture–dislocation of the shoulder, which often requires surgical correction. Plain radiographs of the shoulder demonstrate the inferior subluxation (Fig. 4-42, *left*) but show no evidence of anterior or posterior displacement (Fig. 4-42, *center*). In case of doubt, the proper diagnosis can be made on repeat radiographs with the arm elevated in a sling after arthrocentesis has been performed to remove blood from the joint (Fig. 4-42, *right*). In addition to being a sequela of trauma, the drooping shoulder appearance can be seen in patients with acute hemarthroses secondary to coagulation defects in hemophilia and in patients with neurologic injuries of the brachial plexus, especially those involving the axillary nerve.

BIBLIOGRAPHY

Laskin RS, Schreiber S: Inferior subluxation of the humeral head: The drooping shoulder. Radiology 98:585–586, 1971

FIG. 4-42. *(Top)* Anteroposterior radiograph of the right shoulder demonstrates a fracture of the surgical neck of the humerus with inferior subluxation of the humeral head. *(Center)*. Axillary view following injection of 2 ml of 1% lidocaine into the glenohumeral joint. There is no evidence of anterior or posterior displacement. *(Bottom)* Anteroposterior radiograph following arthrocentesis of the glenohumeral joint and removal of 19 ml of nonclotted blood. The humeral head is relocated in the glenoid fossa. (Laskin RS, Schreiber S: Inferior subluxation of the humeral head: The drooping shoulder. Radiology 98:585–586, 1971)

FIG. 4-43. Lateral view of the elbow demonstrates the normal appearance of the anterior fat pad closely applied to the anterior surface of the distal end of the humerus. The posterior fat pad cannot be identified. (Forrester DM, Brown JC, Nesson JW: The Radiology of Joint Disease. Philadelphia, WB Saunders, 1978)

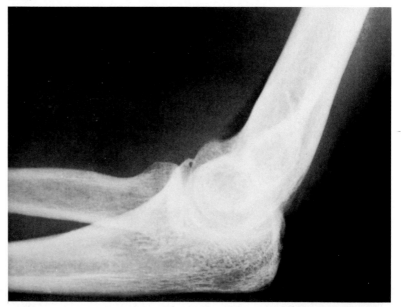

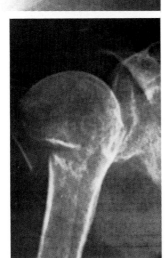

Elbow Fat Pad Sign

The elbow joint contains pads of fat that are intracapsular but extrasynovial in position. On lateral views of the elbow, the anterior fat pad appears as a radiolucency closely applied to the anterior surface of the distal end of the humerus (Fig. 4-43). The posterior fat pad is normally hidden in the depths of the olecranon fossa and should not be visible on standard lateral views of the elbow. Any process producing synovial or hemorrhagic effusion within the elbow joint displaces the fat pads (fat pad sign; Figs. 4-44 and 4-45). The normally hidden posterior fat pad is posteriorly displaced by an effusion and becomes visible as a crescentic lucency behind the lower end of the humerus (Fig. 4-46). The anterior fat pad becomes more rounded and further separated from the underlying bones (Fig. 4-47). The posterior fat pad sign is by far the more sensitive indicator of an elbow joint effusion. Its presence on lateral view in a patient with elbow trauma is strongly suggestive of a fracture, especially of the radial head, and indicates the need for oblique views to be obtained if no fracture is seen on standard projections.

BIBLIOGRAPHY

Bledsoe RC, Izenstark JL: Displacement of fat pads in disease and injury of the elbow: A new radiographic sign. Radiology 73:717–724, 1959

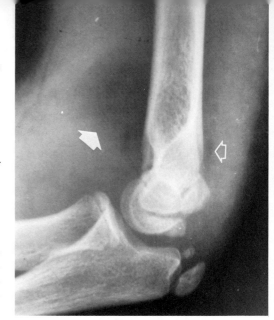

FIG. 4-44. The anterior fat pad (**closed arrow**) is clearly lifted from its fossa as a result of a large joint effusion in this child with a supracondylar fracture. The normally hidden posterior fat pad is posteriorly displaced by the effusion (**open arrow**).

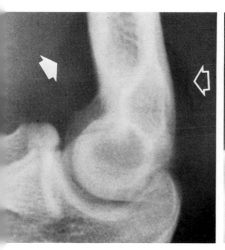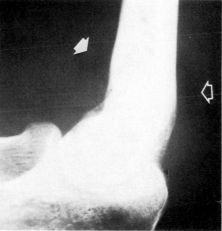

FIG. 4-45.   **FIG. 4-46.**

FIG. 4-45. Displacement of the anterior fat pad (**closed arrow**) and posterior fat pads (**open arrow**) in a patient with a nondisplaced fracture of the radial head.

FIG. 4-46. The posterior fat pad, displaced by an effusion secondary to a fracture of the radial head, is visible behind the lower end of the humerus (**open arrow**). The anterior fat pad has become more rounded and is elevated from its fossa (**closed arrow**).

FIG. 4-47.

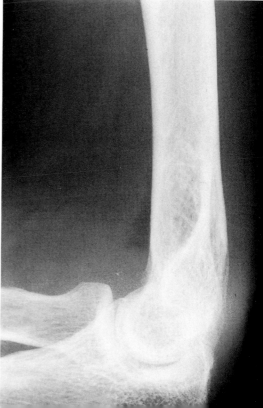

FIG. 4-47 A large joint effusion secondary to the inflammation of rheumatoid arthritis lifts the anterior fat pad from its fossa. Involvement of the olecranon bursa has resulted in a shallow erosion of the posterior olecranon. (Forrester DM, Brown JC, Nesson JW: The Radiology of Joint Disease. Philadelphia, WB Saunders, 1978)

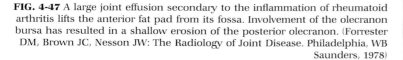

Fabella Sign

The fabella is a small sesamoid bone located within the posterior portion of the joint capsule of the knee. It is present in 10% to 20% of the population. The fabella sign, which represents posterior displacement of this bone, has been reported as an indication of synovial effusion or intrasynovial mass (Fig. 4-48). The fabella sign can be used even when inflammation, post-traumatic edema, or poor film technique obliterates the extrasynovial fat lines, which would otherwise define the extent of the joint capsule. Because the fabella normally moves posteriorly as the knee is flexed, tables are available indicating the appropriate position of the fabella for various angles of knee flexion.

BIBLIOGRAPHY
Friedman AC, Naidich TP: The fabella sign: Fabella displacement in synovial effusion and popliteal fossa masses. Radiology 127:113–121, 1978

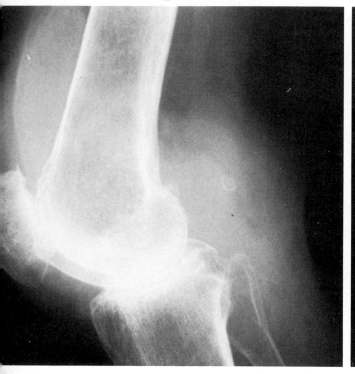 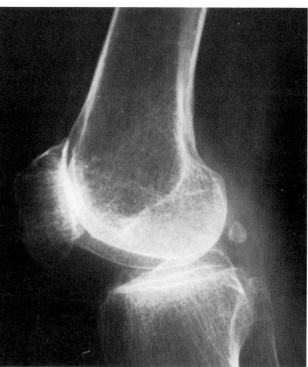

FIG. 4-48. *(Left)* Lateral view of the right knee in a patient with rheumatoid arthritis demonstrates a large synovial effusion distending the joint capsule and clearly displacing the fabella posteriorly. *(Right)* Normal position of the fabella in the contralateral knee. (Friedman AC, Naidich TP: The fabella sign: Fabella displacement in synovial effusion and popliteal fossa masses. Radiology 127:113–121, 1978)

FIG. 4-50. Solitary chip of cortical bone (**arrow**) lies in the dependent portion ▶ of an intramedullary lesion of the humerus. The presence of this bone fragment in an isolated position 3cm to 5cm below the fracture site from which it gravitated provides irrefutable evidence that the lesion is a true cyst. (Reynolds J: The "fallen fragment sign" in the diagnosis of unicameral bone cyst. Radiology 92:949–953,1969)

FIG. 4-51. Following fracture of a large unicameral bone cyst of the humerus, ▶ a fragment of cortical bone projects into the lumen of the cyst at a sharp angle, a position it could not assume were the cyst a solid intramedullary lesion. (Reynolds J: The "fallen fragment sign" in the diagnosis of unicameral bone cyst. Radiology 92:949–953,1969)

Fallen Fragment Sign

A solitary unicameral bone cyst is a fluid-filled intramedullary cavity lined by a thin layer of connective tissue. Although a unicameral bone cyst classically presents as a centrally located radiolucent metaphyseal lesion in a long bone with elongation in the direction of the shaft, a similar radiographic appearance may be seen with such solid intramedullary lesions as fibrous dysplasia and enchondroma. Disruption of the wall of a bone cyst by a pathologic fracture may result in a cortical bone fragment lying free within the cyst space (Fig. 4-49). Because the fluid contents of the cyst offer no resistance, fragments of cortical bone are free to fall down to the dependent portion of the cyst (Fig. 4-50), thus permitting differentiation of a bone cyst from radiographically similar solid processes that have a firm tissue consistency.

A variant of the fallen fragment sign occasionally occurs when the fracturing force causes fragmentation of the thin shell of the cyst but fails to completely dislodge any of these fragments from the adherent periosteal membranes. Under such circumstances, a fragment may become largely detached yet remain joined to the periosteum along one margin so that it tilts into the lumen of the cyst like a door on a hinge (Fig. 4-51). Because a fragment of cortical bone could not easily project in this way if the lucent lesion were not cystic, this appearance has the same diagnostic significance as the fallen fragment sign.

BIBLIOGRAPHY
Reynolds J: The "fallen fragment sign" in the diagnosis of unicameral bone cyst. Radiology 92:949–953, 1969

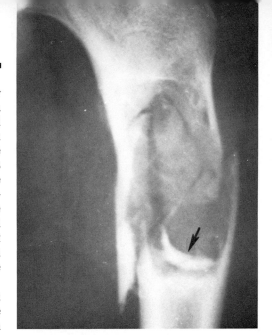

FIG. 4-49. Cortical bone fragment (**arrow**) lying free within the cyst space following a comminuted pathologic fracture of a subtrochanteric unicameral cyst. (Reynolds J: The "fallen fragment sign" in the diagnosis of unicameral bone cyst. Radiology 92:949–953,1969)

FIG. 4-51.

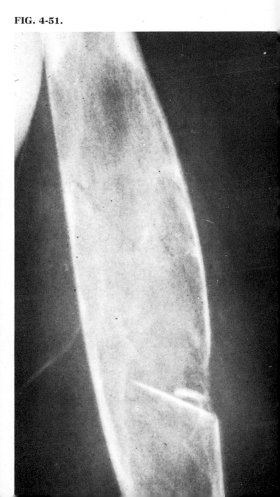

FIG. 4-50.

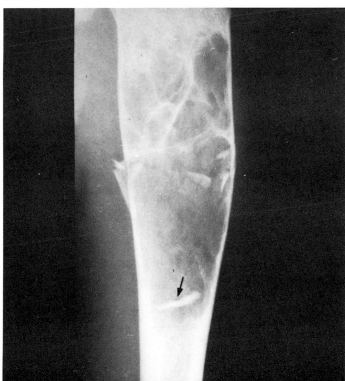

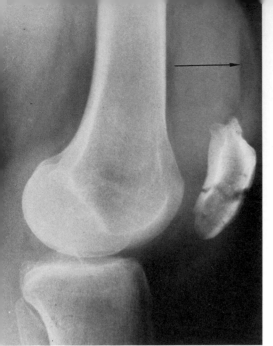

FBI Sign

Traumatic lipohemarthrosis may occur in any joint in which an intracapsular fracture has occurred, allowing blood and fat to extrude into the joint space. On recumbent radiographs using a horizontal beam, a fat–blood interface (FBI sign) can be demonstrated (Fig. 4-52). The FBI sign is most frequently seen in the knee joint, which is composed of bones with abundant fatty marrow and which after trauma is more commonly examined by a horizontal x-ray beam than are other limb joints (Fig. 4-53). A similar appearance has been described on erect views in patients with simple shoulder fractures (Fig. 4-54) and even following simple dislocations of the shoulder without an associated intra-articular fracture.

BIBLIOGRAPHY
Arger PH, Oberkircher PE, Miller WT: Lipohemarthrosis. AJR 121:97–100, 1974
Saxton HM: Lipohaemarthrosis. Br J Radiol 35:122–127, 1962
Wenzel WW: The FBI sign. Rocky Mount Med J 69:71–72, 1972

FIG. 4-52. In this patient with a patellar fracture, a fat–blood interface (**arrow**) is demonstrated within a large suprapatellar effusion on a recumbent radiograph obtained using a horizontal beam. (Wenzel WW: The FBI sign. Rocky Mount Med J 69:71–72, 1972)

FIG. 4-54. *(Top)* Radiograph and *(bottom)* corresponding line drawing demonstrate a fat–blood interface (**arrow**) on the upright view in a patient with a fracture dislocation of the right shoulder and a large collection of fat in the joint. (Saxton HM: Lipohaemarthrosis. B J Radiol 35:122–127,1962)

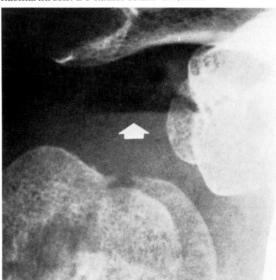

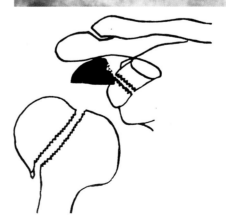

FIG. 4-53. *(Left)* Subtle fracture of the lateral tibial plateau (**arrow**). The lesion was almost overlooked. *(Right)* A positive FBI sign (**arrow**) seen on the cross-table lateral view led the physician to take a second look and subsequently detect the tibial plateau fracture. (Wenzel WW: The FBI sign. Rocky Mount Med J 69:71–72,1972)

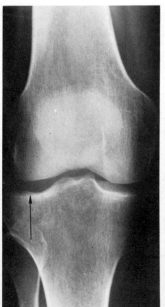

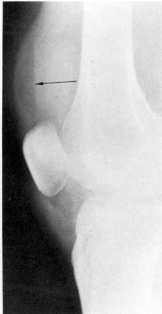

Fish Vertebra

Biconcave deformities of the vertebral bodies seen on lateral view (fish vertebrae; Fig. 4-55) are characteristic of disorders in which there is diffuse weakening of bone. Most common in the lower thoracic and upper lumbar spine, this appearance is frequently seen in osteoporosis (Fig. 4-56). A similar pattern can often be demonstrated in osteomalacia, Paget's disease, hyperparathyroidism, sickle cell disease (Fig. 4-57), and neoplasms. Expansile pressure of the adjacent intervertebral disks causes arch-like indentations on both the superior and inferior margins of the vertebral bodies and the characteristic fish-like appearance.

BIBLIOGRAPHY
Resnick D, Niwayama G: Diagnosis of Bone and Joint Disorders. Philadelphia, WB Saunders, 1981

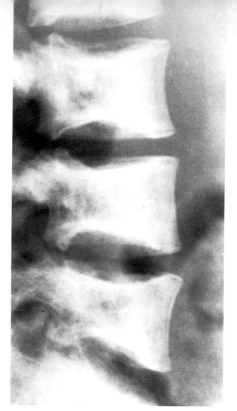

FIG. 4-55. Lateral view of the lumbar spine demonstrates typical biconcave deformities of the vertebral bodies.

FIG. 4-55.

FIG. 4-56. Severe osteoporosis of the thoracic spine in a patient on high-dose steroid therapy for dermatomyositis. Note the thinning of cortical margins and the fish vertebrae configuration.

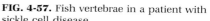

FIG. 4-57. Fish vertebrae in a patient with sickle cell disease.

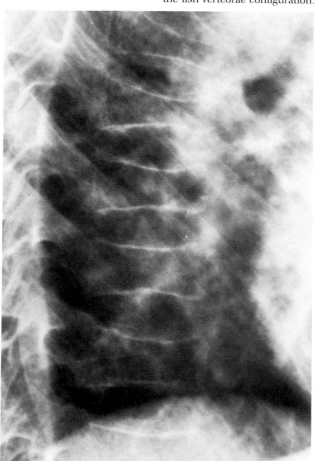

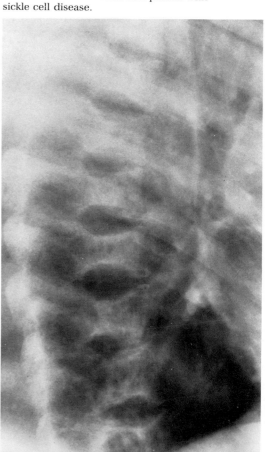

Flared Mandible Sign

A flail mandible is a serious post-traumatic condition in which fractures destroy the ability of the mandible to maintain forward support for the tongue, often resulting in airway obstruction. Fractures of the condylar neck, ramus, and symphysis of the mandible cause the anterior portions of the body of the mandible to be retracted inward and the angles of the mandible to protrude outward (flared mandible sign; Fig. 4-58 and 4-59). This flared appearance of the mandible following facial trauma indicates an unstable, dangerous complex of multiple mandibular fractures which, if not stabilized, can lead to complete airway obstruction and suffocation (Fig. 4-60).

BIBLIOGRAPHY
Gerlock AJ: The flared mandible sign of the flail mandible. Radiology 117:299–300, 1976

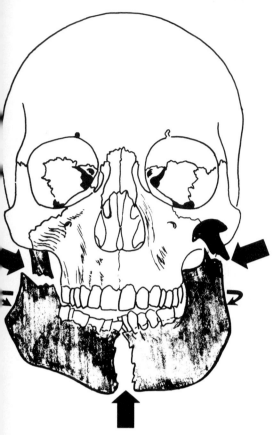

FIG. 4-59. Diagrammatic representation of flaring of the bodies of the mandible as a result of fractures of the condylar neck, ramus, and symphysis menti (**straight arrows**). **Curved arrows** indicate the internal rotation of the mandibular bodies. (Gerlock AJ: The flared mandible sign of the flail mandible. Radiology 117:299–300)

FIG. 4-58. Anteroposterior view of the skull shows flaring of the mandibular bodies. Note the fractures of the condylar neck, symphysis menti region, and ramus of the mandible (**solid arrows**). Malocclusion is also present (**open arrow**). (Gerlock AJ: The flared mandible sign of the flail mandible. Radiology 117:299–300, 1976)

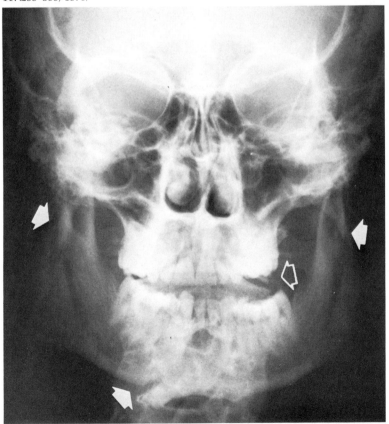

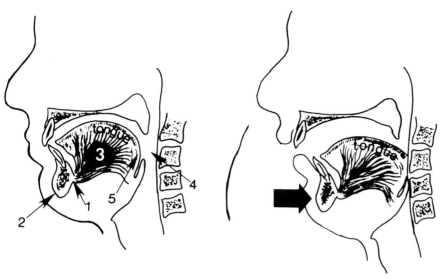

FIG. 4-60. *(Left)* The normal position of the tongue with the oropharynx non-obstructed. *1* = mental spine; *2* = symphysis menti region of the mandible; *3* = genioglossi muscles; *4* = posterior pharyngeal wall; *5* = base of the tongue.

(Right) Posteriorly displaced fracture fragment of the mandible (**arrow**) results in occlusion of the space between the posterior pharyngeal wall and the base of the tongue. (Gerlock AJ: The flared mandible sign of the flail mandible. Radiology 117:299–300, 1976)

Floating Tooth Sign

Circumscribed cyst-like areas around mandibular teeth caused by peridontal destruction can produce a characteristic floating tooth pattern (Fig. 4-61). This appearance is typically found in the reticuloendothelioses, especially eosinophilic granuloma and histiocytosis X, though it has also been reported in such conditions as neuroblastoma and Burkitt's lymphoma.

BIBLIOGRAPHY
Greenfield GB: Radiology of Bone Diseases. Philadelphia, JB Lippincott, 1980

FIG. 4-61. Diffuse periodontal destruction about the mandibular incisors produces the floating tooth appearance in a patient with Hand–Schueller–Christian disease. (Greenfield GB: Radiology of Bone Diseases. Philadelphia, JB Lippincott, 1980)

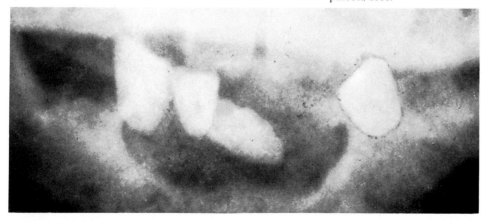

Floppy Thumb Sign

Radial subluxation or dislocation at the interphalangeal joint of the thumb is a characteristic deformity in patients with dermatomyositis or polymyositis (Fig. 4-62).

BIBLIOGRAPHY
Bunch TW, O'Duffy JD, McLeod RA: Deforming arthritis of the hands in polymyositis. Arthritis Rheum 19:243–248, 1976

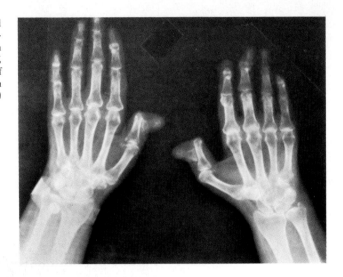

FIG. 4-62. Frontal radiographs of the hand and wrist demonstrate dislocation at the interphalangeal joint of the thumb bilaterally in this patient with polymyositis. (Bunch TW, O'Duffy JD, McLeod RA: Deforming arthritis of the hands in polymyositis. Arthritis Rheum 19:243–248, 1976)

Ghost Vertebrae Sign

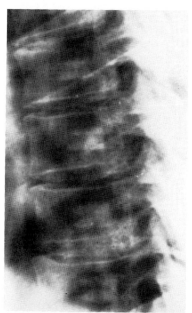

Ghost vertebrae, radiographic densities of infantile vertebrae and pelvis within adult bones, have been demonstrated in adults who received intravenous Thorotrast during early childhood (Fig. 4-63). The size of these ghost vertebrae corresponds to that appropriate for the time at which the intravenous Thorotrast was administered; the anterior notch in the contour of the ghost vertebrae corresponds to the expected shape of infantile vertebral bodies. In most patients with this appearance, reticular or dense opacification of the liver, spleen, or lymph nodes offers confirmatory evidence of previous Thorotrast injection.

BIBLIOGRAPHY

Teplick JG, Head GL, Kricun ME et al: Ghost infantile vertebrae and hemipelves within adult skeleton from thorotrast administration in childhood. Radiology 129:657–660, 1978

FIG. 4-63. Two examples of persistence of radiographic densities of infantile vertebrae within adult bones in adults who received intravenous Thorotrast during early childhood. (Teplick JG, Head GL, Kricun ME et al: Ghost infantile vertebrae and hemipelves within adult skeleton from thorotrast administration in childhood. Radiology 129:657–660, 1978)

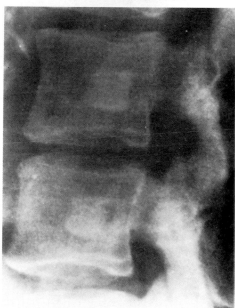

Gull Wing Sign

In a patient with multiple injuries, a lateral view of the entire pelvis may be of value in the diagnosis of fracture–dislocation of the posterior acetabular rim or dislocation of the femoral head. A double curved gull wing shadow, which simulates the silhouette of a flying gull, may be produced by the intact and fractured portions of the acetabulum, each of which forms one of the "wings" in the sign (Fig. 4-64).

BIBLIOGRAPHY

Berkebile RD, Fischer DL, Albrecht LF: The gull-wing sign: Value of the lateral view of the pelvis in fracture–dislocation of the acetabular rim and posterior dislocation of the femoral head. Radiology 84:937–939, 1965

FIG. 4-64. *(Left)* Frontal view of the pelvis demonstrates a fracture in the femoral neck and widening of the joint. *(Right)* On the lateral view, a double curved gull wing shadow is produced. The *inset* is a diagrammatic representation. (Berkebile RD, Fischer DL, Albrecht LF: The gull-wing sign: Value of the lateral view of the pelvis in fracture–dislocation of the acetabular rim and posterior dislocation of the femoral head. Radiology 84:937–939, 1965)

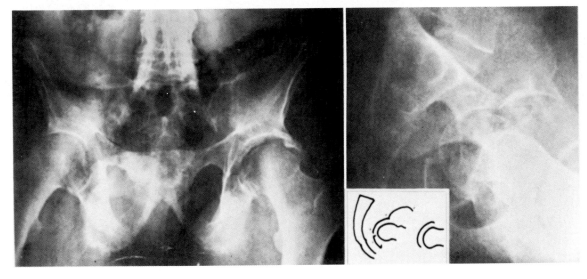

Hair-on-End Sign

In severe congenital hemolytic anemias, marked new bone formation perpendicular to the tables of the skull produces a radial hair-on-end appearance (Fig. 4-65). Although most commonly seen in patients with thalassemia (Fig. 4-66), the hair-on-end pattern may also be produced in patients with sickle cell disease or spherocytosis, as well as in some persons with iron-deficiency anemia. A similar appearance has been described in cyanotic congenital heart disease, childhood polycythemia vera, and metastases from neuroblastoma. When widening of the calvarium and the hair-on-end appearance are of hematologic origin, the occipital bone inferior to the internal occipital protuberance is not involved as a result of lack of marrow in this area. This finding can be used as a basis for differentiation between hematologic and nonhematologic causes of the hair-on-end appearance.

BIBLIOGRAPHY
Greenfield GB: Radiology of Bone Disease. Philadelphia, JB Lippincott, 1980

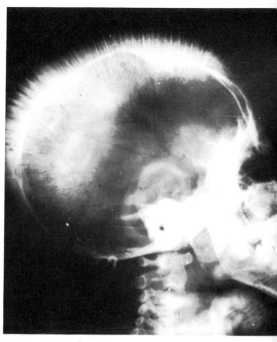

FIG. 4-65. Hair-on-end appearance in a patient with advanced sickle cell anemia. Note that there is no involvement inferior to the internal occipital protuberance. (Greenfield GB: Radiology of Bone Diseases. Philadelphia, JB Lippincott, 1980)

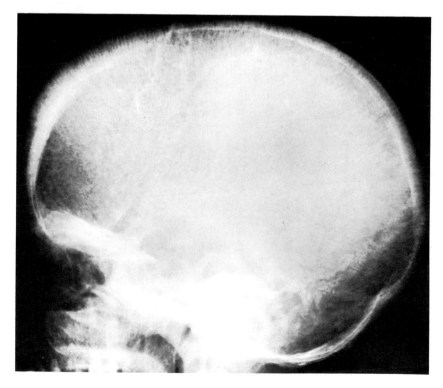

FIG. 4-66. Thickening of the calvarium has caused the hair-on-end appearance in this patient with thalassemia major. There is no involvement of the skull inferior to the internal occipital protuberance. The paranasal sinuses other than the ethmoids show lack of development, a characteristic feature in thalassemia. (Greenfield GB: Radiology of Bone Diseases. Philadelphia, JB Lippincott, 1980)

Hill–Sachs Sign

The Hill–Sachs sign consists of a large defect or groove in the posterolateral aspect of the head of the humerus occurring in patients with repeated or "chronic" anterior dislocation of the shoulder (Fig. 4-69). Best seen on internal rotation views, the indentation is probably produced by small compression fractures of this weakest portion of the humeral head as it impinges against the anterior rim of the glenoid fossa.

BIBLIOGRAPHY

Hill HA, Sachs MD: The grooved defect of the humeral head: A frequently unrecognized complication of dislocations of the shoulder joint. Radiology 35:690–700, 1940

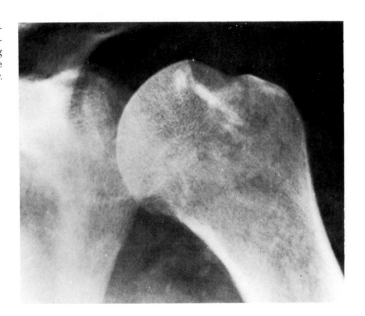

FIG. 4-69. Frontal view of the shoulder demonstrates a V-shaped defect in the posterolateral aspect of the humeral head resulting from repeated anterior dislocations of the shoulder.

Hole-Within-a-Hole Pattern

In patients with histiocytosis X, enlarging osteolytic lesions may demonstrate endosteal scalloping, a multilocular appearance, or bone expansion. A characteristic finding is a peculiar beveled contour of the lesion with multiple undulating contours of the margin, which may produce a three-dimensional hole-within-a-hole effect (Fig. 4-70).

BIBLIOGRAPHY
Greenfield GB: Radiology of Bone Diseases. Philadelphia, JB Lippincott, 1980

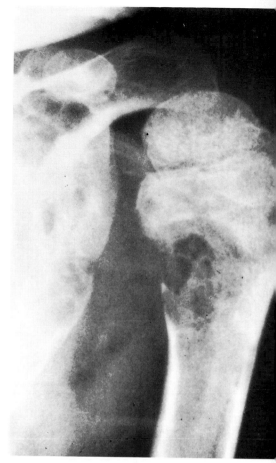

FIG. 4-70. Hole-within-a-hole appearance of a metaphyseal lesion of the humerus in a patient with Hand–Schueller–Christian disease. Destructive changes in the scapula may also be seen. (Greenfield GB: Radiology of Bone Diseases. Philadelphia, JB Lippincott, 1980)

Inverted Napoleon Hat Sign

In patients with congenital spondylolisthesis, the anterior edge of the last lumbar vertebral body may be markedly displaced downward and forward on the sacrum, producing the shadow of an inverted "Napoleon's hat" over the upper sacrum (Fig. 4-73).

BIBLIOGRAPHY

Gehweiler JA, Osborne RL, Becker RF: The Radiology of Vertebral Trauma. Philadelphia, WB Saunders, 1980

FIG. 4.73. *(Left)* Frontal view demonstrates abnormal foreshortening of the lumbar spine due to spondylolisthesis. The contours of the caudally displaced vertebral body present an inverted curvilinear density resembling an "inverted Napoleon's hat." *(Right)* Lateral view clearly demonstrates the anterior and downward displacement of the lumbar spinal column with respect to the sacrum. Note the marked wedge-shaped deformity of the L-5 vertebral body. (Gehweiler JA, Osborne RL, Becker RF: The Radiology of Vertebral Trauma. Philadelphia, WB Saunders, 1980)

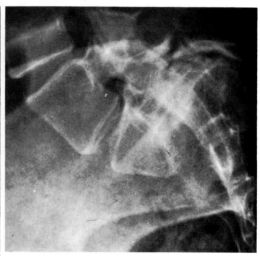

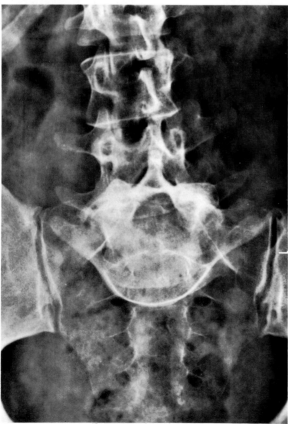

Ivory Vertebra Sign

A uniform increase in the density of an isolated vertebral body with no changes in the intervertebral disk is most likely caused by osteoblastic metastases (Fig. 4-74), Hodgkin's disease (Fig. 4-75), or the sclerotic stage of Paget's disease (Fig. 4-76). In contrast to osteoblastic metastases, Hodgkin's disease may demonstrate erosion or scalloping of the anterior margin of the vertebral body due to associated lymphadenopathy. Paget's disease causes enlargement of the vertebral body and cortical thickening, which more commonly produce a picture-frame appearance in the combined lytic and sclerotic phase of the disease. A similar ivory vertebra pattern has also been described as a very rare finding in multiple myeloma.

BIBLIOGRAPHY

Dennis JM: The solitary dense vertebral body. Radiology 77:618–621, 1961
Greenfield GB: Radiology of Bone Diseases. Philadelphia, JB Lippincott, 1980
Ochsner HC, Moser RH: Ivory vertebra. AJR 29:635–637, 1933

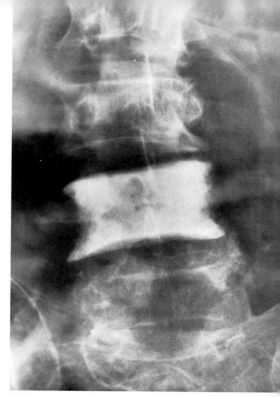

FIG. 4-74. Ivory vertebra in a patient with osteoblastic metastases from carcinoma of the prostate.

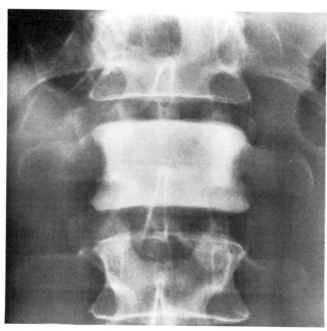

FIG. 4-75. Ivory vertebra in a patient with Hodgkin's disease.

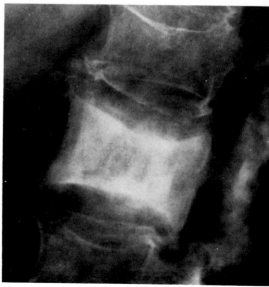

FIG. 4-76. Ivory vertebra in a patient with Paget's disease. Note the enlargement of the vertebral body and cortical thickening. (Edeiken J: Roentgen Diagnosis of Diseases of Bone. Baltimore, Williams & Wilkins, 1981. Copyright 1981. Reproduced by permission)

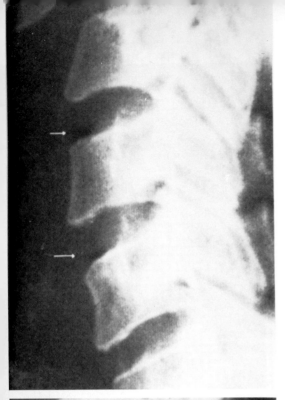

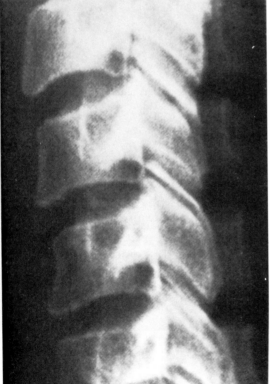

Lucent Cleft Sign

A small, smooth, lucent cleft that is adjacent to the vertebral body end-plate anteriorly and is seen only on the extension lateral view may be the only radiographic sign of cervical injury or disease (Fig. 4-79). Although an injury to the neck can completely avulse a disk and rupture the anterior longitudinal ligament, less severe trauma may partially avulse the disk and only attenuate the ligament. With the injured cervical spine in extension, the potential space where the disk is partially avulsed from the cartilaginous end-plate is pulled apart, much like a joint under stress. This decrease in pressure permits gas (mostly nitrogen) to enter the potential space. A lucent cleft is unlikely with complete avulsion of the disk and rupture of the anterior longitudinal ligament because of associated local hemorrhage, which fills the cleft with blood. The lucent cleft sign must be differentiated from the vacuum phenomenon of disk degeneration, which has ragged borders, often extends into the degenerated disk, is not confined solely to the region adjacent to the end-plate, and is associated with hypertrophic bony changes, disk narrowing, and sclerosis.

BIBLIOGRAPHY

Reymond RD, Wheeler PS, Perovic M et al: The lucent cleft, a new radiographic sign of cervical disc injury or disease. Clin Radiol 23:188–192, 1972

FIG. 4-79. *(Top)* Extension lateral view shows two lucent clefts adjacent to the vertebral end-plates anteriorly **(arrows)**. *(Bottom)* On the flexion lateral view, the lucent clefts can no longer be identified. (Reymond RD, Wheeler PS, Perovic M et al: The lucent cleft, a new radiographic sign of cervical disc injury or disease. Clin Radiol 23:188–192, 1972)

FIG. 4-80. Fractures of both mandibular necks, allowing medial angulation of both mandibular heads and lateral displacement of both ascending rami, and a fracture of the horizontal ramus near the midline make the lower jaw appear too large for the upper jaw. (Tratnell DH: The "magnification sign" of triple mandible fracture. Br J Radiol 50:97–100, 1977)

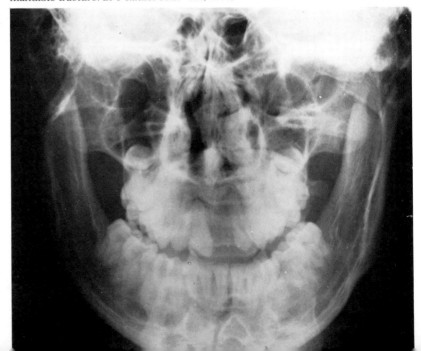

Magnification Sign

Double and triple fractures of the mandible are common, because the bone is a rigid structure connected to the skull by a firm joint at each end and often behaves as if it were a complete bony ring. The radiographic appearance on a standard postero-anterior projection of a mandible that appears "too wide" for the upper jaw indicates the presence of a triple mandibular fracture (magnification sign; Fig. 4-80). Two factors contribute to the production of this appearance. First, the two angles of the mandible are abnormally widely separated from each other, and the ascending rami and the part of the horizontal ramus that is attached to them are "opened out." Second, as a result of this separation, the mandibular molar teeth are displaced lateral to the corresponding teeth in the upper jaw. Lateral displacement of the angle of the mandible and associated teeth producing the magnification sign can occur only if there are fractures of both mandibular necks—thus effectively disconnecting the mandible from the skull base—as well as a third fracture somewhere in the otherwise rigid horizontal ramus, usually near the midline (Fig. 4-81).

BIBLIOGRAPHY

Tratnell DH: The "magnification sign" of triple mandible fracture. Br J Radiol 50:97–100, 1977

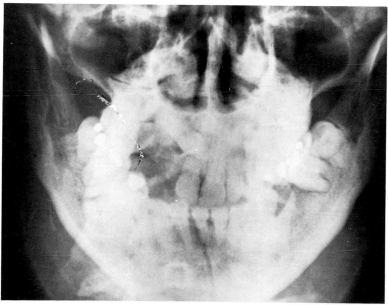

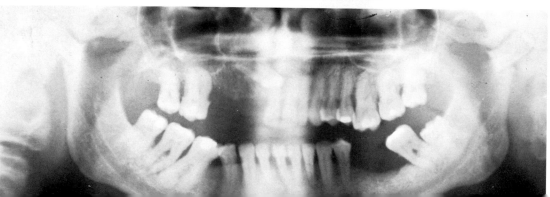

FIG. 4-81. *(Top)* Frontal view of the mandible demonstrates the magnification sign, due to triple fractures. *(Bottom)* Panorex view of the same patient shows the fractures of the mandibular neck on each side and a horizontal ramus fracture near the midline. (Tratnell DH: The "magnification sign" of triple mandible fracture. Br J Radiol 50:97–100, 1977)

Obturator Sign

The obturator sign, an increase in the size of the obturator internus muscle on one side relative to the other, was originally described as a specific indication of infectious arthritis of the hip joint. However, a prominent obturator muscle shadow is more frequently a manifestation of trauma and subsequent hemorrhage. On frontal radiographs, the obturator sign is seen as a bulge of soft-tissue density along the inner pelvic wall with medial displacement of the normal fat line (Fig. 4-92).

BIBLIOGRAPHY

Hefke HW, Turner VC: Obturator sign as earliest roentgenographic sign in diagnosis of septic arthritis and tuberculosis of the hip. J Bone Joint Surg 24:857–869, 1942

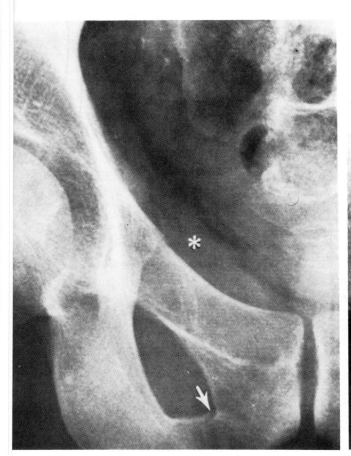
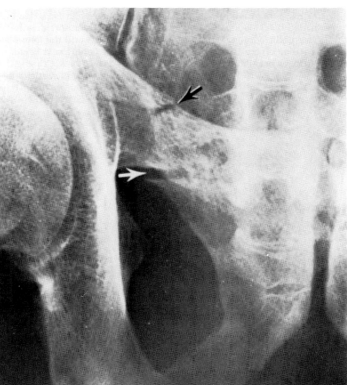

FIG. 4-92. *(Left)* Following right hip injury, a frontal view demonstrates a fracture at the junction of the inferior ramus and the body **(arrow)** of the right pubis. No fracture is seen in the superior ramus, but the abnormal prominence of the shadow of the obturator internus muscle (*) is indicative of adjacent subperiosteal hemorrhage and suggestive of a fracture of the superior ramus. *(Right)* The right anterior oblique projection clearly demonstrates the superior ramus fracture **(arrows).** (Harris JH, Harris WH: The Radiology of Emergency Medicine. Baltimore, Williams & Wilkins, 1981. Copyright 1981. Reproduced by permission)

Signs of Osteopetrosis

Osteopetrosis is a rare hereditary bone abnormality characterized radiographically by symmetric generalized increase in bone density and lack of tubulation. Some patients demonstrate increased density limited to the end-plates, resulting in a *sandwich vertebrae* pattern (Fig. 4-93). Other patients demonstrate the appearance of a miniature inset in each vertebral body, causing a *bone-within-a-bone* pattern (Fig. 4-94). The somewhat similar appearance of ghost infantile vertebrae within the adult skeleton may develop in persons who received Thorotrast in childhood (see Fig. 4-63) and in patients with Gaucher's disease (see Fig. 4-129).

BIBLIOGRAPHY

Pincus JB, Gittleman IF, Kramer B: Juvenile osteopetrosis. Am J Dis Child 73:458–472, 1947

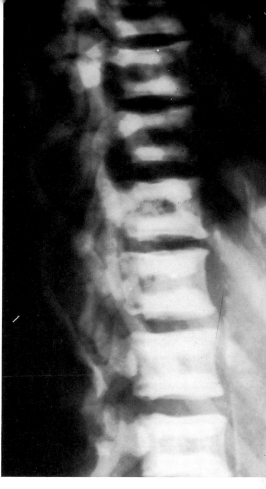

FIG. 4-93. Increased density limited to the end-plates produces the sandwich vertebrae appearance in a patient with osteopetrosis. The spine otherwise appears normal. Note the marked calcification of the abdominal vasculature. (Greenfield GB: Radiology of Bone Diseases. Philadelphia, JB Lippincott, 1980)

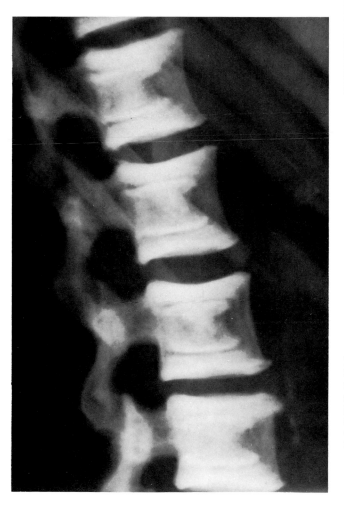

FIG. 4-94. A miniature inset is seen in each lumbar spine vertebral body, giving a bone-within-a-bone appearance in this patient with osteopetrosis tarda. Sclerosis at the end-plates and calcification in the abdominal aorta may also be seen. (Greenfield GB: Radiology of Bone Diseases. Philadelphia, JB Lippincott, 1980)

Phalangeal Sign

In normal patients, the total length of the distal and proximal phalanges of the fourth finger equals the length of the fourth metacarpal, the standard deviation being 2 mm. In patients with gonadal dysgenesis, the total length of the distal and proximal phalanges exceeds by 3 mm or more the length of the fourth metacarpal (phalangeal sign; Fig. 4-98).

BIBLIOGRAPHY

Kosowicz J: The roentgen appearance of the hand and wrist in gonadal dysgenesis. AJR 93:354–361, 1965

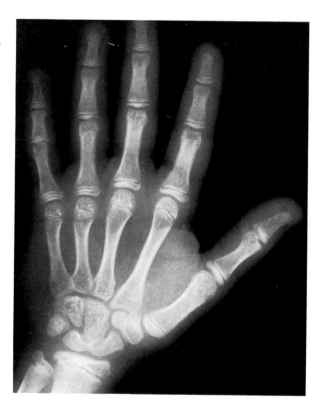

FIG. 4-98. Disproportionate length of the phalanges of the fourth finger (proximal + distal = 4.4 cm) compared to the length of the fourth metacarpal (3.9 cm).

FIG. 4-99. (A) Normal hips in a 19-year-old male. (B) Effect of traction. Note the clarity of the articular cartilage, which measures 3 mm at its thickest point, and the ligamentum teres (**arrow**). The maximum vertical height of the gas gap is 13 mm. (Martel W, Poznanski AK: The value of traction during roentgenography of the hip. Radiology 94:497–503, 1970)

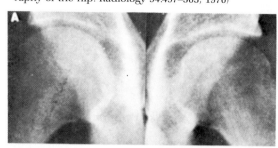
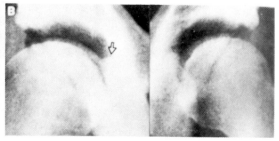

Pneumoarthrogram Sign

A pneumoarthrogram is a type of "vacuum phenomenon" in which traction on a joint causes spontaneous intra-articular release of gas. This presents radiographically as a thin radiolucent band clearly outlining the articular cartilage of the joint (Fig. 4-99). The importance of the pneumoarthrogram sign is that it will not be produced if a joint effusion is present (Fig. 4-100). One can test the presence of a joint effusion by attempting to produce a pneumoarthrogram through applying a traction force on one member of the joint while the other is held fixed. Although most often seen in the hip, a pneumoarthrogram can also be produced in the shoulder or knee (Fig. 4-101).

BIBLIOGRAPHY

Martel W, Poznanski AK: The value of traction during roentgenography of the hip. Radiology 94:497–503, 1970

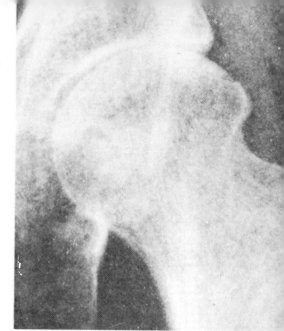

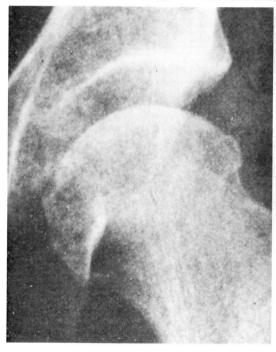

FIG. 4-100. *(Top)* Left hip in a 62-year-old woman with chronic bilateral hip disease, the nature of which was not clear. *(Bottom)* Traction caused marked widening of the interosseous space (10-mm increment) with no gas present to outline the articular cartilage. This indicated the presence of a joint effusion, which was corroborated by needle aspiration. Arthroplasty of the right hip revealed histologic findings compatible with osteoarthritis. (Martel W, Poznanski AK: The value of traction during roentgenography of the hip. Radiology 94:497–503, 1970)

FIG. 4-101. Example of the pneumoarthrogram sign (**arrow**) in a normal knee with no evidence of joint effusion.

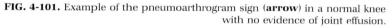

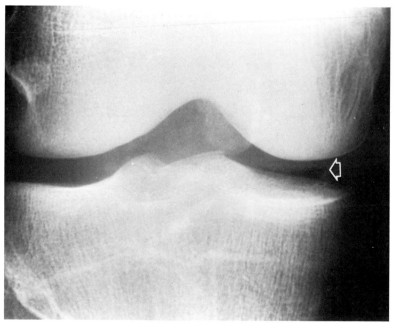

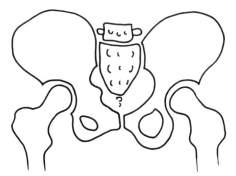

FIG. 4-105. Line drawing. The right side of the pelvis demonstrates relative iliac flaring, an apparent widening of the sacrosciatic notch, decrease in the vertical height of the pubic component of the pelvis, and relative narrowing of the obturator foramen. (Arcomano JP, Stunkle G, Barnett JC et al: Muscle group signs and pubic varus as a manifestation of hip disease in children. AJR 89:966–969, 1963. Copyright 1963. Reproduced by permission)

Pubic or Ischial Varus Sign

A relative iliac flare and an apparent widening of the sacrosciatic notch have been described as a manifestation of hip disease in children (Fig. 4-105). This appearance is a manifestation of the spasm and shortening phenomenon, associated with a variety of diseases of the hip in children, that causes axial rotation of the pubic bones and produces a decrease in the vertical height of the entire affected pubic component of the pelvis with relative narrowing of the obturator foramen (Figs. 4-106 and 4-107).

BIBLIOGRAPHY
Arcomano JP, Stunkle G, Barnett JC et al: Muscle group signs and pubic varus as a manifestation of hip disease in children. AJR 89:966–969, 1963

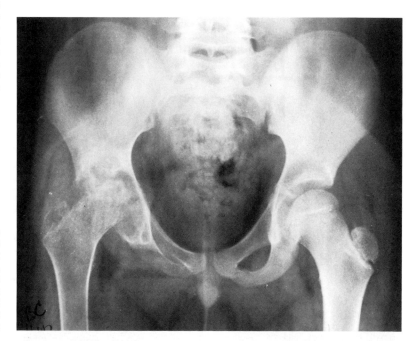

FIG. 4-106. Advanced destructive change in the right hip secondary to tuberculosis. Note the obliteration of all muscle groups about the hip and the prominent pubic varus sign. (Arcomano JP, Stunkle G, Barnett JC et al: Muscle group signs and pubic varus as a manifestation of hip disease in children. AJR 89:966–969, 1963. Copyright 1963. Reproduced by permission)

FIG. 4-107. Ewing's sarcoma. The pubic varus sign is on the left. (Arcomano JP, Stunkle G, Barnett JC et al: Muscle group signs and pubic varus as a manifestation of hip disease in children. AJR 89:966–969, 1963. Copyright 1963. Reproduced by permission)

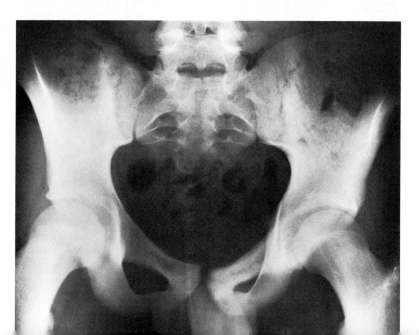

Rim Sign

A greater than normal distance between the humeral head and the anterior rim of the glenoid has been reported as a useful sign of posterior dislocation (positive rim sign; Fig. 4-108). Normal patients have a space of no more than 6 mm between the head of the humerus and the anterior glenoid rim on anteroposterior views using a 36-inch to 40-inch target-film distance. Unfortunately, both false-negative and false-positive rim signs may occur. An impacted fracture of the humeral head may permit the humeral head to move more medially, producing a false-negative sign; effusions in the glenohumeral joint space may cause lateral displacement of the humeral head and a false-positive rim sign. Nevertheless, a positive rim sign should suggest the possibility of posterior dislocation and the need to obtain axillary or transthoracic lateral views.

BIBLIOGRAPHY

Arndt JH, Sears AD: Posterior dislocation of the shoulder. AJR 94:639–645, 1965

FIG. 4-108. *(Left)* Positive rim sign. The joint space (↔) measures 12 mm. A compression fracture of the internally rotated humeral head **(arrows)** is evident. *(Right)* Postreduction transthoracic lateral radiograph demonstrates the restored glenohumeral relationship and the normal broad scapulohumeral arch **(arrows).** (Arndt JH, Sears AD: Posterior dislocation of the shoulder. AJR 94:639–645, 1965. Copyright 1965. Reproduced by permission)

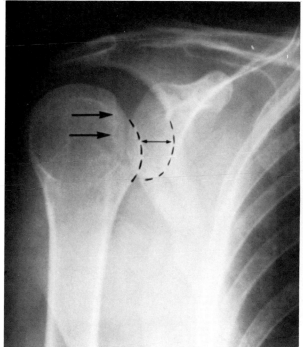
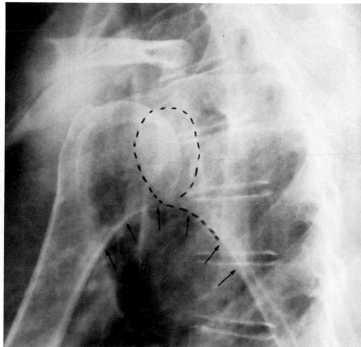

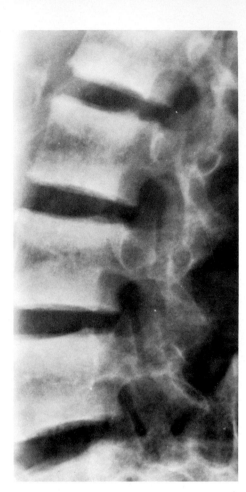

Rugger Jersey Sign

Thick bands of increased density (osteosclerosis) adjacent to the superior and inferior margins of vertebral bodies produce the rugger jersey spine (Fig. 4-109), so named because the horizontal-striped appearance is similar to the design on shirts worn by rugby players. The rugger jersey spine is characteristic of secondary hyperparathyroidism due to renal failure, though a similar appearance may also be seen occasionally in patients with primary hyperparathyroidism.

BIBLIOGRAPHY

Dent CE, Hodson, CJ: General softening of bone due to metabolic causes. II. Radiologic changes associated with certain metabolic bone diseases. Br J Radiol 27:605–618, 1954

Vaughan BF, Walters MNI: Sclerotic banded vertebrae (rugger-jersey spine). J Coll Radiol Aust 7:87–92, 1963

FIG. 4-109. Lateral view of the lumbar spine demonstrates osteosclerosis of the superior and inferior margins of the vertebral bodies producing a rugger jersey appearance in this patient with secondary hyperparathyroidism due to renal failure.

Saber Shin Sign

Marked cortical thickening, often irregular, is a radiographic finding in both congenital and acquired syphilitic osteomyelitis. Involvement of the anterior tibial cortex produces the classic saber shin appearance (Fig. 4-110).

BIBLIOGRAPHY
Greenfield GB: Radiology of Bone Diseases. Philadelphia, JB Lippincott, 1980

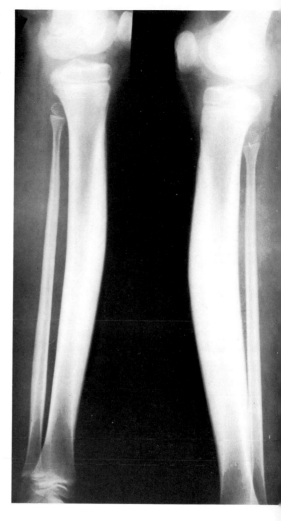

FIG. 4-110. Marked cortical thickening, particularly of the left anterior tibial cortex, giving a characteristic saber shin appearance in a patient with congenital syphilis. (Greenfield GB: Radiology of Bone Diseases. Philadelphia, JB Lippincott, 1980)

Scotty Dog Sign

On oblique views of the lumbar spine, the appearance of the posterior elements has been likened to that of a scotty dog. The pedicle and transverse process form the eye and nose; the superior and inferior articular processes form the ear and leg; and the pars interarticularis forms the neck (Fig. 4-114). A defect in the pars interarticularis (spondylolysis) thus appears as a fracture through the neck of the scotty dog (Fig. 4-115).

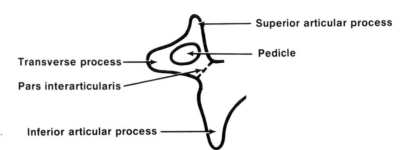

FIG. 4-114. Diagram of the scotty dog sign.

FIG. 4-115. Oblique view of the lumbar spine demonstrates a defect in the pars interarticularis (spondylolysis) appearing as a fracture through the neck of the scotty dog (**arrow**).

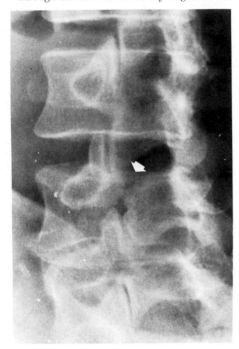

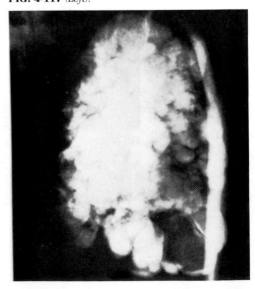

FIG. 4-117 (*Left*).

Sedimentation Sign

Massive periarticular calcifications may occur in metabolic disturbances with an increased calcium phosphate product (*e.g.*, renal insufficiency, hyperparathyroidism, vitamin D intoxication, milk–alkali syndrome). Identical massive deposits of calcium may be found in patients with tumoral calcinosis who have normal calcium metabolism and a normal skeleton. Tumoral calcinosis is a rare disease in which the periarticular calcified tumors are honeycomb-like clusters of cysts in a dense fibrous capsule (Fig. 4-116). The cysts are filled with a granular, pasty, or liquid material. Tumoral calcinosis can be differentiated from an abnormality of calcium metabolism by the demonstration on upright views of sedimentation of calcium phosphate crystals in the liquid-filled cysts (Fig. 4-117).

BIBLIOGRAPHY

Hug I, Guncaga J: Tumoral calcinosis with sedimentation sign. Br J Radiol 47:734–736, 1974

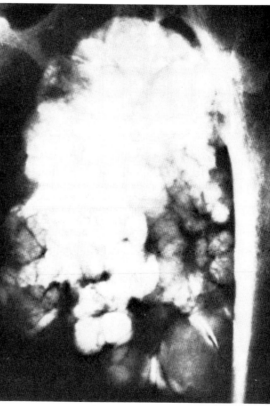

FIG. 4-116. *(Left)* coned and *(right)* full supine views of a mass of tumoral calcification in the proximal thigh demonstrate homogeneous density of the cysts at the lower pole and amorphous deposits at the upper pole of the mass. (Hug I, Guncaga J: Tumoral calcinosis with sedimentation sign. Br J Radiol 47:734–736, 1974)

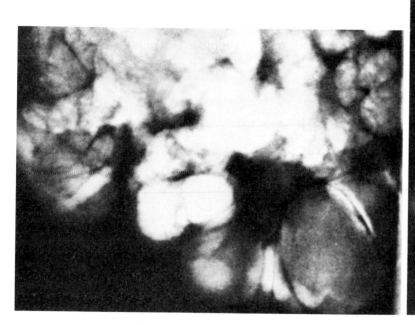

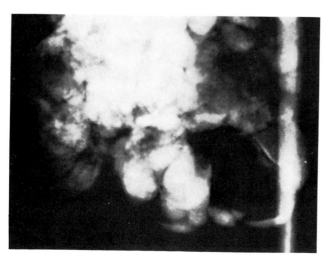

FIG. 4-117. *(Left)* Full and *(right)* coned upright views demonstrate sedimentation in the liquid-filled cysts with increased translucency of the liquid material. No sedimentation is noted in the amorphous gritty deposits. (Hug I, Guncaga J: Tumoral calcinosis with sedimentation sign. Br J Radiol 47:734–736, 1974)

Shoulder Pad Sign

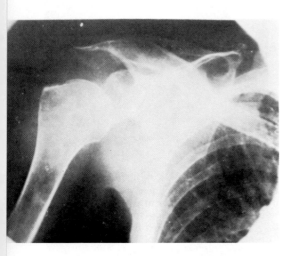

Bilateral soft-tissue swelling about the shoulders with inferior displacement of the humeral heads and widening of the joint spaces has been described in patients with amyloid arthropathy (Fig. 4-120). The radiographic pattern correlates with the physical finding of massively enlarged shoulders with a rubbery hard consistency mimicking the appearance of a football player wearing shoulder pads (Fig. 4-121).

BIBLIOGRAPHY
Katz GA, Peter JB, Pearson CM et al: The shoulder-pad sign—A diagnostic feature of amyloid arthropy. N Engl J Med 288:354–355, 1973

FIG. 4-120. Frontal view of the right shoulder demonstrates the shoulder pad sign in a patient with amyloid arthropathy. (Katz GA, Peter JB, Pearson CM et al: The shoulder-pad sign — A diagnostic feature of amyloid arthropathy. N Engl J Med 288:354–355, 1973)

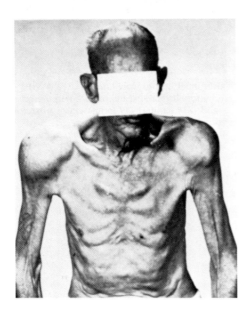

FIG. 4-121. Photograph of a 78-year-old man with biopsy-proved amyloid deposition demonstrates massively enlarged shoulders mimicking the appearance of a football player wearing shoulder pads. (Katz GA, Peter JB, Pearson CM et al: The shoulder-pad sign — A diagnostic feature of amyloid arthropathy. N Engl J Med 288:354–355, 1973)

Sickle Sign

The sickle sign, a crescent-shaped deformity of the sacrum with a large concave defect on the involved side, is characteristic of anterior sacral meningocele (Fig. 4-122). The combination of a presacral mass and typical sacral deformity strongly suggests this diagnosis, which may be confirmed by myelography demonstrating the size and extent of the communicating sac.

BIBLIOGRAPHY
Werner JL, Taybi H: Presacral masses in childhood. AJR 109:403–410, 1970

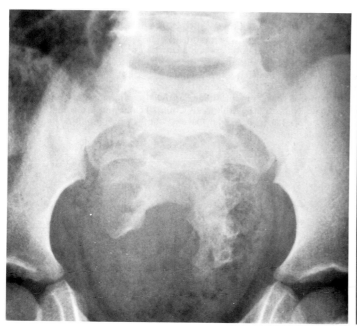

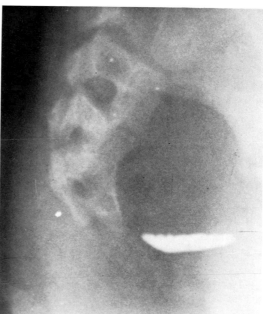

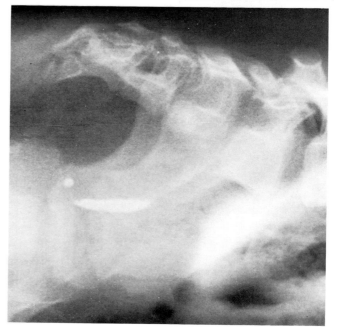

FIG. 4-122. (*Top, left*) A sickle-shaped defect of the sacrum is seen in this patient with anterior sacral meningocele and imperforate anus. (*Top, right*) Upright and (*bottom*) prone views from a Pantopaque myelogram demonstrate the size of the meningocele. (Werner JL, Taybi H: Presacral masses in childhood. AJR 109:403–410, 1970. Copyright 1970. Reproduced by permission)

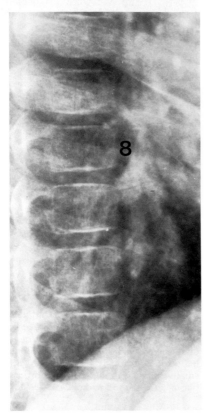

Step-Off Vertebral Body Sign

A step-like central depression of multiple vertebral end-plates is usually considered virtually pathognomonic of sickle cell anemia and its variants (Fig. 4-127). However, scattered reports have demonstrated a similar step-off sign occurring in other conditions, especially Gaucher's disease (Fig. 4-128). In sickle cell anemia, the step-off sign is probably caused by circulatory stasis and ischemia, which retard growth in the central portion of the vertebral cartilaginous growth plate; the periphery of the growth plate has a different blood supply and thus continues to grow at a more normal rate. In Gaucher's disease, there is an initial collapse of the entire vertebral body with subsequent growth recovery peripherally. This is often associated with horizontal and vertical sclerosis, giving a bone-within-a-bone appearance (Fig. 4-129).

BIBLIOGRAPHY

Hansen GC, Gold RH: Central depression of multiple vertebral end-plates: A "pathognomonic" sign of sickle hemoglobinopathy in Gaucher's disease. AJR 129:343–344, 1977

Schwartz AM, Homer MJ, McCauley RGK: "Step-off" vertebral body: Gaucher's disease versus sickle cell hemoglobulinopathy. AJR 132:81–85, 1979

FIG. 4-127. *(Top)* Normal spine at age 7 and *(bottom)* multiple areas of typical central depression at age 14 in a patient with sickle cell β-thalassemia. (Schwartz AM, Homer MJ, McCauley RGK: "Step-off" vertebral body: Gaucher's disease versus sickle cell hemoglobinopathy. AJR 132:81–85, 1979. Copyright 1979. Reproduced by permission)

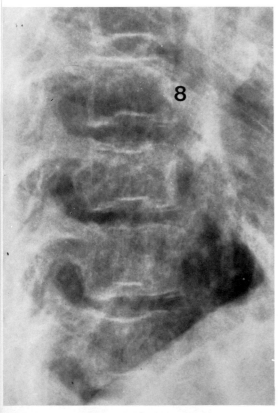

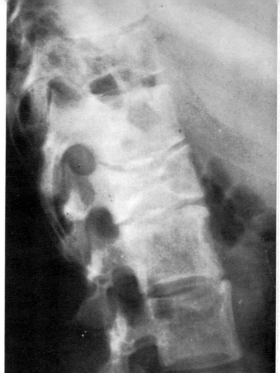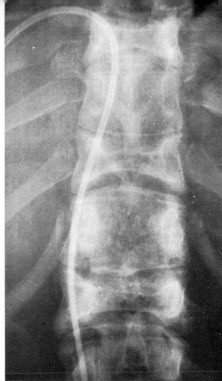

FIG. 4-128. *(Left)* Lateral and *(right)* frontal views of the lower thoracic and upper lumbar vertebrae showing step-like central depressions of the superior and inferior end-plates of the ninth and 11th thoracic and first lumbar vertebrae. The inferior surface of the expanded 12th thoracic vertebra protrudes into a depression left in the adjacent first lumbar vertebra, signifying a slowly progressive, expansile, destructive process that began in early life. The disk spaces are well preserved. The catheter in the hepatic vein is a result of angiography performed to exclude Budd–Chiari syndrome. (Hansen GC, Gold RH: Central depression of multiple vertebral end-plates: A "pathognomonic" sign of sickle hemoglobinopathy in Gaucher's disease. AJR 129:343–344, 1977. Copyright 1977. Reproduced by permission)

FIG. 4-129. Bone-within-a-bone appearance caused by sclerotic densities parallel to vertebral contours of T-12 in the same patient as seen in Figure 4-128 at age 14 1/2. (Schwartz AM, Homer MJ, McCauley RGK: "Step-off" vertebral body: Gaucher's disease versus sickle cell hemoglobinopathy. AJR 132:81–85, 1979. Copyright 1979. Reproduced by permission)

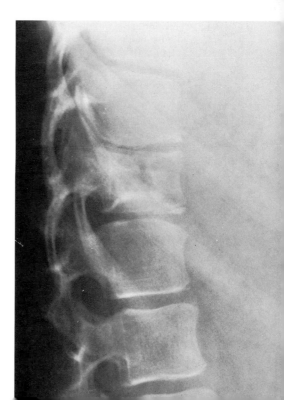

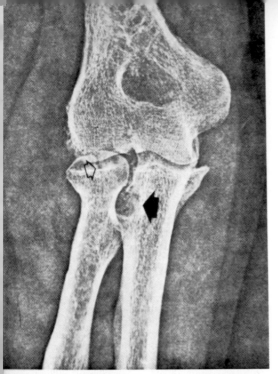

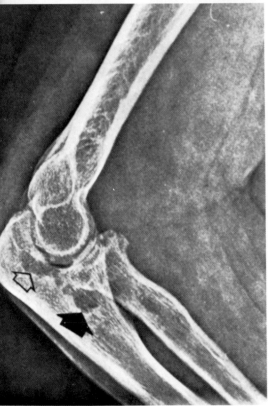

Supinator Notch Sign

A juxta-articular erosion of the ulna producing a notch-like appearance in the region of the supinator groove has been reported as a characteristic and common sign of rheumatoid arthritis involving the elbow joint (Fig. 4-133, *left*). The shallow notch, which is seen opposite the neck of the radius, probably results from surface erosion of bone by the inflammatory synovium. The lesion is usually best shown on standard frontal views, though shallow erosions may be evident only on oblique projections. On lateral radiographs, the lesion is viewed *en face* (Fig. 4-133, *right*) and may be difficult to demonstrate unless the margin is well corticated.

BIBLIOGRAPHY

Foster DR, Park WM, McCall IW et al: The supinator notch sign in rheumatoid arthritis. Clin Radiol 31:195–199, 1980

FIG. 4-133. *(Top)* Anteroposterior projection demonstrates a deep erosion with an irregular margin (**solid arrow**) in a patient with rheumatoid arthritis. The fracture line in the radial head (**open arrow**) resulted from an injury that had occurred 1 year previously. *(Bottom)* Lateral view demonstrates the supinator notch *en face* (**solid arrow**). A subarticular erosion related to the trochlear notch is also identified (**open arrow**). (Foster DR, Park WM, McCall IW et al: The supinator notch sign in rheumatoid arthritis. Clin Radiol 31:195–199, 1980)

FIG. 4-134. Swan neck deformity in a patient with systemic lupus erythematosus. In addition to the alignment abnormalities, diffuse osteoporosis is present. (Forrester DM, Brown JC, Nesson JW: The Radiology of Joint Disease. Philadelphia, WB Saunders, 1978)

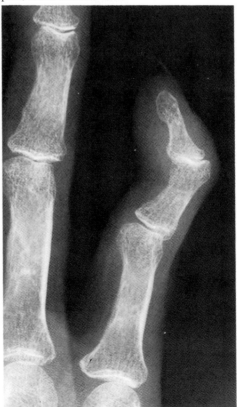

Swan Neck Deformity

The combination of flexion of the distal interphalangeal joint and hyperextension of the proximal interphalangeal joint results in a swan neck deformity (Fig. 4-134). This sign is characteristically seen in systemic lupus erythematosus (Fig. 4-135) but can also appear in other arthritic conditions such as scleroderma (Fig. 4-136).

BIBLIOGRAPHY
Forrester DM, Brown JC, Nesson JW: The Radiology of Joint Disease. Philadelphia, WB Saunders, 1978

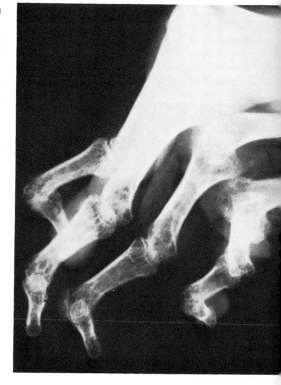

FIG. 4-135. Oblique view of the hand of a patient with systemic lupus erythematosus demonstrates a classic wedge of swans. (Forrester DM, Brown JC, Nesson JW: The Radiology of Joint Disease. Philadelphia, WB Saunders, 1978)

FIG. 4-136. Swan neck deformities of the fingers accompanied by subluxation of the metacarpophalangeal joints in a patient with scleroderma. The deformities are suggested by the overlapping shadows on *(left)* frontal projection but are best evaluated on *(right)* the oblique view. The presence of subcutaneous calcification in the second digit and wrist is typical of scleroderma. (Forrester DM, Brown JC, Nesson JW: The Radiology of Joint Disease. Philadelphia, WB Saunders, 1978)

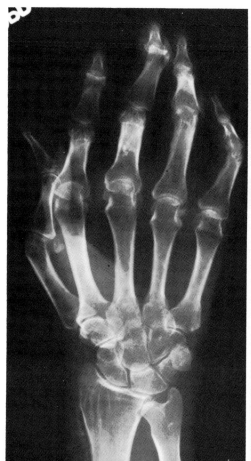

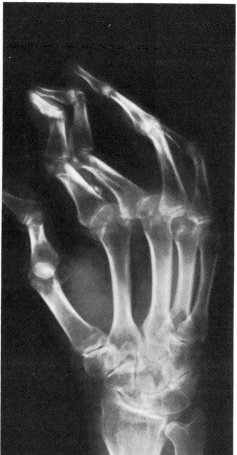

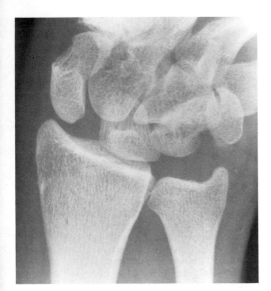

Terry-Thomas Sign

Subluxation of the carpal navicular involves backward rotation of the proximal pole and forward rotation of the distal pole. Frontal radiographs of the wrist in rotary subluxation of the navicular demonstrate a gap between the navicular and lunate (Fig. 4-139). This gap has been colorfully compared to the upper central dental diastema of the famous British comedian Terry-Thomas (Fig. 4-140).

BIBLIOGRAPHY
Frankel VH: The Terry-Thomas sign. Clin Orthop 129:321–322, 1977

FIG. 4-139. Radiograph of the hand demonstrates rotational subluxation of the navicular resulting in a wide gap between the navicular and lunate.

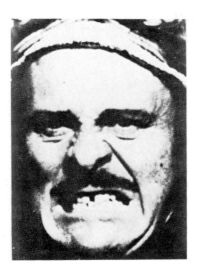

FIG. 4-140. Central dental diastema of the British comedian Terry-Thomas. (Frankel VH: The Terry-Thomas sign. Clin Orthop 129:321–322, 1977)

Tibiotalar Slant Sign

Tibiotalar angulation in black patients has been reported to be strongly suggestive of sickle cell anemia (Fig. 4-141). It is thought that the wedge-shaped angulation deformity results from chronic hyperemia complicated by asymmetric epiphyseal growth, bony and synovial ischemia, or progressive joint cartilage destruction. Tibiotalar angulation deformities have also been described in patients with hemophiliac arthropathy (Fig. 4-142), juvenile rheumatoid arthritis, and epiphyseal dysplasia multiplex (Fig. 4-143).

BIBLIOGRAPHY

Forrester DM, Brown JC, Nesson JW: The Radiology of Joint Disease. Philadelphia, WB Saunders, 1978

Shaub MS, Rosen R, Boswell W et al: Tibiotalar slant: A new observation in sickle cell anemia. Radiology 117:551–552, 1975

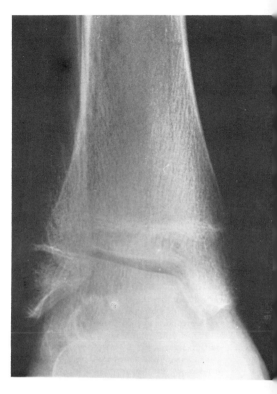

FIG. 4-141. Tibiotalar angulation in a patient with sickle cell anemia. (Greenfield GB: Radiology of Bone Diseases. Philadelphia, JB Lippincott, 1980)

FIG. 4-142. Tibiotalar angulation (**arrow**) in a patient with hemophiliac arthropathy. Destruction of the joint and erosions of the articular bones are similar to the changes seen in rheumatoid arthritis. (Forrester DM, Brown JC, Nesson JW: The Radiology of Joint Disease. Philadelphia, WB Saunders, 1978)

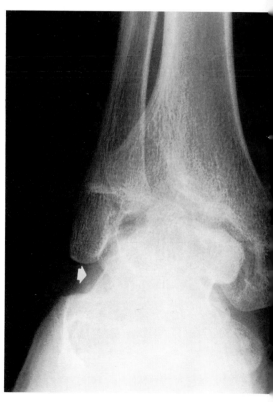

FIG. 4-143. Tibiotalar angulation in a patient with epiphyseal dysplasia multiplex (Fairbank's disease). Note the irregularity of the distal tibial epiphyses, bilaterally and symmetrically, with deficiency of the ossification center at the lateral aspects. (Greenfield GB: Radiology of Bone Diseases. Philadelphia, JB Lippincott, 1980)

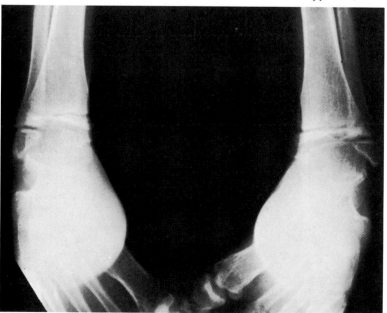

Triangular Sign

In the normal adolescent hip, a portion of the diaphysis of the femoral neck inferomedially is intra-articular and overlies the posterior wall of the acetabulum on frontal view, creating a dense triangular appearance (Fig. 4-146). In most cases of slipped capital femoral epiphysis, this dense triangle is lost as that portion of the neck moves lateral to the acetabulum (Fig. 4-147). Therefore, for the dense triangle to be absent on one side when it is clearly present on the opposite side suggests the diagnosis of slipped capital femoral epiphysis.

BIBLIOGRAPHY
Scham SM: The triangular sign in the early diagnosis of slipped capital femoral epiphysis. Clin Orthop 103:16–17, 1974

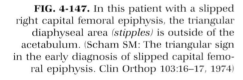
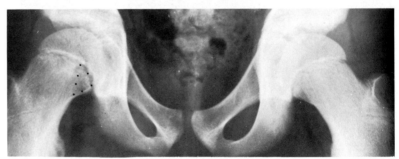

FIG. 4-146. The *stipples* delineate the triangular diaphyseal area overlying the acetabular shadow in a normal right hip. (Scham SM: The triangular sign in the early diagnosis of slipped capital femoral epiphysis. Clin Orthop 103:16–17, 1974)

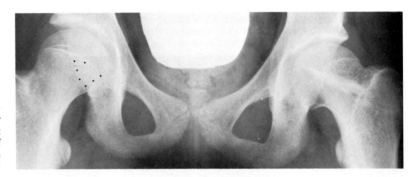

FIG. 4-147. In this patient with a slipped right capital femoral epiphysis, the triangular diaphyseal area *(stipples)* is outside of the acetabulum. (Scham SM: The triangular sign in the early diagnosis of slipped capital femoral epiphysis. Clin Orthop 103:16–17, 1974)

FIG. 4-148. Classic *ivory osteoma* in an 18-year-old male whose ulcer had been present for 1 year. There is also cortical thickening of the tibia on the side opposite the ulcer (**black arrow**). Medullary resorption is starting at the inner margin of the osteoma, and the solid cortex is beginning to show a trabecular pattern (**white arrow**). (Kolawole TM, Bohrer SP: Ulcer osteomas — Bone response to tropical ulcer. AJR 109:611–618, 1970. Copyright 1970. Reproduced by permission) ▶

FIG. 4-149. Two examples of *cancellous ulcer osteomas* in children, both of whom had had their ulcers for more than 5 years. Note the loss of overlying soft tissue (**arrows** are at the skin surface) and the distal osteoporosis. (Kolawole TM, Bohrer SP: Ulcer osteomas — Bone response to tropical ulcer. AJR 109:611–618, 1970. Copyright 1970. Reproduced by permission) ▶

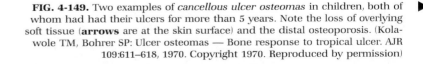

Signs of Tropical Ulcers

Tropical ulcers, extremely common throughout much of Africa, are often associated with lesions in the underlying bone (ulcer osteoma). The earliest finding is periosteal reaction localized to the bone beneath the ulcer, which is usually fusiform but occasionally has a sunburst or onion peel appearance. Later, the periosteal new bone blends with the cortex to produce a thickened sclerotic cortex, which can become over 1 inch thick and give rise to the classic *ivory osteoma* (Fig. 4-148). *Cancellous ulcer osteoma* is an even more common sequela, resulting from osteoporosis distal to the ulcer with subsequent bulbous expansion of the medullary cavity toward the ulcer and thinning of the cortex in this region (Fig. 4-149). A complication of tropical ulcers is malignant transformation, which occurs in about 2% of patients and should be suspected if the ulcer begins to increase in size and radiographs demonstrate destruction of the cortex of the osteoma and a soft-tissue mass (Fig. 4-150).

BIBLIOGRAPHY
Kolawole TM, Bohrer SP: Ulcer osteoma—Bone response to tropical ulcer. AJR 109:611–618, 1970

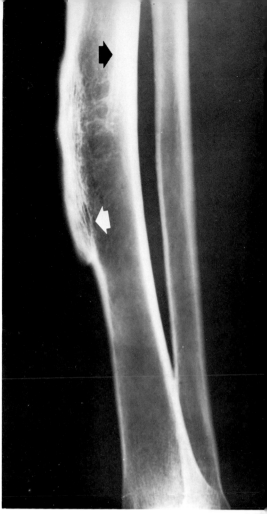

FIG. 4-148.

FIG. 4-149.

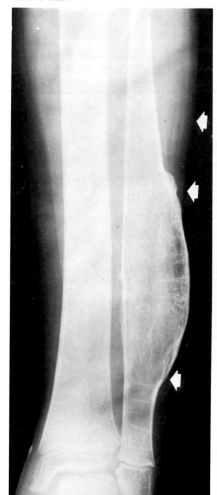 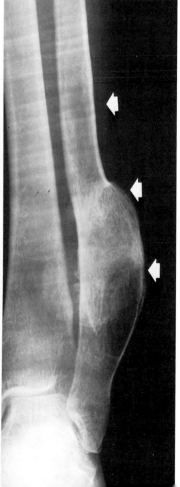

Tumbling Bolt Sign

The development of a deep soft-tissue abscess may result in extrusion of the side compression bolt following Richards' fixation for hip fracture. Sequential radiographs may demonstrate the freely mobile bolt at some distance from its insertion site, indicating that it lies free within an abscess cavity (Fig. 4-152).

BIBLIOGRAPHY
Naimark A, Lander P: The tumbling bolt: A new sign of deep soft-tissue abscess following Richards fixation. Radiology 129:30, 1978

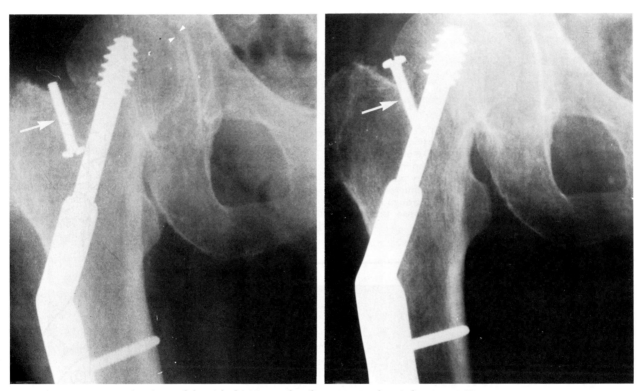

FIG. 4-152. Anteroposterior views of the right hip 2 months after surgery, taken 9 days apart. Note the compression bolt (**arrows**) tumbling freely in the deep soft-tissue abscess. The joint space is thinned (**arrowheads**), a sign of pyarthrosis. (Naimark A, Lander P: The tumbling bolt: A new sign of deep soft-tissue abscess following Richards fixation. Radiology 129:30, 1978)

Tumbling Bullet Sign

The *fallen fragment sign* of a bone fragment falling to the dependent portion of a cyst has been described as pathognomonic of a unicameral bone cyst (see Fig. 4-49). One case has been reported of a bullet entering the medullary cavity without splintering or obviously fracturing the cortex and subsequently moving freely with gravity, thus serving as a reliable sign of the cystic nature of the resultant post-traumatic lesion (Fig. 4-153).

BIBLIOGRAPHY

Taxin RN, Feldman F: The tumbling bullet sign in a post-traumatic bone cyst. AJR 123:140–143, 1975

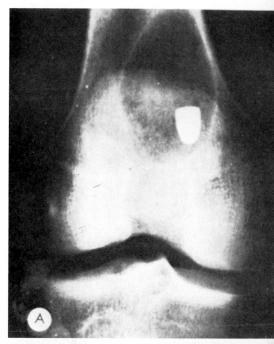

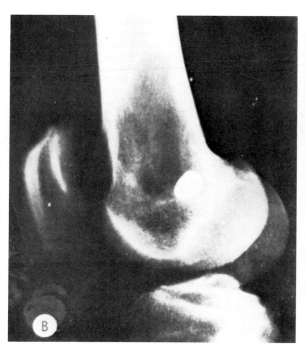

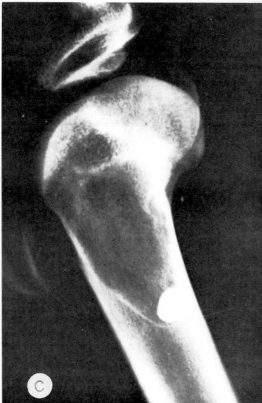

FIG. 4-153. (A) Frontal and **(B)** lateral upright radiographs obtained 16 months after injury demonstrate the opaque bullet at the inferior margin of a large radiolucent lesion with well-defined borders. **(C)** On a lateral view with the femur elevated, the bullet falls to the superior margin of the lesion, which in this position becomes its most dependent portion, thereby demonstrating its cystic nature. (Taxin RN, Feldman F: The tumbling bullet sign in a post-traumatic bone cyst. AJR 123:140–143, 1975. Copyright 1975. Reproduced by permission)

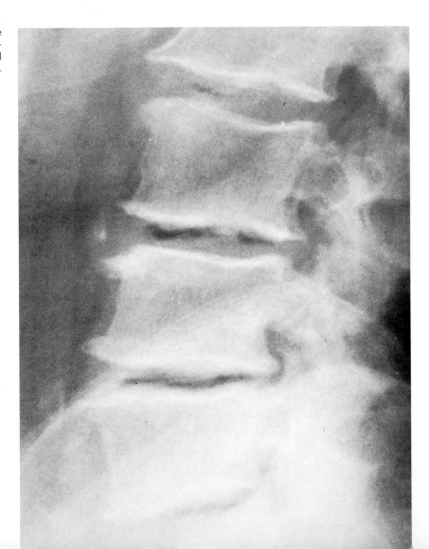

Vacuum Phenomenon

The appearance of linear or circular radiolucent collections overlying the intervertebral disks (vacuum phenomenon) has been described as a reliable indicator of degenerative disk disease (Fig. 4-154). However, a similar pattern has also been reported in such disorders as vertebral osteomyelitis, Schmorl node formation, spondylosis deformans, and vertebral collapse with osteonecrosis. The lucent areas are produced by gas (90% nitrogen), which accumulates within diskal clefts. This phenomenon arises during extension, in which distraction of the intervertebral disk increases the diskal space and attracts gas from the surrounding extracellular fluid. In flexion, the space is obliterated and the gas resorbed. The vacuum phenomenon related to disk degeneration is usually associated with loss of height of the intervertebral disk space and reactive sclerosis (Fig. 4-155).

BIBLIOGRAPHY

Ford LT, Gilula LA, Murphy WA et al: Analysis of gas in vacuum lumbar disc. AJR 128:1056–1057, 1977

Knutsson F: The vacuum phenomenon in the intervertebral discs. Acta Radiol 23:173–179, 1942

Resnick D, Niwayama G, Guerra J et al: Spinal vacuum phenomena: Anatomical study and review. Radiology 139:341–348, 1981

FIG. 4-154. Vacuum phenomenon at the L5-S1 level (**arrow**) in a patient with degenerative disk disease.

FIG. 4-155. Vacuum phenomenon at multiple levels of the lower lumbar spine. Note the associated hypertrophic spurring, intervertebral disk space narrowing, and reactive sclerosis.

Wasp Waist Sign

Anterior and posterior constriction at the junction of the fused vertebral bodies has been described as the single most useful sign for determining that a cervical fusion is congenital rather than acquired (Fig. 4-156). This characteristic indentation at the site of the absent disk between congenitally fused vertebral bodies probably represents cessation of growth at the disk level while the remainder of the vertebral bodies continued to grow normally.

BIBLIOGRAPHY

Brown MW, Templeton AW, Hodges FJ: The incidence of acquired and congenital fusion in the cervical spine. AJR 92:1255–1259, 1964

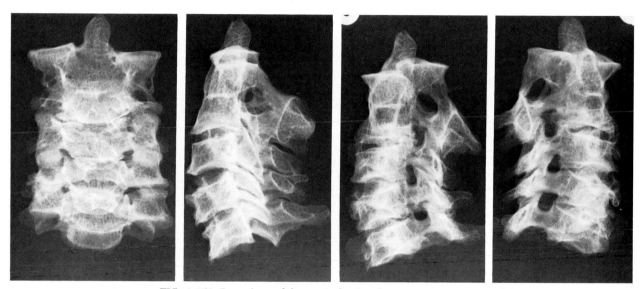

FIG. 4-156. Four views of the cervical spine demonstrating a congenital fusion at the C2-C3 level. There is a line of increased density and a slight constriction (wasp waist) where the disk space should be. The intervertebral foramina at this level are smooth and round. The laminae are fused posteriorly. (Brown MW, Templeton AW, Hodges FJ: The incidence of acquired and congenital fusions in the cervical spine. AJR 92:1255–1259, 1964. Copyright 1964. Reproduced by permission)

Whiskering Effect

In patients with ankylosing spondylitis, irregular proliferative new bone formation at sites of muscular attachments or points of stress causes a whiskering effect (Fig. 4-157). This sign is sometimes associated with reactive sclerosis. It most commonly involves the ischial tuberosities, iliac margins, and calcaneus.

BIBLIOGRAPHY
Greenfield GB: Radiology of Bone Diseases. Philadelphia, JB Lippincott, 1980

FIG. 4-157. Whiskering effect along the inferior pubic ramus.

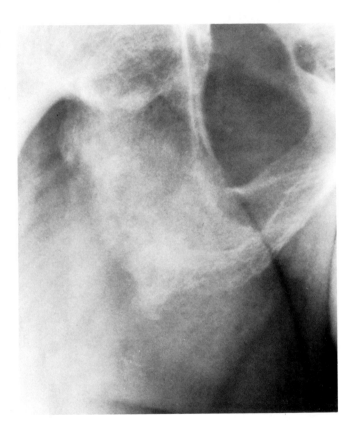

FIG. 4-159. *(Left)* On a flexion lateral radiograph of a patient with cervical hyperextension injury, there is suggestion of widening of the C3-C4 intervertebral disk. *(Right)* with extension, the C3-C4 disk space is obviously widened. (Cintron E, Gilula LA, Murphy WA et al The widened disk space: A sign of cervical hyperextension injury. Radiology 141:639–644,1981)

Widened Disk Space Sign

Cervical hyperextension sprain injuries result when the traumatic force is dissipated through the soft tissues only, with no evidence of the bone injury that occurs in the more common fracture–dislocations associated with cervical hyperextension. Hyperextension force ruptures the anterior longitudinal ligament, detaches or tears the intervertebral disk, and injures the remaining posterior ligaments. The musculoskeletal injury may be accompanied by a neurologic injury when the spinal cord is pinched between the posterior inferior margin of the retroluxing vertebral body and the lamina of the subjacent vertebrae. Because the spine flexes and often returns to a neutral position when the hyperextension force ends, this potentially unstable cervical spine injury may be difficult to diagnose. An isolated wide disk space (Fig. 4-158) is a sign of cervical hyperextension injury that may either be clearly evident on initial radiographs or require a carefully positioned extension view (Fig. 4-159).

BIBLIOGRAPHY
Cintron E, Gilula LA, Murphy WA et al: The widened disk space: A sign of cervical hyperextension injury. Radiology 141:639–644, 1981

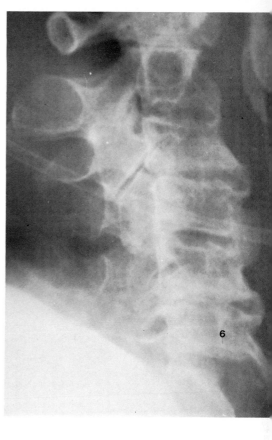

FIG. 4-158. Neutral lateral radiograph in a patient with cervical hyperextension injury shows marked widening of the C6-C7 intervertebral disk space. (Cintron E, Gilula LA, Murphy WA et al: The widened disk space: A sign of cervical hyperextension injury. Radiology 141:639–644, 1981)

FIG. 4-159.

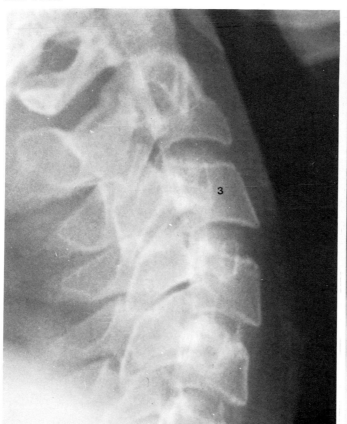

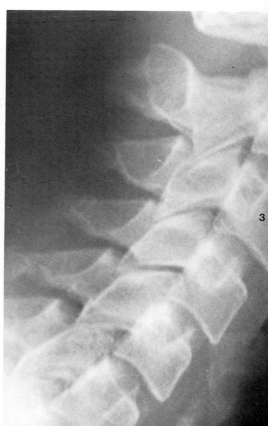

Widened Interspinous Distance Sign

Anterior dislocation of the cervical spine may be detected reliably in the supine frontal projection by evaluation of the cervical spinous processes. A widened interspinous distance that measures both more than 1½ times the interspinous distance above and more than 1½ times the interspinous distance below indicates anterior cervical dislocation at the level of the abnormal widening (Fig. 4-160). This sign is specific for anterior cervical dislocation. It is of no value for diagnosing posterior cervical dislocation, rotary subluxations, or the unstable cervical spine that has not yet dislocated.

BIBLIOGRAPHY

Naidich JB, Naidich TP, Garfein C et al: The widened interspinous distance: A useful sign of anterior cervical dislocation in the supine frontal projection. Radiology 123:113–116, 1977

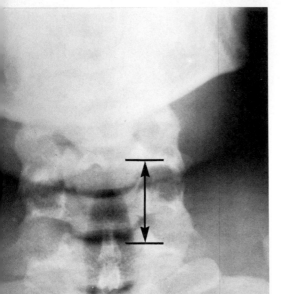

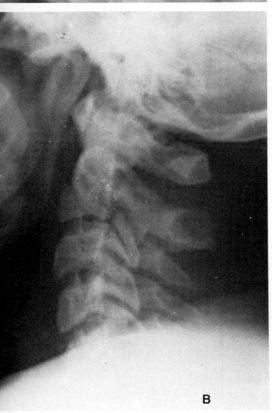

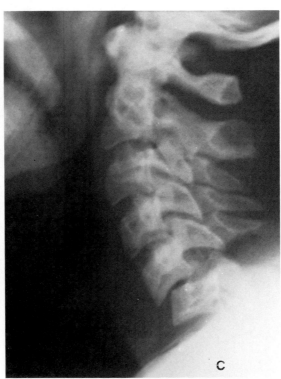

FIG. 4-160. (A) Supine frontal projection shows marked separation of the spinous processes of C5-C6 (arrows). (B) On the supine (crosstable) lateral projection, the shoulders obscure the site of injury. (C) on an erect lateral projection, the position of the shoulders is lower, and the anterior dislocation of C5-C6 can be clearly identified. The erect lateral projection was considered necessary and safe for diagnosis because the referring physician had seen no abnormality on radiograph A or B. The significance of the widened C5-C6 interspinous distance was not appreciated. The patient escaped neurologic injury. (Naidich JB, Naidich TP, Garfein C et al: The widened interspinous distance: A useful sign of anterior cervical dislocation in the supine frontal projection. Radiology 123:113–116,1977)

Widened Suture Sign

Abnormal widening of sutures is a sign of increased intracranial pressure in children (Fig. 4-161). The coronal and sagittal sutures are the ones most often widened. Separation of the interdigitating portions of sutures by more than 2 mm is considered abnormal in children older than 3. Widened sutures are most commonly caused by hydrocephalus; a similar pattern may occur in cases of acquired subdural hematoma or effusion, brain tumor or abscess, meningitis or encephalitis, and deprivation and malnourishment. Although sutural widening often develops only with long-standing raised intracranial pressure, it has been demonstrated as early as 2 days after the onset of acute meningitis.

BIBLIOGRAPHY

Holmes RD, Kuhns LR, Oliver WJ: Widened sutures in childhood meningitis: Unrecognized sign of an acute illness. AJR 128:977–979, 1977

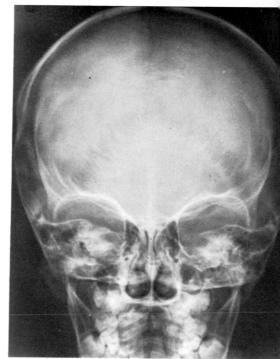

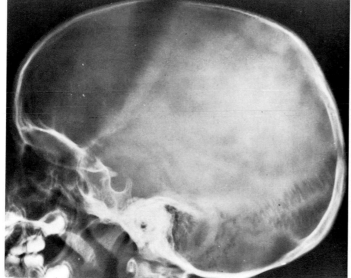

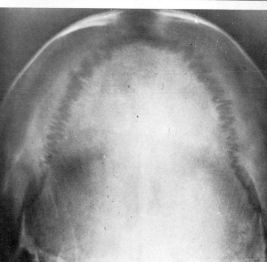

FIG. 4-161. Three views of the skull of a 3-year-old child demonstrate definite widening of all of the sutures due to increased intracranial pressure. (Taken from the Diagnostic Radiological Health Sciences Learning Laboratory, as developed by the Radiological Health Sciences Education Project, University of California at San Francisco, under contract with the Bureau of Radiological Health, Food and Drug Administration, and in cooperation with the American College of Radiology)

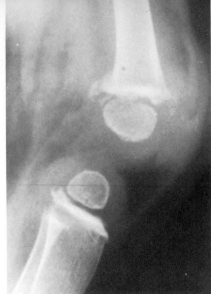

Wimberger's Sign of Scurvy

Wimberger's sign of scurvy is a dense, sharply demarcated, marginal ring of calcification about the epiphyseal ossification centers and ossification centers of small bones (Fig. 4-162).

BIBLIOGRAPHY
Greenfield GB: Radiology of Bone Diseases. Philadelphia, JB Lippincott, 1980

FIG. 4-162. Lateral radiographs of both knees demonstrate Wimberger's sign in a patient with scurvy. Note also the characteristic marginal spur formation (Pelken's spur).

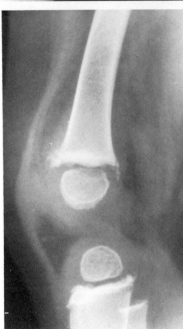

Wimberger's Sign of Syphilis

In moderately severe cases of congenital syphilis, destructive lesions initially involve the corners of the metaphysis adjacent to the cartilage plate, partially sparing the widened zone of provisional calcification. This process most characteristically produces symmetric involvement of the medial aspects of the proximal tibial metaphyses (Fig. 4-163).

BIBLIOGRAPHY

Edeiken J: Roentgen Diagnosis of Diseases of Bone. Baltimore, Williams & Wilkins, 1981

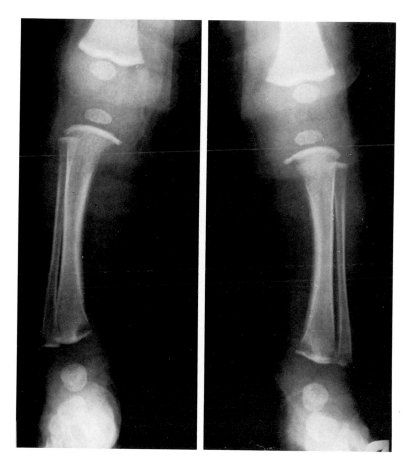

FIG. 4-163. The symmetric destruction at the medial border of the tibias (Wimberger's sign) is almost pathognomonic of syphilis. Note also the destructive areas at the distal ends of the tibias and fibulae and the increased density at the juxtaepiphyseal areas of bone. (Edeiken J: Roentgen Diagnosis of Diseases of Bone. Baltimore, Williams & Wilkins. 1981. Copyright 1981. Reproduced by permission)

5

Angiography

and

Myelography

6

Ultrasound

Disruptive Diaphragmatic Echo Sign

On routine ultrasound scans of the right upper quadrant, the right hemidiaphragm is usually seen as a strong echogenic curvilinear line superior and adjacent to the liver (Fig. 6-10). Disruption or interruption of the right hemidiaphragmatic echoes may be caused by such conditions as tumor invasion from direct extension or distal metastases and diaphragmatic rupture secondary to infection or trauma (Fig. 6-11).

BIBLIOGRAPHY
Worthen NJ, Worthen WF: Disruption of the diaphragmatic echoes: A sonographic sign of diaphragmatic disease. J Clin Ultrasound 10:43–45, 1982

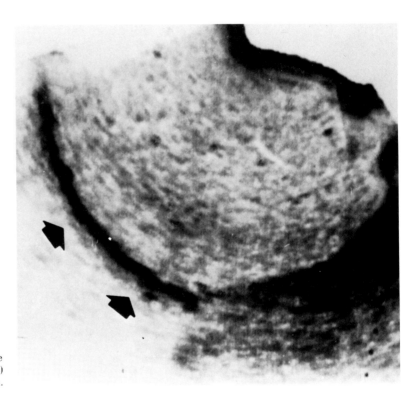

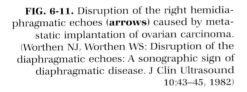

FIG. 6-10. Strong echogenic curvilinear line superior and adjacent to the liver (**arrows**) represents the right hemidiaphragm.

FIG. 6-11. Disruption of the right hemidiaphragmatic echoes (**arrows**) caused by metastatic implantation of ovarian carcinoma. (Worthen NJ, Worthen WS: Disruption of the diaphragmatic echoes: A sonographic sign of diaphragmatic disease. J Clin Ultrasound 10:43–45, 1982)

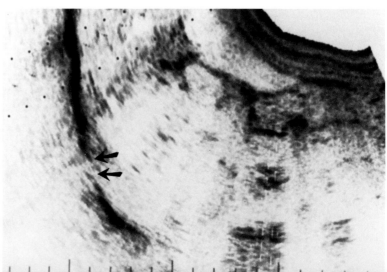

Double-Arc-Shadow Sign

The double-arc-shadow sign is an ultrasound indication of stones within a contracted gallbladder. The sign consists of two parallel arcuate echogenic lines spearated by a thin anechoic space with distal acoustic shadowing (Fig. 6-12). The proximal arc represents the near wall of the gallbladder. The anechoic space represents bile in the gallbladder lumen, and the distal arc represents the gallstone(s) responsible for the acoustic shadowing. In patients in whom the gallbladder lumen cannot be identified by static sonography, the double-arc-shadow sign indicates the presence of stones within a contracted gallbladder.

BIBLIOGRAPHY

Raptopoulos V, D'Orsi C, Smith E et al: Dynamic cholecystosonography of the contracted gallbladder: The double-arc-shadow sign. AJR 138:275–278, 1982

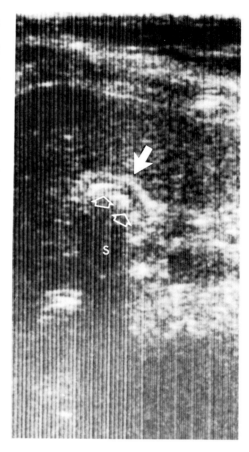

FIG. 6-12. Real-time sonographic image of a patient with cholelithiasis and a contracted gallbladder demonstrates the double arc shadow sign. The proximal arc (**solid arrow**) represents the near wall of the gallbladder; the distal arc (**open arrows**) represents the gallstones responsible for the acoustic shadowing *(s)*. (Raptopoulos V, D'Orsi C, Smith E et al: Dynamic cholecystosonography of the contracted gallbladder: The double-arc-shadow sign. AJR 138:275–278. Copyright 1978. Reproduced by permission)

Mickey Mouse Sign

In ultrasound evaluation of suspected biliary obstruction, it is important to assess the size of the main bile duct (common hepatic or common bile duct). The easiest way to identify this structure is by a transverse view, in which the configuration of the portal vein, main bile duct, and hepatic artery resembles the cartoon character Mickey Mouse (Fig. 6-23). The portal vein forms the head, the main bile duct is the right ear, and the hepatic artery is the left ear. Although Mickey's head is sometimes tipped a little to one side and his left ear often varies in size, the overall relationship is generally quite constant.

BIBLIOGRAPHY

Bartrum RJ, Crow HC: Inflammatory disease of the biliary system. Semin Ultrasound 1:102–112, 1980

FIG. 6-23. *(Left)* Line drawing and *(right)* ultrasound scan of the porta hepatis resembling Mickey Mouse. *BD* = main bile duct; *HA* = hepatic arteries; *PV* = portal vein.

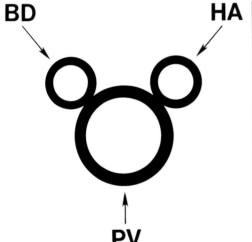

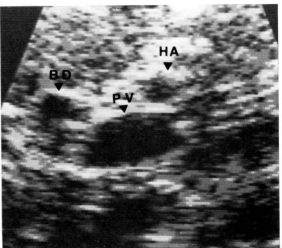

Moon Crescent Sign

A thin, crescent-shaped sonolucent strip adjacent to the liver is a sign of a small juxtahepatic effusion. Although the sign is most frequently identified between the liver and the right perirenal fat, a similar appearance may be seen between the liver and abdominal wall or between the inferior aspect of the liver and adjacent intestinal loops. The moon crescent sign may be due to ascites (Fig. 6-24), fluid of inflammatory origin (Fig. 6-25), blood, or fluid caused by pancreatic autolysis (Fig. 6-26).

BIBLIOGRAPHY
Weill FS: Ultrasonography of Digestive Diseases. St. Louis, CV Mosby, 1982

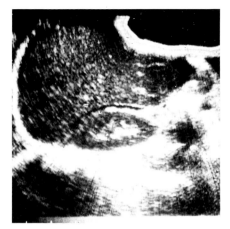

FIG. 6-24. Moon crescent sign between the liver and perirenal fat in a patient with ascites. Fluid is also visible between the diaphragm and dome of the liver and below the inferior edge of the liver. (Weill FS: Ultrasonography of Digestive Diseases. St. Louis, CV Mosby, 1982)

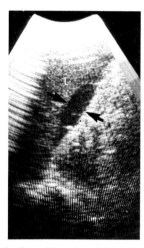

FIG. 6-25. Moon crescent sign **(arrows)** between the liver *(L)* and perirenal fat representing inflammatory intraperitoneal fluid in a patient with acute cholecystitis. (Weill FS: Ultrasonography of Digestive Diseases. St. Louis, CV Mosby, 1982)

FIG. 6-26. Small moon crescent sign **(arrows)** indicating a small volume of intraperitoneal fluid caused by pancreatic autolysis. (Weill FS: Ultrasonography of Digestive Diseases. St. Louis, CV Mosby, 1982)

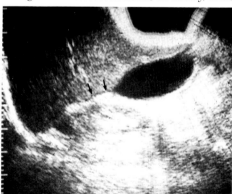

Sulcus Sign

Nonvisualization of the gallbladder on ultrasound in a fasting patient is strongly suggestive of pathology. To be certain that appropriate ultrasound sections have been obtained, it is important to identify structures that have specific and reliable anatomic relationships with the gallbladder. The sulcus sign, a linear echo connecting the gallbladder to the right or main portal vein, represents a portion of the main lobar fissure of the liver (Fig. 6-43). This sign is reported to be a reliable anatomic indicator of the location of the gallbladder.

BIBLIOGRAPHY

Callen PW, Filly RA: Ultrasonographic localization of the gallbladder. Radiology 133:687–691, 1979

FIG. 6-43. Two examples of linear echoes (**arrows**) connecting the gallbladder to portal venous structures in patients with *(top)* single and *(bottom)* multiple gallstones.

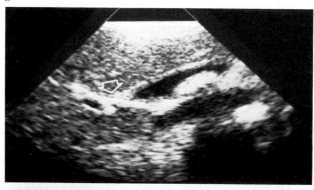

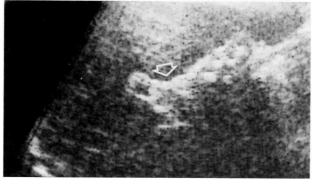

Target Sign

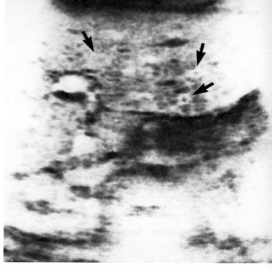

Ultrasound of the liver may demonstrate a target appearance caused by anechoic spherical structures containing internal echoes (Fig. 6-44). The target sign is a nonspecific finding that has been described in patients with metastatic lesions and hepatic microabscesses.

BIBLIOGRAPHY

Callen PW, Filly RA, Marcus FS: Ultrasonography and computed tomography in the evaluation of hepatic microabscesses in the immunosuppressed patient. Radiology 136:433–434, 1980

Scheible W, Gosink BB, Leopold GR: Gray scale echographic patterns of hepatic metastatic disease. AJR 129:983–987, 1977

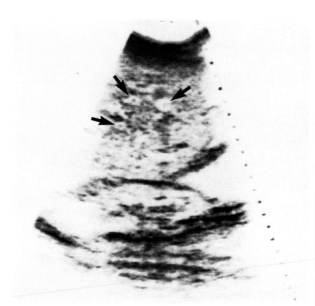

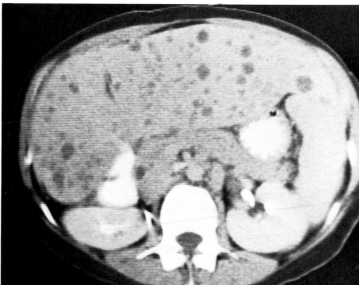

FIG. 6-44. *(Top)* Transverse and *(bottom, left)* longitudinal sonograms through the liver demonstrate numerous rounded fluid-filled lesions (**arrows**) with a target appearance. *(Bottom, right)* CT scan of the midabdomen demonstrates numerous low-density lesions in the liver and spleen. Postmortem examination showed a massively enlarged liver, enlarged spleen, and multiple abscesses containing *Candida albicans* throughout both organs. (Callen PW, Filly RA, Marcus FS: Ultrasonography and computed tomography in the evaluation of hepatic microabscesses in the immunosuppressed patient. Radiology 136:433–434, 1980)

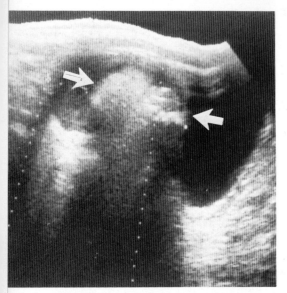

FIG. 6-48. Sagittal sonogram demonstrates only the near wall of a dermoid because of acoustic shadowing from the hairball (**arrows**) producing the tip of the iceberg sign.

Tip of the Iceberg Sign

Benign cystic ovarian teratomas (dermoids) frequently demonstrate highly reflective irregular solid components due to hair and sebum within the tumor. This appearance may be mistaken for bowel gas and be responsible for a false-negative interpretation. The resulting acoustic shadowing often totally obscures the back wall of a large, clinically evident mass. This tip of the iceberg sign is suggestive of ovarian dermoid (Fig. 6-48). The most common false-positive tip of the iceberg sign has been reported with hemorrhagic ovarian cysts, which can be differentiated from ovarian dermoids on the basis of their attenuation characteristics.

BIBLIOGRAPHY
Guttman PH: In search of the illusive benign cystic ovarian teratoma: Application of the ultrasound "tip of the iceberg" sign. J Clin Ultrasound 5:403–406, 1977

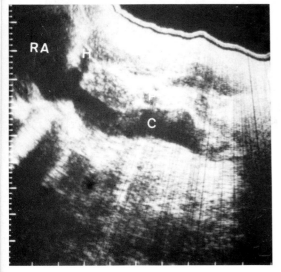

FIG. 6-49. Longitudinal sonogram shows marked dilatation of the vena cava *(C)* in this patient with right-sided cardiac insufficiency. The junction of the vena cava with the enlarged right atrium *(RA)* is visible. *H* = hepatic vein; *P* = portal vein. (Weill FS: Ultrasonography of Digestive Diseases. St. Louis, CV Mosby, 1982)

Vena Cava Sign

Congestion of the inferior vena cava with loss of respiratory variability has been reported as a reliable sign of hepatomegaly of cardiac origin (Fig. 6-49). Respiratory variability reappears at subsequent examinations with therapeutic improvement. One exception to this otherwise pathognomonic sign of right cardiac insufficiency is thrombosis of the inferior vena cava, in which respiratory variability may also be lost.

BIBLIOGRAPHY
Weill FS: Ultrasonography of Digestive Diseases. St. Louis, CV Mosby, 1982

7

Computed

Tomography

Cracked Walnut Sign ▬▬▬▬▬▬▬▬▬▬▬

Normal aging and a multitude of degenerative diseases may cause generalized enlargement of sulci, fissures, and ventricles, giving the brain a "cracked walnut" appearance on computed tomography (Fig. 7-1). In patients over 65, there is no relationship between dementia and measurements of ventricle or sulcus size. However, in young and middle-aged persons, the cracked walnut appearance is strongly suggestive of degenerative disease.

BIBLIOGRAPHY
Huckman MS: Computed tomography in the diagnosis of degenerative brain disease. Radiol Clin North Am 20:169–183, 1982

FIG. 7-1. *(Left)* Large ventricles are seen in this demented 88-year-old man with Alzheimer's disease. *(Right)* Prominence of the cortical sulci in the high convexity region shows the typical cracked walnut appearance of Alzheimer's disease. (Huckman MS: Computed tomography in the diagnosis of degenerative brain disease. Radiol Clin North Am 20:169–183, 1982)

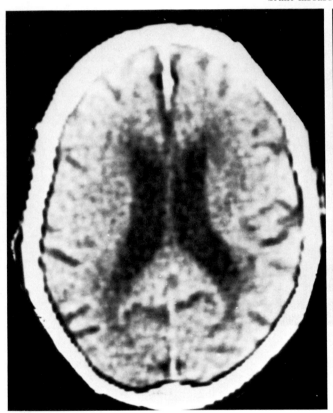 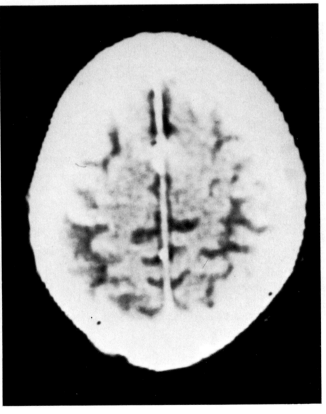

Displaced Crus Sign

Fluid collections in the lower pleural cavity and upper abdominal cavity sometimes appear similar on computed tomography (CT). The crura of the diaphragm are usually imaged by CT as obliquely oriented curvilinear structures passing posterolaterally from the aorta toward the posterior thoracic wall closely applied to the vertebral column. Lateral displacement of the diaphragmatic crus and interposition of fluid between the crus and vertebral column indicate the presence of intrapleural fluid (Fig. 7-2). Intraperitoneal collections produce fluid anterior to the crus without displacement, so that the normal relationship of the crus to the vertebral column is maintained.

BIBLIOGRAPHY

Callen PW, Filly RA, Korobkin M: Computed tomographic evaluation of the diaphragmatic crura. Radiology 126:413–416, 1978

Dwyer A: The displaced crus: A sign for distinguishing between pleural fluid and ascites on computed tomography. J Comp Asst Tomogr 2:598–599, 1978

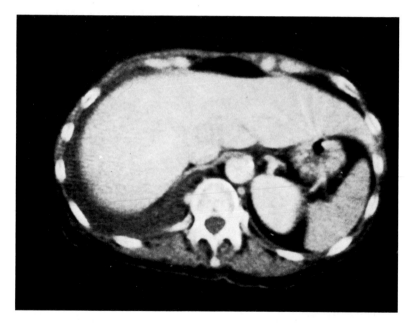

FIG. 7-2. Displaced crus sign. (Dwyer A: The displaced crus: A sign for distinguishing between pleural fluid and ascites on computed tomography. J Comp Assist Tomogr 2:598–599, 1978)

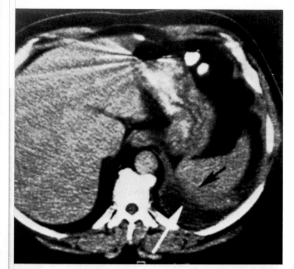

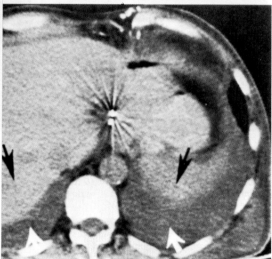

Interface Sign

Free intraperitoneal fluid (ascites) is generally easy to recognize on CT scans because of its low CT number and its location. It typically accumulates around the liver and spleen, often displacing these structures from the lateral walls. Sometimes, however, pleural effusions filling the deep lateral and posterior recesses of the pleural cavity and displacing the liver or spleen may be confused with ascites on upper abdominal sections. The character of the interface between the fluid collection and the liver or spleen has been reported as an aid to discrimination between pleural and peritoneal fluid collections. When the fluid collection is pleural, the interface with the liver or spleen is hazy and unsharp (Fig. 7-13). In contrast, with ascitic fluid the interface with these organs is very sharp (Fig. 7-14). Because the lateral and posterior pleural recesses virtually never extend below L-2 and usually end at L-1, free fluid seen in the middle or lower abdomen is always intraperitoneal and shows a sharp interface with adjacent organs.

BIBLIOGRAPHY
Teplick JG, Teplick SK, Goodman L et al: The interface sign: A computed tomographic sign for distinguishing pleural and intra-abdominal fluid. Radiology 144:359–362, 1982

FIG. 7-13. Two examples of the hazy, unsharp interface between pleural fluid collections (**white arrows**) and the liver and spleen (**black arrows**). (Teplick JG, Teplick SK, Goodman L et al: The interface sign: A computed tomographic sign for distinguishing pleural and intra-abdominal fluid. Radiology 144:359–362, 1982)

FIG. 7-14. Sharp interface between the free intraperitoneal fluid collection (**white arrow**) and the entire liver margin (**black arrow**) in a patient with ascites. (Teplick JG, Teplick SK, Goodman L et al: A computed tomographic sign for distinguishing pleural and intra-abdominal fluid. Radiology 144:359–362, 1982)

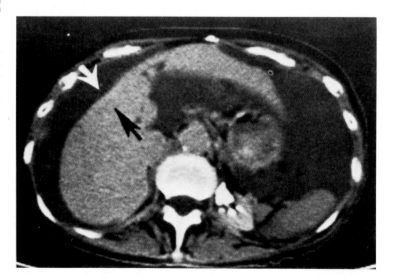

Intraosseous Gas Sign

Demonstration on CT scans of gas within the medullary cavity
has been reported as a sign of osteomyelitis of the involved bone
(Fig. 7-15). The presence of intraosseous gas on CT scans is an
early sign that may be seen even when plain radiographs reveal
no bone abnormally (Fig. 7-16).

BIBLIOGRAPHY
Ram PC, Martinez S, Korobkin M et al: CT detection of intraosseous gas: A new
    sign of osteomyelitis. AJR 137:721–723, 1981

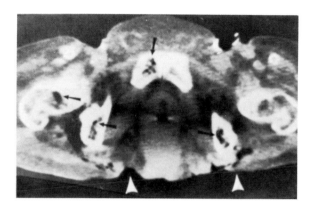

FIG. 7-15. Gas bubbles (**arrows**) are seen in
the right pubic ramus, both ischial bones,
and right femoral neck in a patient with diffuse pelvic osteomyelitis. Gas is also seen in
soft tissues surrounding the ischial bones and
adjacent to decubitus ulcers (**arrowheads**).
(Ram PC, Martinez S, Korobkin M et al: CT
detection of intraosseous gas: A new sign of
osteomyelitis. AJR 137:721–723, 1981. Copyright 1981. Reproduced by permission)

FIG. 7-16. Gas bubbles are seen within the
medullary cavity of the fibula (**arrows**) and in
soft tissues surrounding the fibular cortex in
a patient with osteomyelitis of the fibula.
Plain radiographs of the right calf showed air
bubbles within the soft tissues but no evidence of osteomyelitis. (Ram PC, Martinez S,
Korobkin M et al: CT detection of intraosseous gas: A new sign of osteomyelitis. AJR
137:721–723, 1981. Copyright 1981. Reproduced by permission)

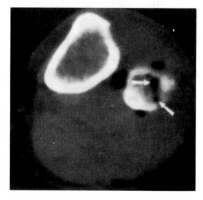

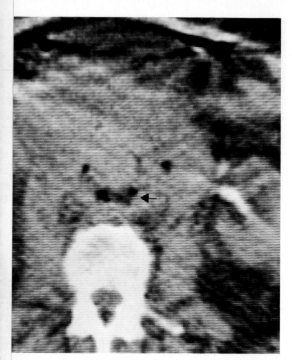

FIG. 7-19. CT scan demonstrates small gas pockets (**arrow**) posteriorly in the para-aortic region in a patient with an infected aortic graft. (Haaga JR, Baldwin GN, Reich NE et al: CT detection of infected synthetic grafts: Preliminary report of a new sign. AJR 131:317–320, 1978, Copyright 1978. Reproduced by permission)

Pockets of Gas Sign

Infected prostheses are a serious complication of vascular surgery that are associated with high mortality and morbidity rates. Successful surgical management of this problem depends on early and accurate diagnosis of the presence of infection. An early sign of infected synthetic grafts on CT scans is demonstration of small pockets of gas located posteriorly within the aortic bed around the prosthesis (Fig. 7-19). Use of intravenous contrast material demonstrates that the pockets of gas are external to the lumen of the graft. The gas noted on the CT scan may reflect infection by gram-negative gas-forming organisms (especially *Escherichia coli*) or aortoenteric fistulae, which are a potential source of perivascular gas. The pockets of gas sign must be distinguished from the single pocket of gas that can be identified anteriorly in the area of the aortic bed within a week of surgery (Fig. 7-20). Unlike the normal postsurgical pocket of gas, "infected" gas collections are multiple, located posteriorly, and first apparent more than 10 days after surgery.

BIBLIOGRAPHY
Haaga JR, Baldwin GN, Reich NE et al: CT detection of infected synthetic grafts: Preliminary report of a new sign. AJR 131:317–320, 1978

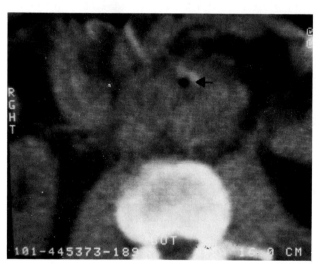

FIG. 7-20. CT scan 7 days after surgery for aneurysm repair demonstrates a single pocket of gas (**arrow**) anteriorly in a noninfected patient. (Haaga JR, Baldwin GN, Reich NE et al: CT detection of infected synthetic grafts: Preliminary report of a new sign. AJR 131:317–320, 1978. Copyright 1978. Reproduced by permission.

Splenic Pedicle Sign

The splenic vascular pedicle serves as a useful landmark for differentiating between tumors arising from the tail of the pancreas and tumors arising from the adrenal gland. Masses located behind the splenic pedicle and displacing it anteriorly have their origin in the adrenal gland (Fig. 7-21). Masses arising anterior to the splenic pedicle and displacing it posteriorly arise from the body or tail of the pancreas (Fig. 7-22).

BIBLIOGRAPHY

Haaga J, Reich NE: Computed Tomography of Abdominal Abnormalities. St. Louis, CV Mosby, 1978

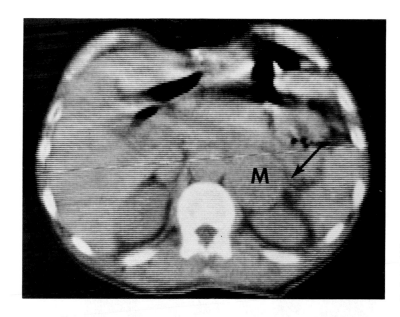

FIG. 7-21. A large, left-sided adrenal mass *(M)* lies behind the splenic pedicle (**arrow**) and displaces it anteriorly. (Haaga J, Reich NE: Computed Tomography of Abdominal Abnormalities. St. Louis, CV Mosby, 1978)

FIG. 7-22. A pancreatic mass *(M)* is located anterior to the splenic vascular pedicle (**arrow**). (Haaga J, Reich NE: Computed Tomography of Abdominal Abnormalities. St. Louis, CV Mosby, 1978)

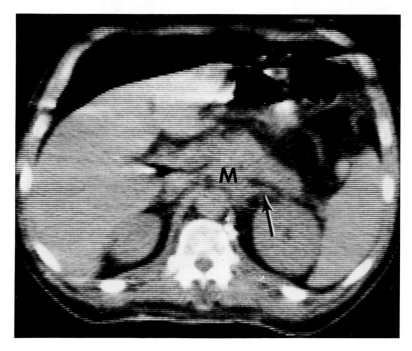

Thickened Sclera Sign

Orbital pseudotumor, a histologically benign but often clinically severe inflammatory condition of unknown origin, is one of the most common causes of unilateral exophthalmos. Two major differential diagnoses in this disorder are true neoplasms of the orbit and unilateral Graves' disease, especially in euthyroid patients. Thickening of the scleral uveal rim seen on CT scans with contrast enhancement has been reported as a sign of inflammatory involvement of the rim and adjacent tissues (Fig. 7-25). In a patient with no recent history of trauma or surgery, scleral uveal rim thickening suggests the presence of an orbital pseudotumor (Fig. 7-26). Because this disease usually responds well to steroid therapy, a prompt and accurate diagnosis is extremely important.

BIBLIOGRAPHY

Bernadino ME, Zimmerman RD, Citrin CM et al: Scleral thickening: a CT sign of orbital pseudotumor. AJR 129:703–706, 1977

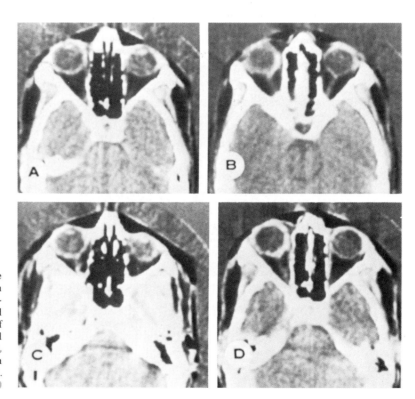

FIG. 7-25. (A) and **(B)** CT scans demonstrate thickening of the left scleral uveal rim with exophthalmos in a patient with orbital pseudotumor. No retrobulbar mass is seen. **(C)** and **(D)** Scans obtained after administration of contrast show enhancement of the left scleral uveal rim. (Bernardino ME, Zimmerman RD, Citrin CM et al: Scleral thickening: A CT sign of orbital pseudotumor. AJR 129:703–706, 1977. Copyright 1977. Reproduced by permission)

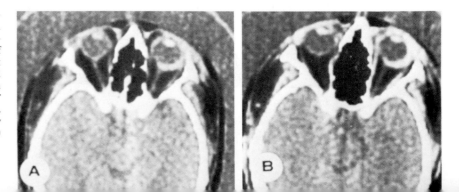

FIG. 7-26. (A) CT scan demonstrates thickening of the right posterior lateral scleral uveal rim and minimal thickening of the right lateral rectus muscle. **(B)** Scan after injection of contrast shows enhancement of the right scleral uveal rim in a patient with an orbital pseudotumor. (Bernardino ME, Zimmerman RD, Citrin CM et al: Scleral thickening: A CT sign of orbital pseudotumor. AJR 129:703–706, 1977. Copyright 1977. Reproduced by permission)

Twinkling Star Sign

Pulmonary vessels that parallel the long axis of the body may appear on CT scans as nodules that may be difficult to distinguish from true parenchymal lesions. Pulmonary vessels produce radial linear artifacts (twinkling star sign; Fig. 7-27) whereas true pulmonary nodules do not (Fig. 7-28). Therefore, visualization of such radial artifacts on a single CT section provides evidence that the structure in question simply represents a vessel seen on end rather than a nodule. In contrast to the usual evaluation of pulmonary parenchyma, which is performed at a 400-HU window width, the twinkling star sign is best appreciated at a 100-HU to 200-HU window width (Fig. 7-29).

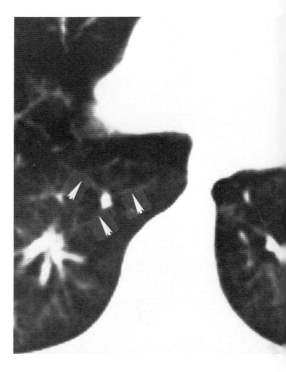

BIBLIOGRAPHY
Kuhns LR, Borlaza G: The "twinkling star" sign: An aid in differentiating pulmonary vessels from pulmonary nodules on computed tomograms. Radiology 135:763–764, 1980

FIG. 7-27. Faint opaque linear artifacts (**arrowheads**) emanate from a pulmonary vessel that has been imaged axially. Numerous other vessels with radial artifacts are also seen. (Kuhns LR, Borlaza G: The "twinkling star" sign: An aid in differentiating pulmonary vessels from pulmonary nodules on computed tomograms. Radiology 135:763–764, 1980)

FIG. 7-28. Absence of radial artifacts around a surgically proved metastatic nodule (**arrow**). (Kuhns LR, Borlaza G: The "twinkling star" sign: An aid in differentiating pulmonary vessels from pulmonary nodules on computed tomograms. Radiology 135:763–764, 1980)

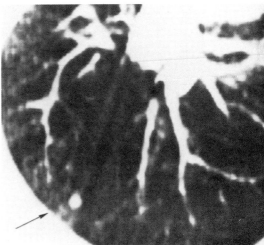

FIG. 7-29. (Top) CT scan imaged at a window width of 100 HU demonstrates radial artifacts around a pulmonary vessel (**arrow**) far better than on Figure 7-27, which used a wide (400 HU) window setting. (Bottom) CT scan obtained 1.5 cm caudal to the area shown in the (top) figure reveals a metastatic lesion (**arrow**) without radial linear artifacts. A window width of 100 HU was also used for this scan. Presence of the metastatic lesion was confirmed at surgery. (Kuhns LR, Borlaza G: The "twinkling star" sign: An aid in differentiating pulmonary vessels from pulmonary nodules on computed tomograms. Radiology 135:763–764, 1980)

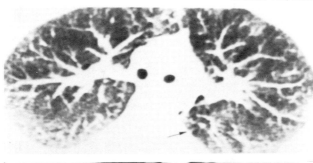

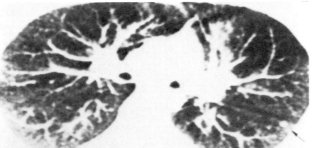

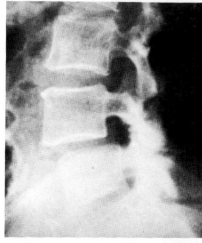

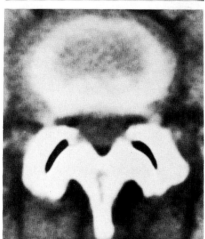

Vacuum Facet Sign

A lens-shaped lucency within a lumbar facet joint (vacuum facet sign) has been reported as a CT sign of degenerative spondylolisthesis (Fig. 7-30). In this condition, breakdown of the cartilage lining the apophyseal joint permits anterior subluxation of the upper vertebrae and overriding of the facets. In this form of spondylolisthesis, in contrast to other forms, the pars interarticularis remains free of spondylolysis, and the bony configuration of the neural arch is preserved. Consequently, traction between opposing articular facets occurs, allowing development of a vacuum phenomenon. Conversely, when spondylolysis or acute trauma involving the pars interarticularis results in spondylolisthesis, it is not associated with traction between adjacent articular facets and does not lead to the vacuum phenomenon.

BIBLIOGRAPHY

Lefkowitz DM, Quencer RM: Vacuum facet phenomenon: A computed tomographic sign of degenerative spondylolisthesis. Radiology 144:562, 1982

FIG. 7-30. *(Top)* Lateral view of the lumbar spine demonstrates anterior spondylolisthesis of L4 on L5. The frontal view demonstrated degenerative changes of apophyseal joints at this level. *(Bottom)* CT scan (−190 HU) demonstrates gas within the widened facet joints of L4-L5. (Lefkowitz DM, Quencer RM: Vacuum facet phenomenon: A computed tomographic sign of degenerative spondylolisthesis. Radiology 144:562, 1982)

White Matter Buckling Sign

Superficially situated extra-axial masses usually preserve the gray–white interface and tend to compress or buckle adjacent edematous white matter (Fig. 7-31). Because this does not occur with superficially situated intra-axial lesions, the white matter buckling sign is essentially diagnostic of an extra-axial mass. This appearance is almost invariably associated with extracerebral fluid collections (Fig. 7-32). It is less often seen in association with meningioma. The sign is of major value in correct localization to the extra-axial compartment of isodense subdural hematomas or atypical meningiomas, conditions that otherwise might not be correctly diagnosed (Fig. 7-33). It is postulated that the white matter buckling sign reflects the relative resistance of gray matter to edema in conjunction with the destruction of the gray–white interface by the infiltration of intra-axial lesions.

BIBLIOGRAPHY

George AE, Russell EJ, Kricheff II: White matter buckling: CT sign of extraaxial intracranial mass. AJR 135:1031–1036, 1980

FIG. 7-31. *(Left)* Normal transverse axial CT scan at the centrum semiovale above the lateral ventricles. Fronds of central white matter *(black area)* insinuate themselves into the cortical gray matter *(G). s* = subarachnoid space; *K* = skull; *sl* = sulcus. The border between the white and gray matter is the gray-white interface. The central white matter describes the shape of a porcupine, its belly directed medially. *(Right)* CT gray-white matter changes associated with a laterally placed extra-axial mass *(T).* The gray matter and the gray-white interface are preserved. White matter fronds **(arrows)** are crowded together. The white matter is compressed, despite the presence of edema, and buckled adjacent to the lesion. (George AE, Russell EJ, Kricheff II: White matter buckling: CT sign of extraaxial intracranial mass. AJR 135:1031–1036, 1980. Copyright 1980. Reproduced by permission)

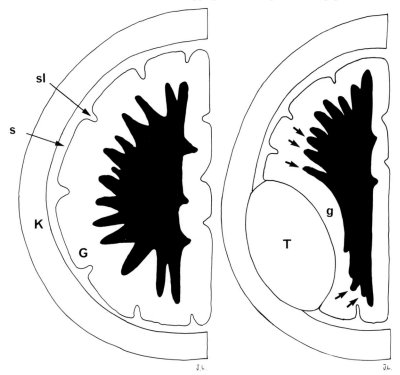

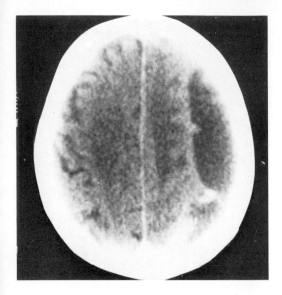

FIG. 7-32. Typical noncontrast scan demonstrates a chronic right convexity subdural hematoma in a 70-year-old man with mild left hemiparesis. The white matter is clearly compressed, though the gray-white interface is maintained. (George AE, Russell EJ, Kricheff II: White matter buckling: CT sign of extraaxial intracranial mass. AJR 135:1031–1036, 1980. Copyright 1980. Reproduced by permission)

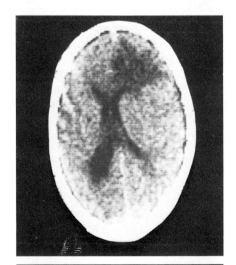

FIG. 7-33. Contrast scans of an isodense subdural hematoma. *(Top)* A right frontal contusion of undetermined age is seen at the lateral ventricle level. Compression of the right lateral ventricle and a right-to-left shift are evident. *(Bottom)* At the convexity level, compression and medial displacement of the central white matter (**arrows**) are seen. This finding is consistent with an extracerebral mass. Presence of a large right subdural hematoma was confirmed by arteriography. (George AE, Russell EJ, Kricheff II: White matter buckling: CT sign of extraaxial intracranial mass. AJR 135:1031–1036, 1980. Copyright 1980. Reproduced by permission)

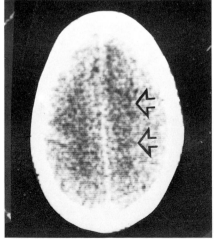

General Index

angiofibroma, juvenile, of nasopharynx
antral bowing sign, 301-302
ankle joint effusion
teardrop sign (ankle), 386
ankylosing spondylitis
whiskering effect, 400
aorta
abdominal, lesions of
floating aorta sign, 471
aneurysm
due to chest trauma
apical cap sign, 187
dissecting
mucosal stripe sign, 64
twisted tape sign, 428
coarctation
figure 3 and figure E signs,
213-214
thoracic, rupture due to trauma
esophageal tube displacement
sign, 210
aortic arch, trachea and, adhesions
between
aortic swallowing sign, 186
appendicitis
dilated transverse colon sign, 25
psoas sign, 71
reverse 3 sign, 75
arrythmia(s)
cardiac blur sign, 195
arteriovenous malformation
bag of worms sign, 408
arthritis
infectious, of hip joint
obturator sign, 358
psoriatic, arthritis mutilans
main en lorgnette *deformity*
(opera glass hand), 352
rheumatoid
boutonniere *deformity, 307*
main en lorgnette *deformity*
(opera glass hand), 352
metacarpal sign, 354
scallop sign, 371
sternal cupping sign, 382
supinator notch sign, 384
tibiotalar slant sign, 389
tuberculous
kissing sequestra sign, 348
asbestosis
shaggy heart sign, 271-272
Ascaris infestation
Medusa locks sign, 61

hump sign, 50
ascites
ground-glass sign, 44
Hellmer's sign, 46
moon crescent sign, 449
peripheral bubble sign, 66
vs ovarian cyst
curvature sign, 437
vs pleural effusion
displaced crus sign, 467
interface sign, 474
thickened gallbladder wall sign,
463
urinary, in abdomen
perirenal P and subcapsular C
signs, 155-156
vascular cut-off sign, 292
aspergillosis
air crescent (meniscus) sign, 182-
183
target sign, 281
asplenia
symmetric liver sign, 94
atresia
colonic
hook sign, 48
windsock sign, 109
duodenal
double bubble sign, 28
esophageal
coiled tube sign, 20
gastric
single bubble sign, 83
jejunal
triple bubble sign, 102
atrium, left, enlargement
deviated descending thoracic
aorta sign, 204
double contour sign, 205
third mogul sign, 283
auditory canal, internal, acoustic
neuroma blocking
fickle finger sign, 415-416

basal cell nevus syndrome
metacarpal sign, 354
Beckwith-Wiedemann syndrome
metacarpal sign, 354
bile duct, common
distended
distended common bile duct
sign, 26

filling defect of, vs impacted
stone
pseudocalculus sign, 69
stone, impacted
Poppel's sign, 68
bile duct obstruction
Mickey Mouse sign, 448
bladder
distended
bladder sign, 119
herniation
bladder ear sign, 120
outlet obstruction
pine tree (Christmas tree)
bladder, 157
shotgun wound
sinking pellet sign, 168
spastic, neurogenic
pine tree (Christmas tree)
bladder, 157
tumor
white line sign, 177
bladder neck contracture
acorn deformity, 113
toothpaste sign, 174
blighted ovum
tennis racquet sign, 462
blood
juxtahepatic
moon crescent sign, 449
subarachnoid, in interhemis-
pheric fissure
falx sign, 470
blowout fracture of orbit
teardrop sign (blowout fracture),
387
bowel. *See* intestine.
brachial plexus, neurologic injuries
drooping shoulder sign, 328
brain. *See also* skull
abscess
padlock sign, 477
ripple sign, 421
degenerative disease
cracked walnut sign, 466
extra-axial mass
white matter buckling sign,
485-486
metastases to
padlock sign, 477
subarachnoid blood in inter-
hemispheric fissure
falx sign, 470

ventricles
  compression
    squeezed ventricle sign, 480
  dermoid cyst leakage into
    floating Myodil sign, 472
bronchiectasis
  gloved finger shadow sign, 217
  sentinel lines sign, 270
  tram line sign, 288
  vascular plethora sign, 294
bronchitis, chronic
  leafless tree sign, 237
bronchus(i)
  asymmetric narrowing in malig-
    nant disease
    rat tail narrowing sign, 257
  dilatation
    gloved finger shadow sign, 217
  sputum inspissation
    mucoid impaction signs, 245
Burkitt's lymphoma
  floating tooth sign, 335

calcinosis, tumoral, vs calcium metabolism abnormalities
  sedimentation sign, 373
calculus, ureteral
  Bergman's sign, 118
capital femoral epiphysis, slipped
  triangular sign, 392
carcinoid tumor, intestinal
  tacked-down sign, 95
carcinoma
  bronchioalveolar
    indrawn pleura sign, 230
    leafless tree sign, 237
    pleuropulmonary tail signs,
     254-255
  bronchogenic
    rat tail narrowing sign, 257
    S sign of Golden, 264
    stretched (bent) bronchus sign,
     280
    tumor track sign, 289
  esophageal
    thickened posterior tracheal
     stripe sign, 282
  of hypopharynx
    vallecular sign, 107
  of intestinal tract
    sonographic bull's-eye sign,
     459

metastatic to skull
  button sequestrum sign, 311
of pancreas
  Frostberg's inverted 3 sign, 38-
   40
  struggling antrum sign, 93
renal
  beak sign, 115
  dimple sign, 131
  renal vein compromise with
    collateral vein sign, 124
  thick wall sign, 174
in retroperitoneal space
  renal halo (perirenal fat) sign,
   160-161
of stomach
  Carman meniscus sign, 18
  trapped air sign, 100
  whalebone in a corset sign,
   108
ureteral
  Bergman's sign, 118
carcinomatosis
  ascites due to
    peripheral bubble sign, 66
  peritoneal, diffuse
    tacked-down sign, 95
cardiomyopathy
  third mogul sign, 283
cardiophrenic angle fat pads
  cardiac blur sign, 195
Caroli's disease
  lollipop-tree sign, 58
carpal navicular, rotatory subluxation
  cortical ring sign (navicular), 318
cecum, volvulus
  coffee bean (kidney bean) sign, 19
celiac sprue
  gallbladder inertia sign, 42
  moulage sign, 63
cervical spine
  anterior dislocation
    widened interspinous distance
     sign, 402
  clay shoveler's fracture
    double spinous process sign,
     326
  extension–flexion injuries of
    double outline sign, 325
  flexion injury to
    acute kyphosis sign, 300
    divergent spinous processes
     sign, 324

fused vertebral bodies, congenital vs acquired
  wasp waist sign, 399
hyperextension sprain of
  widened disk space sign, 401
injury or disease
  displaced spinolaminar line
   sign, 323
  lucent cleft sign, 350
  nasopharyngeal soft-tissue
   sign, 356
cholangiohepatitis
  arrowhead sign, 13
cholecystitis
  thickened gallbladder wall sign, 463
choledochal cyst
  rim sign, 77-78
chronic obstructive pulmonary
  disease
  saber sheath trachea sign, 265
chronic obstructive uropathy. *See*
  uropathy, chronic ob-
  structive
clay shoveler's fracture
  double spinous process sign, 326
coarctation of aorta
  figure 3 and figure E signs, 213-
   214
colitis
  Crohn's
    thumbprinting, 97-98
    transverse stripe sign, 99
  infectious
    thumbprinting, 97-98
  ischemic
    lumen with a lumen sign, 60
    thumbprinting, 97-98
  pseudomembranous
    thumbprinting, 97-98
  ulcerative
    thumbprinting, 97-98
colon
  appearance, in renal absence vs
    renal disease
    colon sign, 125
  atresia
    hook sign, 48
    windsock sign, 109
  diverticula
    border sign, 15
  hemorrhage
    thumbprinting, 97-98
  ischemia
    thumbprinting, 97-98

gastric outlet obstruction in newborn
single bubble sign, 83
gastric ulcer(s)
benign
crescent (quarter moon) sign,
24
ellipse sign, 31
malignant
Carman meniscus sign, 18
whalebone in a corset sign, 108
gastrointestinal tract. *See specific*
parts
Gaucher's disease
osteopetrosis signs, 359
step-off vertebral body sign, 380-
381
gestational sac
tennis racquet sign, 462
glenohumeral joint space effusion
rim sign, 367
glioma
padlock sign, 477
gonadal dysgenesis
carpal sign, 312
metacarpal sign, 354
phalangeal sign, 362
granulomatous disease
clear space sign, 199
lymph nodes in
eggshell calcification, 206-207
pulmonary
air crescent (meniscus) sign,
182-183
pleuropulmonary tail signs,
254-255
Rigler notch sign, 261
thickened posterior tracheal
stripe sign, 282

hematoma
adjacent to uterus
indefinite uterus sign, 444
vs hemoperitoneum following
splenic trauma
drowned hilus sign, 442
renal, hypertension due to
Page kidney, 148
in retroperitoneal space
renal halo (perirenal fat) sign,
160-161

of stomach
gastric cannonball sign, 43
subdural
hematocrit effect, 473
squeezed ventricle sign, 480
white matter buckling sign,
485-486
hematuria
spaghetti sign, 169
hemoperitoneum vs hematoma following splenic trauma
drowned hilus sign, 442
Hemophilus influenzae, pneumonia
due to
bulging fissure sign, 192
hemorrhage
adrenal, neonatal
rim sign, 164
of colon, *thumbprinting, 97-98*
hepatic vein, junction with inferior
vena cava
Playboy bunny sign, 453
hepatitis, viral
thickened gallbladder wall sign,
463
hepatocellular carcinoma
in portal or hepatic vein
thread and streaks sign, 424
hepatomegaly
benign vs metastatic
edge sign, 443
of cardiac origin
vena cava sign, 464
signs of, 446
vascular cut-off sign, 292
hereditary angioneurotic edema
thumbprinting, 97-98
hernia
diaphragmatic, congenital
absent liver sign, 5
Morgagni
sign of the cane, 194
umbilical
incomplete border sign, 51
ureteral
curlicue ureter sign, 129
hip joint
congenital dislocation, forcible
reduction of, epiphysitis
after
sagging rope sign, 370
deep soft-tissue abscess
tumbling bolt sign, 396

disease, in children
pubic or ischial varus sign,
366
effusion
pneumoarthrogram sign, 363
infectious arthritis of
obturator sign, 358
nonspecific inflammatory disease of
ileopsoas–gluteus medius sign,
344
trauma and hemorrhage
obturator sign, 358
histiocytosis X
floating tooth sign, 335
hole-within-a-hole pattern, 343
Hodgkin's disease
ivory vertebra sign, 347
humerus, head
impacted fracture of
rim sign, 367
inferior subluxation of, vs frac-
ture-dislocation of shoulder
drooping shoulder sign, 328
necrosis
crescent sign, 320
posterior dislocation
half-moon sign, 340
rim sign, 367
trough line sign, 395
hydromyelia
collapsing cord sign, 411-412
hydronephrosis
noninfected
pelvocalyceal wall opacification
sign, 152-153
in renal duplication
drooping lily sign, 133
hydropneumoperitoneum
peripheral bubble sign, 66
hypernephroma, renal
hypernephroma halo sign, 138-
139
hyperparathyroidism
black pleura sign, 191
fish vertebra, 333
rugger jersey sign, 368
hypertension
Page kidney, 148
portal venous
bull's-eye falciform ligament
sign, 436

osteomalacia of thoracic and
    lumbar spine
  fish vertebra, 333
osteomyelitis
  intraosseous gas sign, 475
  saber shin sign, 369
  serpiginous tract sign, 374
  vacuum phenomenon, 398
osteoporosis of thoracic and lum-
    bar spine
  fish vertebra, 333
ovary
  dermoid of
    halo (wall) sign, 175
    tip of the iceberg sign, 464
  hemorrhagic
    tip of the iceberg sign, 464
  mass in, vs distended bladder
    bladder sign, 119
  rim sign, 165-166
  vs massive ascites
    curvature sign, 437
  teratoma of
    indefinite uterus sign, 444

Paget's disease
  blade of grass sign, 305
  brim sign, 308
  cotton wool sign, 319
  ivory vertebra sign, 347
  shepherd's crook sign, 375
pancreas
  antral pad sign, 11
  autolysis, fluid due to
    moon crescent sign, 449
  carcinoma
    *Frostberg's inverted 3 sign, 38-
      40*
    struggling antrum sign, 93
  ectopic
    bull's-eye sign, 17
  gas abscess of, 2-3
  mass, vs nonpancreatic retroper-
      itoneal mass
    mesenteric vein sign, 447
  pseudocyst, infected
    fuzzy fluid level sign, 41
  tail, tumor, vs adrenal tumor
    splenic pedicle sign, 479

pancreatitis
  acute
    *abdominal fat necrosis sign, 2-
      3*
    colon cut-off sign, 21
    *dilated transverse colon sign,
      25*
    *Frostberg's inverted 3 sign, 38-
      40*
    gasless abdomen sign, 42
    Poppel's sign, 68
    *renal halo (perirenal fat) sign,
      160-161*
papilla of Vater, enlargement, sec-
    ondary to acute pancrea-
    titis
  Poppel's sign, 68
parietal foramina, enlarged
  Catlin mark, 313
pars interarticularis defect
  scotty dog sign, 372
patella, degenerative changes
  tooth sign, 390
pericallosal plexus, vascular blush
    due to hemispheric mass
  smile sign, 422
Perthes' disease
  sagging rope sign, 370
pertussis
  shaggy heart sign, 271-272
pheochromocytoma
  apical sign, 114
  ring sign, 167
pituitary, adenoma
  bulging tumor sign, 309
pneumomediastinum
  continuous diaphragm sign, 201
  extrapleural air sign, 212
  pericardial line sign, 251
  rocker-bottom thymus sign, 262
  spinnaker sail sign, 279
pneumopericardium
  halo sign, 220
  pericardial line sign, 251
pneumoperitoneum
  double wall sign, 30
  falciform ligament sign, 32
  football sign, 37
  inverted V sign, 55
  lucent liver sign, 59
  peripheral bubble sign, 66
  triangle sign, 101

urachal sign, 105
pneumothorax
  *anterior sulcus (double dia-
      phragm) sign, 184*
  clicking pneumothorax sign, 200
  deep sulcus sign, 203
  *herniated mediastinal pleural sac
      sign, 223*
  hyperlucent hemithorax sign, 226
  medial stripe sign, 240
  migrating staple sign, 243
  pericardial fat tag sign, 250
  scallop sign, 267
  sharp edge sign, 273
  V sign, 291
polycythemia vera, childhood
  hair-on-end sign, 339
polymyositis
  floppy thumb sign, 336
polyps, colonic
  border sign, 15
  bowler hat sign, 16
  target sign, 96
polysplenia
  symmetric liver sign, 94
prostate, hypertrophy of
  fishhook (J-shaped) ureter, 136
prostatectomy, vesicle neck con-
    tracture in
  toothpaste sign, 174
prostheses in vascular surgery, in-
    fection
  pockets of gas sign, 478
pseudopseudohypoparathyroidism
  metacarpal sign, 354
pseudotumor of orbit
  thickened sclera sign, 482
pulmonary artery
  vs calcified lymph node
    monocle sign, 244
  enlarged
    hilum convergence sign, 224
pulmonary infarction
  Hampton's hump sign, 221-222
  melting sign, 241
pulmonary venous return, anoma-
    lous
    partial, 268
    type 1 total, 278
pyloric stenosis, hypertrophic
  pyloric string sign, 72
  pyloric tit sign, 73

Index of Signs

If two or more signs have the same name, the anatomical area or body system to which each sign refers follows the sign in parentheses. For example, crescent sign (bone); crescent sign (genitourinary). Signs are also followed by the following abbreviations: An = angiography; CT = computed tomography; My = myelography; US = ultrasound.